COMMUNITY HEALTH NURSING PRACTICE

RUTH B. FREEMAN, R.N., Ed.D.

Professor of Public Health Administration
The Johns Hopkins University
School of Hygiene and Public Health

W. B. SAUNDERS COMPANY   Philadelphia, London, Toronto

W. B. Saunders Company: West Washington Square
                          Philadelphia, Pa.   19105

                          12 Dyott Street
                          London WC1A   1DB

                          1835 Yonge Street
                          Toronto 7, Ontario

Community Health Nursing Practice   SBN 0–7216–3876–7

Print Number: 2   3   4   5   6   7   8   9

Preface

Dramatic changes in the technical and social nature of health services are demanding equally dramatic changes in professional practice in all of the health disciplines.

This imperative is reflected in nursing education and nursing practice in many ways. The nursing curriculum appears to be shifting from a disease, or categorical, orientation to a generic nursing approach. Sophisticated and vocal student nurses are challenging traditional educational patterns, and as graduates they are carrying this independent, questing, challenging spirit to the community health field. The public is pressing a disorganized and creaking health system to find solutions to the problem of providing comprehensive care to all segments of the population, and administrators are responding with new and unorthodox uses of personnel of all types.

These developments have changed the character of public health, or community, nursing practice and have placed new responsibilities on the community health nurse practitioner. This book is intended to take account of these changes. Community health nursing is seen as a population-based obligation, realized through a multidisciplinary, ecologically oriented effort and utilizing concepts and skills that derive both from generic nursing and from public health practice. It focuses on nursing the community, in contradistinction to nursing *in* the community. Family nursing care is seen as an essential aspect of health care of the population, and the community health nurse's responsibility is seen as encompassing but not being limited to this aspect of the program.

In the chapters concerned with process, the attempt is to demonstrate the integral nature of community health nursing and its parent disciplines. Later chapters are designed to provide students and practitioners with a ready reference to community health aspects of nursing care of certain subgroups of the population—those in a specific developmental period, or in a particular locale, or with a particular kind of health or illness problem. Throughout, the emphasis is on the need for the beginning as well as the experienced community health nurse to engage in management as well as ministration, to concern himself or herself with policy setting and planning as well as with direct patient care, to see the nursing system in the context of the community health system of which it is a part.

The ephemeral nature of much of the information on which practice in any field is based makes the textbook only a point of departure for independent study and professional growth. For this reason, suggested readings have been selected to introduce the student or practitioner to sources, rather than to provide a definitive bibliography.

Faced with the immensity of the social potential of community health services and with the centrality of nursing effort in the achievement of this potential, any author must feel that even his best efforts produce haunting omissions and inadequacies. However, if this book can convey the excitement of the challenge of community health care and can stimulate dissent, revisions, and rethinking of community nursing purposes and process, it will have served its purpose.

Many people have made this book possible — old friends who supplied ideas or references; the entire nurse faculty of the Johns Hopkins University School of Hygiene and Public Health, who helped in many ways; the students whose penetrating questions and comments provoked new thinking. In particular, I am grateful to Anna Scholl and Edith Wilson, who not only helped clarify ideas but also often took on extra chores to release writing time. Thanks are due to Loretta Peterson, Mary Nori, Peggy Bremer, and Brenda Bailey, all of whom patiently typed and retyped the manuscript; and also to Sandra Elliott for editorial assistance. I am indebted to the staff of W. B. Saunders Company, especially to Robert E. Wright for his continuing support, and to Pamela Herr, who edited the final draft of the manuscript. Most of all I am indebted to Anselm Fisher, who provided exhortation, support, and a judicious amount of nagging during the writing period.

RUTH B. FREEMAN

Contents

Perspectives and Prospects

In virtually every country of the world there is a group of nursing personnel that functions primarily outside the hospital setting. Their function is to provide for the preventive and curative care of a defined population.

They may represent a fully professional group of nurses who have elected this field of practice, or they may be primarily *middle-trained;* that is, having preparation below the professional level but nevertheless prepared in some systematic way over a substantive period of time. They can also be *short-trained* workers: those prepared either on the job or in brief training courses to function in a limited way. Perhaps most often the nursing corps represents a combination of all three of these levels of preparation.

This group of nursing personnel may work under the immediate supervision of a nurse, or they may function with distant nursing supervision and under the immediate direction of a physician or other administrator. They may work under the sponsorship of government agencies of health, welfare, education, or insurance or under the sponsorship of voluntary or private groups.

They may be organized under a countrywide system, or they may function within a multitude of independent services working with varying degrees of coordination. Their "community" may be a village, a neighborhood, a school, an industrial population, a state or province, or the world.

The work of nursing may be done in many ways. The level of care may vary from one in which the majority of personal nursing services stem from untrained indigenous workers to one that offers the most sophisticated professional specialist services in a comprehensive-care center.

Whatever the nature of the staff, the locus, or the services provided, these efforts are welded together by a common purpose based on the principles that (1) nursing be used as a channel for health care and that (2) the community as a whole, rather than solely the individual, be the object of this care.

It is not always easy for those engaged in community health nursing to realize that community health nursing is only one part of nursing and of the community health system, that the community health system is only part of the entire health system, that the health system is only one part of the system for dealing with human needs and resources, and that the system for dealing with human resources is only one part of the total economic and social development program of a particular population group.

Whatever happens to any part of this total system has some effect on every other part of the system. Therefore if the community accepts a concept of human justice that creates new patterns of providing support for the disadvantaged, health-care patterns must also change to conform to this new approach. If the development of the economy is of paramount importance at a given point in time, human services may be pushed back to a minimal level pending greater economic viability. Thus, what happens to the specific community health nursing program will have its roots in the whole structure of community aspirations, needs, values, demands, and capabilities. Community health nursing both reflects and influences these broader concerns and actions.

To understand the development of community health nursing, and to function intelligently within it, it is important to see this field of human service in the context of the broad social and technical developments that set both the opportunities and the limits within which work is done.

HUMAN RIGHTS AND HUMAN HOPES PROVIDE THE FOUNDATION

Perhaps there is no movement more significant for the future of health services than the current worldwide reappraisal of the dimension of human rights. This movement can only be described as revolutionary in its force and in its potential for influencing the course of human history. Its impact will likely be as great as that of the industrial revolution of the last century.

This movement is particularly visible in the United States of America, which is founded on the principle of the right of the individual to "life, liberty, and the pursuit of happiness." However, the concept of these words changes with the times or, more specifically, with the conditions that characterize the times.

The incompatibility of this concept with slavery, with uncontrolled work conditions in an industrial society, and with the subjugation of women constituted the struggles of the last century. The struggle of today has a different focus. The preservation of the dignity of the individual, man's right to equal opportunity as well as a right to protection from overt harm, the incorporation of the concept of redress of previous injustices, and the increasingly frequent application of the phrase "with justice" to the traditional concept of law and order are all facets of today's concerns. This new focus is reflected by the words of

John Gardner, Secretary of Health, Education, and Welfare during the Johnson administration:

> In this nation today we have begun to explore energetically, seriously, sympathetically, the conditions—all the conditions—that prevent human fulfillment. Through all of these efforts—whether they involve health or racial justice or education or the attack on poverty—run the same great themes—the release of human potential, the enhancement of human dignity, the liberation of the human spirit.[1]

An expanded concept of human rights brings with it many implications for health and for the nurse's participation in community health programs. Perhaps the most striking effect is an *acceleration of the trend toward higher expectations on the part of the public with respect to health care.* Already escalated demands for care of the elderly sick, for the very young, and for the low-income groups are going even higher. Furthermore, these expectations are accompanied by an insistence upon prompt, adequate response. *The rate of upward revision of available care has been sharply increased.* This insistence is particularly strong in, or on behalf of, those whose care in the past has been inadequate in amount or unsuitable in type. The tendency of the health professional to move slowly and soundly into new services may have to be abrogated in favor of faster response with a minimum of desirable quality controls.

The adoption of self-realization as one of the facets of human rights has had a profound effect upon the location of decisional responsibility. The right of individuals, of families, and of communities to help decide the kind and amount of care they require or will accept creates a new imperative for the involvement of the recipient—whether individual, group, or community—in his own care.

Although the principle of maximum self-determination has been upheld in the professional literature of community health for several decades, the traditional concept of what is actually included in the policy of *maximum self-determination* is quite different from that now held by a newly aware recipient group. Decisions—such as the patterns for the delivery of health-care services—formerly considered to require only professional judgment are now believed to require also the special and intimate knowledge of the recipients of care. The practice of being "spoken for," as exemplified by the traditional actions of public-spirited citizens dedicated to the improvement of the human condition, is no longer considered by the recipient group to be adequate involvement. The poor, for example, want to, are ready to, and in today's terms of reference are entitled to decide for themselves what they need.

For these reasons, marked changes must take place in the methods of community health administration and practice. The development of communication skills that will transcend the language of different cultures must be developed. Goal setting that takes into account feelings and readiness as well as medical or technical potentials for care is required. An unwonted subordination of the desires and drives of the professional worker to the human, as well as to the health, needs of the group being served may be necessary.

Moreover, there must be a willingness to see and hear messages that contradict the previously held estimations of both the purveyor and the recipient of health services: a readiness on the part of the health team to understand newly surfaced, and sometimes hostilely expressed, feelings

among the formerly "happy feckless poor"; and a willingness on the part
of a population eager to get more and better health care to understand
the problems of the health team in providing service. The concept of
health planning as an essentially rational science-based operation may to
some degree have to give way to the concept of health planning as one
of the ways in which fallible humans try to secure their future in a
manner that does not threaten their present.

As noted, the changing concept of human rights sets new requirements upon the provision of community health care and also brings into
view new and dazzling possibilities for the potential of care. The pros-
pect of a truly integrated patient-community-professional effort on behalf of health care makes credible an intensification of programs currently hampered by public apathy. The recipient's involvement in his own
care would permit an unparalleled group of health disciples knowledgeable enough to help others, as well as themselves, toward better health
care.

The press to get something done "yesterday if not before" may
provide the impetus needed for exciting innovation. It may even lead to
a clearer definition of the theory underlying community health practice
as it pertains to nursing, medicine, and social work.

HEALTH IS THE DREAM

Health for all is the dream of both the health professional and the
public. What constitutes *health,* however, is a matter of little agreement.

The oft-quoted definition of the World Health Organization describes
health as a state of complete physical, mental, and social well-being and
not merely the absence of disease or infirmity. Ever since the publication of that definition in 1945, there have been many efforts to bring into
focus a definition of health that is related to the modern condition and
that could serve as a basis for establishing health goals and for evaluating health programs.

For some the approach has been that of a spectrum. A few have
defined health in terms of levels. The term health may imply the degree
to which the individual is able to carry on his usual activities or the level
the individual can achieve within the limits of preëxisting disease, disability, or genetic endowment. Some attempt the definition in theoretical
or ideal terms and envision man as living out his biologic span of 120 or
130 years unencumbered with illness or disability. Still others seek an
operational definition: one that can be the basis for realistic planning
here and now; a definition that is achievable.

The definition of health that serves as the goal will undoubtedly be
influenced by what is possible as well as by what is desirable. The
degree to which health, by any definition, is perceived as achievable or
desirable will depend upon the place of health in the total hierarchy of
values. Qualitative and quantitative aspects of health will be involved in
the definition.

In defining health, it is important to establish what one considers
nonhealth and whether one is speaking of individual health, family
health, or community health. As noted, health is a relative term; it may

mean different things to different individuals or to different governments, and it can mean different things at different points in time. Dr. William Stewart, Surgeon General of the United States Public Health Service, recently said, "It is out of date to think of health in solely negative terms—as the absence of disease and disability. The healthy individual is not merely un-sick. He is strong, aware of his powers and eager to use them. Therefore, in our approach to the environment we need to be conscious of sanity as well as sanitation. We should be as concerned with ugliness and loneliness as we are concerned with carcinogens. A truly healthful environment is not merely safe but stimulating."[2]

If applied to the past, and also currently in some developing countries with massive health problems and limited resources for health care, Dr. Stewart's concept may have little reality. In such cases, the presence of health conditions that cause premature death and disability may represent the public concept of a nonhealth state.

In current terms and in highly industrialized countries, however, health is increasingly seen as involving four levels of concern:

1. Prevention of premature death.
2. Amelioration of disease and disability.
3. Prevention of disease, disability, or threats to health.
4. Promotion of health and vigor.

Dr. Stewart's statement indicates an acceptance of all four levels as pertinent to today's health planning.

A recent Canadian report also reflects an acceptance of this broad concept. It defines the goal of comprehensive care to include "all services, preventive, diagnostic, curative and rehabilitative, that modern medical and other sciences can provide."[3] However, despite this general acceptance of the concept of health as a condition that maximizes the individual's capacity to live happily and productively, the services actually provided may lag considerably behind the declaration of intent.

It is more and more apparent that health must always be seen in comparative terms rather than in absolute terms; health for some persons will be less than perfect functioning. The very actions which resolve one health problem may produce new ones. As we find ways to keep older people alive longer, the problems of accident prevention and personal care for those with reduced vital strength assume a new importance. Some of the children who survive as a result of improved maternal and child care practices may suffer from illnesses or impairments that constitute new health problems. In certain cases, "therapeutic health" is the best that can be achieved; an example is health dependent upon frequent dialysis or on constant medication for glaucoma or diabetes. Dubos points out that the struggle for health must be seen as a continuing one: the circumstances are ever changing, and the methods must be dynamic rather than static.[4]

PEOPLE—THE PURPOSE AND THE MEDIUM

People are the purpose for which health services, including community health nursing, exist. People are also the major medium through which these services are achieved. It is the human condition that health care seeks to modify, and it is through the behavior and action of people as patients, health workers, taxpayers, legislators, family members, neighbors, and citizens that health programs are largely effected. To understand the "people" dimension of today's health world, it is important to know what changes are occurring with respect to:

1. The size and characteristics of the population.
2. The health or disease conditions from which individuals suffer or die.
3. The way in which people live and act as it affects their health care.

Though the discussion here will be largely limited to trends in the United States, these tendencies might be considered characteristic of many other highly developed industrial nations.

The Growing Population

The population in the United States is growing. In 1967 the population was estimated at 195,857,000 people. This figure places the United States fourth among the 20 most populated countries.[5] It is estimated that the figure may go to 245 million by 1980.[6]

The birth rate (number of live births per 1000 of the population) has declined in the past decade subsequent to an increase in the forties and fifties.[7] During the same period, the *death rate* (number of deaths from all causes per 1000 of the population) has remained constant. This relationship between births and deaths is shown in Figure 1.

The *growth rate* (the annual percentage increase in population), which is dependent upon the relationship between births and deaths and upon immigration and emigration, has varied from 1.95 percent in 1910 to 0.7 percent in 1940. Between 1960 and 1964 there was a steady decline from 1.75 percent to 1.44 percent.[8] This may presage a somewhat slower rate of growth in the future. However, since the excess of births over deaths is still substantial and since immigration and emigration have remained relatively constant, there continues to be a substantial natural increase in the population.

THE CHANGING COMPOSITION OF THE
POPULATION

The composition of the population has also undergone some changes. Some of these changes are illustrated in Figure 2.

In 1900, children under 5 years made up 12.1 percent of the total population, school children aged 5 to 19 constituted 32 percent, and persons 65 years or older made up 4.1 percent. By 1965 these proportions had shifted: the under-five group made up 10.5 percent of the total population, those aged 5 to 19 constituted 29 percent, and persons 65 years and over made up 9.4 percent. The proportion of the population 65 or older has remained fairly constant over the past decade. The under-five group showed a decline in 1964 and 1965. The proportion of females in the population has increased somewhat because of relative

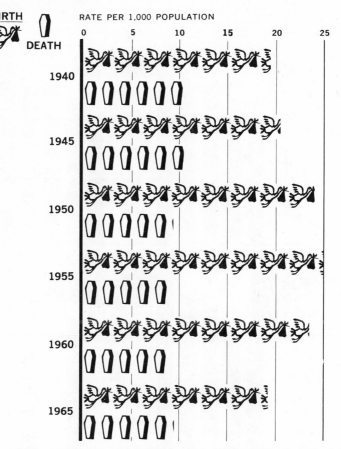

FIGURE 1.   Birth and death rates per 1000 population: 1940 to 1965. (From *Pocket Data Book, U.S.A., 1967*. U.S. Department of Commerce, Bureau of the Census, U.S. Government Printing Office, Washington, D.C., 1967.)

longevity. The nonwhite population constituted 11.8 percent of the population in 1964, compared to 9.8 percent in 1940.[9]

MOBILITY OF THE POPULATION

Most significant for health planning is the increasing movement of people to urban areas. As farms become more and more mechanized, the demand for unskilled labor, and indeed, even the amount of labor needed, is reduced. Subsistence farming and tenant farming have long been known to constitute a poverty occupation. Hence there has been a trek to the cities and a consequent transformation of farm and nonfarm rural areas into metropolitan communities. In 1965, over 70 percent of the total population lived in urban areas, and by the year 2000 it is expected that 80 percent of the population will live in urban communities.[10] The population is exceedingly mobile in other ways: a number of persons equivalent to the total population of Pennsylvania moved

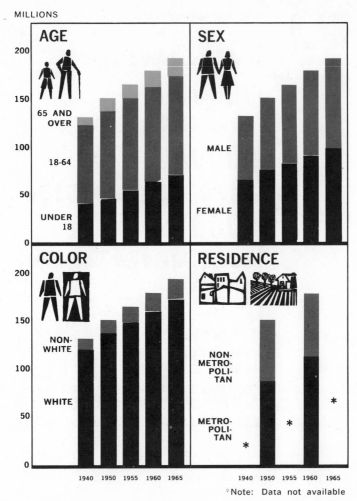

FIGURE 2.   Population characteristics of the United States: 1940 to 1965. (From *Pocket Data Book, U.S.A., 1967*. U.S. Department of Commerce, Bureau of the Census, U.S. Government Printing Office, Washington, D.C., 1967.)

from one state to another between March 1964 and March 1965.[11] Thus it can be said that we are a large and growing population, largely urban, highly mobile, and largely white with a slightly increasing nonwhite component. Almost 46 percent of the population either is under 18 years or is 65 years old and older, two age groups that are very frequent users of health services.

Changing Causes of Death and Illness

As communicable diseases come under control and as acute conditions surrender to more effective and heroic therapies, longterm illnesses and health conditions that are rooted in the behavior of the individual, rather than in specific disease organisms, take center stage.

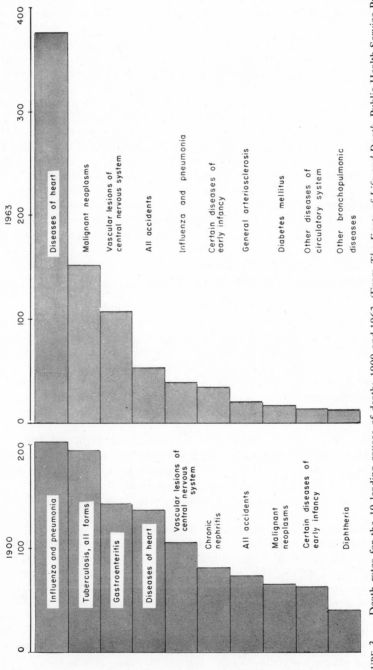

FIGURE 3. Death rates for the 10 leading causes of death: 1900 and 1963. (From *The Facts of Life and Death*. Public Health Service Publication, U.S. Government Printing Office, Washington, D.C., 1965, p. 13.)

THE KILLERS—CAUSES OF DEATH

Although mortality rates alone do not provide a clear picture of the health problems of a community, they are an important index of change. Figure 3 shows the changes in major causes of death in the United States from 1900 to 1963.

In 1900 the five leading causes of death were influenza and pneumonia, tuberculosis, gastroenteritis, diseases of the heart, and vascular lesions of the central nervous system. By 1965 diseases of the heart were in first place, followed by malignant neoplasms, vascular lesions of the central nervous system, and accidents. Yet, even more important than rank is the change in the relative proportion of deaths from certain causes. Deaths caused by diseases of the heart, for example, moved from a rate of 137.4 deaths per 100,000 of the population to 367.4 per 100,000; deaths from cancer and all other malignant neoplasms rose from a rate of 64 deaths per 100,000 of the population in 1900 to 153.5 deaths in 1963. During the same period, deaths from tuberculosis dropped from a rate of 194.4 to 4.1. The magnitude of the shifts, as well as the relative position among the various causes of death, has great implications for the development of community health practice and services.[12]

It is clear that at present the major killers in the United States are heart disease, cancer, stroke, and accidents.

In countries where the stage of economic development resembles our own, the principal causes of death are remarkably similar. A recent World Health Organization report indicated that in 10 highly industrialized nations (Australia, Canada, England, France, West Germany, Hungary, Italy, Poland, Sweden, and the United States), the leading causes of death were diseases of the heart, cancer and stroke (which accounted for about 70 percent of the total deaths), and accidents. In eight developing, or "in-between," countries, on the other hand, the three leading causes of death were gastroenteritis, influenza and pneumonia, and accidents.[13.]

Many Preventable Deaths. However, the principal causes of death are not always the most cogent concerns of public health. In 1963 it was estimated that 101,000 of the approximately 1,800,000 deaths were preventable.[14] Even though this represents a small proportion of the total deaths that year, such human waste is a matter of very real concern.

One major cause of death in which preventability is assumed to be high is accidents, which are leading causes of death in the one through 44 age group. Although the accident rate has declined between 1950 and 1963, as indicated in Table 1, there has been no reduction between 1960 and 1963, and accidents still remain a major control problem.

Infant deaths are also a matter for concern, first because the United States is not in an enviable position with respect to other industrialized countries, and second because the variation in death rates in infancy is very great, particularly among those in different economic groups. In 1965 the infant mortality rate for the country as a whole was 24.7 per 1000 live births. This represented a substantial drop from the 1935 level of 55.7, but the reduction since 1955 (when the rate was 26.4) has been

Table 1.   Deaths From Accidents in the United States: 1950 to 1963*

Year	Number	Rate per 100,000	Rate per 100,000 under 1 year old	Rate per 100,000 65 years and older
1950	91,200	60.6	114.2	210.8
1960	93,800	52.3	93.2	153.6
1961	92,200	50.4	83.9	146.9
1962	97,100	52.3	87.6	154.6
1963	100,700	53.4	86.2	155.3

*From *Health, Education and Welfare Trends,* 1965. U.S. Department of Health, Education and Welfare, U.S. Government Printing Office, Washington, D.C., 1965, p. 5–11.

much less gratifying. Furthermore, the continuing disparity in rates of white and nonwhite infant deaths is particularly disturbing. In 1965 the rate among white infants was 21.5 per 1000 live births compared to 40.3 for nonwhite infants.[15] There is no reason to suppose that this disparity, which is generally ascribed to differences in socioeconomic conditions, is irreversible.

Tuberculosis death rates have declined from 194.4 deaths per 100,000 of the population in 1900 to 4.1 deaths per 100,000 people in 1965. However, there are many who believe that this disease could be completely eradicated or that deaths from this cause should occur rarely or not at all. Furthermore, the fact that the death rates vary considerably by socioeconomic status, race, and locality of residence indicates the need for intensive control measures to eliminate these pockets of resistance.

THE DISABLERS—CAUSES OF DAYS LOST FROM USUAL ACTIVITY

In the United States in 1966 there were almost three billion days on which individuals were not able to carry on their usual activities because of illness or injury; over a billion of these days were spent in bed. This represented almost 425 million work-loss days and over 200 million school-loss days.[16]

The major disablers are, of course, the chronic illnesses, including nervous and mental disorders. In the period from July 1964 to June 1965, 87.3 million people, 46 percent of the population, had one or more chronic diseases, and one in four of these persons was limited in some degree by these conditions.[17] Among the chronic diseases responsible for activity limitation, heart conditions, arthritis, mental and nervous diseases, and hypertension without heart disease were the most frequent causes in 1964. Among acute conditions causing limitation of activity, the most common were respiratory conditions, infective and parasitic diseases, and disorders of the digestive system.[18]

Accidents also account for a large amount of disability. With respect to accidents, the number of people affected—that is, the number who have some kind of accident—far exceeds that of those who either die or are disabled as a result of accidents. It was estimated that in the period from 1959 to 1961, a total of almost 45 million people suffered some kind of accident.[19.]

THE RISK MAKERS—THREATS TO HEALTH

In looking at the health of the community, one must be concerned not only about the diseases that exist in individuals or in populations but also about conditions that make it likely that disease or disability will occur. In other words, conditions that pose a threat to health must be seen in perspective.

These threats may reside in the environment either because the environment in itself is unsafe or because technological advances, good in themselves, create new health hazards. Health threats may also reside in the individual in the form of special vulnerabilities.

Environmental risks to health are assuming new importance. Our exploding population and increasingly sophisticated technology have created new threats. The recent concern about air pollution, water conservation and sanitation, control of radioactive substances, and waste disposal are matched by a concern about a social environment that can also be a serious health threat. Rat proofing of houses still has an important place in health programs, but attention is now also directed toward housing that permits elderly people to see grass outside their windows and that provides children with play facilities and gardens as well as with toilets.

Over 90 percent of the housing in the United States was considered satisfactory and reasonably up-to-date in 1967 (compared to 84 percent in 1960). However, there are still thousands of run-down dilapidated unsanitary houses and apartments in the slums, the ghettos, and the backwoods.[20]

High-speed roadways, with cars to match, represent another environmental hazard. The highway system of the United States increased from 3,313,000 miles in 1950 to 3,644,000 miles in 1964. The percentage of families owning automobiles increased from 59 percent in 1950 to 79 percent in 1965; 24 percent of these families owned two or more cars. In 1964 there were 90,367,000 motor vehicles registered as compared to 49,300,000 in 1950.[21] Thus the automobile becomes one of the risk makers since the number of vehicles exposed to possible accident is greatly increased.

With such a large segment of the population at special risk because of the physical environmental challenge to health, it is appropriate to speak of "the era of sanitation in public health" as a current happening, not as an historic event.

The Social Environment as a Health Threat. There is ample evidence that poverty represents a particular threat to health and that death and illness rates are higher among those living in poverty. In 1964 about 17.6 percent of the families in the United States had incomes less than $3000, the sum then considered to be the poverty level.[22]

Births out of wedlock have increased, and currently about 7 percent of all babies are born to unmarried mothers.[23] It is felt that this situation increases the risks to both mother and baby. One study showed that about half of the unmarried mothers received late or no prenatal care and that premature births and maternal deaths and complications during pregnancy were more frequent in the unmarried group. Infant mortality was twice as high in the unmarried group of mothers.[24]

A large proportion of the population is affected by special personal vulnerabilities, though this is not a well-documented fact. Families of diabetic patients, persons with certain congenital anomalies, the elderly with impaired sensory faculties, and the infant who fails to thrive are examples of this category of health threat. Recently the National Center for Health Statistics has been collecting data on conditions related to health or associated with the development of disease but not actually constituting disease. These data include, for instance, the cholesterol levels of adults, which may identify a group particularly vulnerable to heart disease.[25] Gunn points out that the moneyed, as well as the poor, may have vulnerable groups; for example, the business executive seems to be unusually prone to coronary thrombosis.[26]

Thus in the United States, as in most industrialized countries, the patterns of deaths tell us that the great killers are heart disease, cancer, stroke, and accidents. The first three of these killers are most frequently found in the older members of the population, and a knowledge of disease prevention and cure is still far from complete. Accidents, the fourth main cause of death, affect all age groups to some degree, although the frequency peaks at several points; again, the problem of accident prevention is complex, and the methods are still far from being explicit.

Concerning the causes of death that are somewhat less frequent in the general population, persistent differential rates among certain subgroups would indicate that preventive measures have been unequally effective in securing reductions medically possible with present knowledge. Although much disability is related to longterm illnesses, there is no doubt that a substantial decrease might be effected in some areas if all possible preventive measures were used. Threats to health that arise from the environment are increasing in importance.

Affluence and Technology Create New Ways of Life

The most obvious change in the American socioeconomic scene is the prevalence of relative affluence. This country, as a whole, is an affluent one compared to most other countries in the world. The citizens are proud of their economic growth and productivity and consider it reasonable that the good things of life be made available to them. The television and other communication media make quite clear how many things there are to want, and indeed, they make some of the luxuries sound like necessities. There is ample reason for the confusion of luxury and necessity.

The median family income in the United States in 1964 was $6569 compared to $3013 in 1947; this latter figure is equivalent to $4214 in 1964 dollars. Furthermore, the distribution of income was somewhat improved between those years. Families with an income of $10,000 or more represented 2.7 percent of the total families in 1947. The proportion of families falling in that category had risen to 22.5 percent in 1964. Those with incomes below $3000 dropped from 49.3 percent in 1947 to 17.6 percent in 1964.[27]

Another indication of affluence is the things for which money is spent. In 1947, 33 percent of consumer expenditures went for food and beverages; in 1966 these items represented only 23 percent of the total expenditures.[28]

A cursory glance will show the degree to which sports cars have replaced the "hot rods" of a decade ago, the prevalence of residential swimming pools, and the preponderance of sheer luxury items in mail-order catalogues and department stores.

POVERTY PERSISTS

Within this affluence there are many who live in poverty. In 1964, 6.8 million of the 47.8 million families in the United States were classified as poor; that is, their incomes were at, or below, the amount considered by the Social Security Administration as adequate to provide for a family at a minimum level, which in 1964 was approximately $3100 per year for a family of four.[29] Although a great number of those falling in the poverty classification are white, the proportion of nonwhites is considerably higher. The differential in salaries earned by white and nonwhite families in 1964 was a substantial one — $6858 for white families and $3839 for nonwhite families.[30]

Attention has been focused on the plight of the nonwhite population by problems incident to the implementation of the civil rights legislation. Interest was also directed to the Appalachian region where efforts were made to provide more effective assistance to the very low-income families living in great hardship.

The voice of the poor began to be heard more clearly as leaders and spokesmen emerged. Just as the evils of the industrial revolution became more visible as workers gathered in cities, so the plight of the poor, particularly the nonwhite poor, could no longer be ignored. The isolation of poverty neighborhoods and the alienation of its residents became so apparent that the word "ghetto" came into use to describe the "invisible wall" that kept the poor separated from the rest of the community.

The aroused conscience of the "haves," as well as the sense of injustice among the "have nots," has created an indignant demand for the alleviation of poverty in the midst of affluence. The war on poverty, spearheaded by President Johnson, was launched with the sweeping provisions of the Economic Opportunity Act of 1964. In its declaration of purpose this act states: "It is [therefore] the policy of this nation to eliminate the paradox of poverty in the midst of plenty in this nation, by opening to everyone the opportunity for education and training, the opportunity to work and the opportunity to live in decency and dignity." (Public Law 88-452.) Thus the existence of poverty, which affects a relatively small proportion of the total population, has assumed a major place in the nation's concern and may be expected to take a high priority with respect to health care as well as other human services.

Changing Patterns of Family Living

Although the family is still the primary social unit in American life, family life has been subjected to many stresses and strains. The increasing frequency with which mothers work requires a juggling of the roles of every family member. The trek to the suburbs, though creating an environment favorable in many ways for the children of the family, may in fact lead to absent fathers and frustrated mothers. The rising rate of divorce is also creating new patterns of family living. Family planning, the introduction of many labor-saving devices into the home, the increasing opportunities for a woman to engage in meaningful action while still remaining essentially a homemaker, and the introduction of better transportation into center city which brings father back to his family more quickly are other factors which change the pattern of family living. Greater support for care of the aged may relieve the family of unreasonable burdens and may make the extended family pattern more desirable. For each family there is apt to be a choice, since family roles and family management are individually, not culturally, determined in an increasing number of instances.

People Have More Education

In 1940, about one out of four of those persons 25 years or older had four or more years of high school. By 1966 that proportion had risen to 40 percent. During that same period, those finishing four or more years of college rose from 4.6 percent to 9.9 percent.

In 1957-58, 66 percent of those 15 to 19 years old were in school. In France, only 31 percent and in the United Kingdom, less than 20 percent of this age group were in school.[31]

Prevalent Risk Taking with Respect to Health

Even though it is not possible to estimate the number of people who are behaving in a manner prejudicial to their health, certain problems may be readily identified. Despite the evidence that cigarette smoking is associated with the incidence of lung cancer, chronic bronchitis, and emphysema, as well as with days of illness and disability, it has been estimated that about 49 million adults, approximately 42 percent of the adult population, are smokers.[32] The abuse of alcohol and of hallucinogenic drugs is also sufficiently frequent to occasion great concern.[33] These are problems that can be dealt with only through changing the behavior of individuals.

THE HEALTH SYSTEM — THE MEANS

The health system — the great complex of public policy; private, voluntary, and public facilities; and health manpower — is the means by which the community acts to realize its program for health action. To the degree that this system is adequate, properly related, and viable, the health program is able to move ahead in a strong and orderly way.

Fragmentation and Lack of Coordination

At present the health system in the United States might well be described as a non-system. There is no clearly delineated national policy regarding health. Facilities, for the most part, grew up without much concern for the development of related facilities or for the cultivation of manpower to staff their organizations. Consequently, services are largely fragmented and uncoordinated. According to the report of the National Commission on Community Health Services: "Health programs have become a crazy quilt of disconnected and rambling services . . . the coordination of agency services by the very magnitude and complexity of agencies involved has become like the weather—something to talk about but about which people believe little can be done."[34]

In the literature of community health, there is evidence of considerable concern about this fragmentation and uncontrolled proliferation of services. The passage of the Comprehensive Health Planning and Public Health Services Amendment of 1966 (Public Law 89-749) is one evidence of national concern. This legislation provides for grants to states for comprehensive state health-planning. These grants are subject to certain conditions: there must be a single state agency responsible for the grant; and there must be a state health-planning council which provides for the representation of local and state government health units, of other agencies concerned with health, and of consumers. Although most states have moved to establish such planning agencies, it would appear that the relatively meager allocation of funds and the unavailability of people skilled in methods of planning may weaken the effectiveness of this program.

A Dual Health-Care System

The health-care system in the United States is a dual one: it combines private and public sectors. Although by far the greater part of the care is provided under private systems, the public sector assumes much importance in certain areas: in the large urban centers, for instance. Furthermore, the public sector increasingly provides "backup" services for the private sector. These services have great influence on the total care provided; for example, the health department may offer cancer screening services that identify patients needing follow-up from their private physician.

The health resources of the United States are indeed great. The "health industry" is the third largest of all industries, being exceeded only by agriculture and construction.[35] Expenditures for health and medical care rose from approximately 3 billion 600 thousand dollars in 1928-29 to 38 billion 441 thousand in 1964-65, and the proportion of the gross national product used for health and medical care rose from 3.6 percent to 5.9 percent during that same period.[36]

Trends in the Resources of the Health System

The health industry includes many component parts: a network of hospitals and related institutions; a large number of private practice physicians who work either alone or in groups; the community health structure, including national, state, and local agencies in a variety of government units; and a large and vocal voluntary health action group.

UNPROPORTIONATE INCREASE IN HOSPITAL BEDS

Whereas the number of hospital beds has increased between 1950 and 1965 from 1,456,000 to 1,696,000, the ratio of hospital beds to the population has decreased in that period from 9.6 beds per 1000 people to 8.9 beds per 1000 people.[37, 38] This trend may reflect the practice of shortened hospital stays and a concomitant increase in ambulatory care services. However, this count also includes beds which, in the opinion of hospital personnel, are "inadequate."

INCREASED HEALTH INSURANCE COVERAGE

Another kind of resource is insurance for sickness care. Between 1950 and 1964, the proportion of health and medical care expenditures paid for by consumers covered with insurance increased from 12.1 percent to 33 percent.[39] This trend allows for a greater use of available facilities, since the financial barrier to care is lessened.

FEWER PHYSICIANS IN PRIVATE PRACTICE

The number of physicians has increased approximately 21 percent in the last decade, and the proportion of physicians to the population has also increased from 149 per 100,000 of the population to 153 per 100,000 of the population.[40] The proportion of physicians electing private practice has decreased from 72 percent of the total physicians in 1950 to 63 percent in 1964. The change with respect to the proportion in general practice is even more marked; the proportion dropped from 48 percent in 1950 to 26 percent in 1964.[41]

This trend toward specialization and toward institutional, rather than independent or individual, practice has a profound effect on the health-care pattern. Specialization tends to contribute to fragmentation of care. For the most part, institutions, as well as those in private practice, operate on a specialized organizational system. For some of the population this creates a vacuum with respect to the roles traditionally filled by the family physician: adviser, confidant, and knowledgeable friend. The American Medical Association has proposed a new area of specialty for the family practitioner who would be expected to take on some of these

functions.[42] It is not yet known what attraction this program will hold
for members of the medical profession.

EXPANDED GOVERNMENTAL PUBLIC HEALTH ESTABLISHMENT

During the last decade the government health effort has grown. It has
been in an almost constant state of reorganization and realignment of
responsibilities. Perhaps the best index of what is happening is the
change in local health units. Between 1954 and 1964, there was some
increase in the proportion of the population covered by organized health
units: 88.8 percent of the people were covered in 1954, and 94.8 percent
were covered in 1964.[43] However, all of this progress occurred before
1958. Between 1958 and 1964 there was virtually no change. The *per
capita* expenditure for local health units increased 60 percent during that
time. There were differences in coverage from state to state: 29 states
provided coverage for 100 percent of their population, and 35 states
provided coverage for over 90 percent of the population. There were
only five states with less than half of the population covered.

Personnel employed in local health units increased 31.6 percent between 1954 and 1964: from 37,514 in 1954 to 49,357 in 1964. Despite
this increase, however, the number of full-time personnel serving the
public did not increase proportionately: there were 26.5 health personnel
for each 100,000 of the population in 1954 and only 27.4 per 100,000 in
1964. Morever, in 1964 there were 15,226 people employed by other
than health units to do health work. Of this number about 10,400 were
nurses.

These local efforts are supported by and are responsible to state
health departments (or other comparable authorities) in every state.
Occasionally they are sponsored by a number of nonhealth state
agencies, such as departments of welfare and mental hygiene.

At the national level is another network of agencies that provides
leadership and supportive professional and financial services as well as
some direct services. The Department of Health, Education and Welfare
is the focal point of this network. The Department of Defense, the
Veterans Administration, the Department of Labor, and the Department
of Agriculture are among the related agencies with substantive health
programs.

At the international level, the World Health Organization serves as a
meeting ground for health discussion, planning, and action. It is
supplemented by many other agencies such as the International Labor
Organization, the Food and Agriculture Organization, and the United
Nations International Children's Emergency Fund (UNICEF).

Working within this broad context, in many ways and in many places,
the community nurse fulfills her role.

A STRONG VOLUNTARY HEALTH ORGANIZATION SYSTEM

The presence of a strong tradition of voluntary action in the United
States is reflected in the multitude of voluntary health agencies. Hamlin
estimated that in 1961 there were approximately 100,000 national, re-

gional, or local voluntary agencies with health or welfare, or both, as their principal function.[44] This figure was exclusive of churches and civic or fraternal organizations, many of which carry out health activities. The public contributed over 1.5 billion dollars to these agencies, 570 million dollars of which went to agencies having the promotion of health as their principal function.

SHIFTING RELATIONSHIPS AND ROLES

Perhaps more important than the number of health resources is the present state of confusion that exists concerning the roles and responsibilities of each of the component parts. There is an urgent need to find some resolution to the problems of maldistribution, differential utilization, and lack of coordination.

There appears to be a considerable reshuffling of responsibilities between government and private sectors, especially with respect to the provision of certain medical care services. In some urban centers the emergency room has become, in fact, the family physician of low-income families. Consequently, nonemergency services may exceed the emergency services provided. Preventive services, such as well-child supervision, previously considered to be the responsibility of the community health agency are more and more often being incorporated into the overall program of care afforded either by the private physician or by hospital ambulatory services. With the advent of Medicare and Medicaid, many health departments have become deeply involved with the provision of medical care, both directly, as with the provision of certain home-care services, and indirectly, through the licensing or accreditation of agencies providing care. In many instances, patient-care responsibility is shared with the family physician or with a hospital staff.

A similar realignment of responsibilities appears to be going on with respect to different members of the health team. In some instances public health nurses are assuming higher levels of decisional responsibility in patient-care management, often providing the kind of surveillance previously given by the physician; however the nature of this surveillance is such that it is properly encompassed within nursing practice. Nurses are in turn delegating much patient-care responsibility to short-trained workers, a group that, until recently, rarely provided patient-care service in community health agencies.

New kinds of workers are coming into being: the indigenous neighborhood worker who may undertake many health responsibilities, the general representative in public health, and the medical assistant whose work may also include aspects formerly considered those of the nurse.

Out of this ferment should come not only new alignments but also new insights and new perspectives. As the indigenous worker becomes involved in health decisions and health care, his professional partner benefits from this new and very effective communication channel. The outcome may be the discovery that the professional's seemingly adequate knowledge of what is going on is, in fact, erroneous or incomplete. As attention is focused both on the consumer as an active participant in the health-care system and on the population receiving this care, rather than merely on the institution whose programs are being implemented, new programs and new methods are certain to ensue.

Health Manpower Lagging Behind Public Demands for Service

Although the supply of physicians, nurses, and medical auxiliary personnel has increased both in absolute numbers and in proportion to the general population, as shown in Figure 4, there is a strong feeling of shortage in all health fields. This shortage arises from what seems to be the insatiable demand for health services. A discrepancy between manpower resources and service demands is particularly acute in community health because of a tremendous expansion of commitment to medical care at home and a relatively small increase in the manpower available.

The question has been raised as to whether or not the problems and the commitments of the present day can ever be met by the traditional

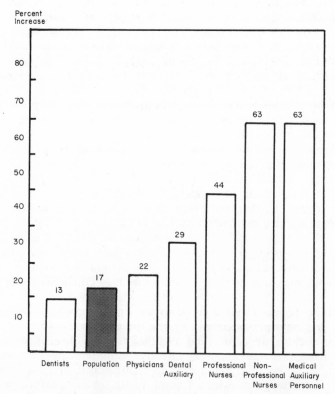

FIGURE 4.   Increases in the number of medical personnel, expressed both in absolute numbers and in proportion to the general population. (Redrawn from *Report of the Health Manpower Commission*. U.S. Government Printing Office, Washington, D.C., 1967.)

use of a staff predominantly made up of professional workers. This question concerns sheer quantitative relationships: the required number of doctors, nurses, and other personnel simply can not be recruited and trained within the present social structure. The aspect of utilization is also involved in this question; the professional-level worker may not be the best person to provide care in certain situations. When the problem is one of longterm care that is essentially custodial and supportive, the use of a short-trained worker may prove more efficient. When there is a problem of cultural distance between worker and client, it may be easier for the worker with short-term training to communicate with the client. There has already been a sharp increase in the use of short-trained personnel both in hospitals and in other community health agencies. This trend seems likely to continue.

INCREASED, BUT STILL INADEQUATE, NUMBER OF NURSES IN COMMUNITY HEALTH

The United States exceeds the ratio of one nurse for every 350 people suggested as an international standard in a recent Pan American Health Organization statement. Moreover, the United States greatly exceeds the ratio of many other "developed countries." France, for example, has one nurse for every 1200 people, and in Europe as a whole, the ratio is one nurse to 850 persons.[45]

However, as shown in Figure 5, the supply of nurses in the United States does not seem likely to meet projected needs. More importantly, the proportion of nurses with baccalaureate degrees or higher academic preparation, from which nurses must be drawn for leadership positions in administration, public health, teaching, and research, is dangerously low. The greatest rate of growth in new admissions to the nursing profession in the United States is in the number of nurses graduated from the relatively new associate degree programs, which do not provide the strong general education base on which to build leadership preparation.

Thus, despite the fact that the proportion of nurses to population has increased from 251 nurses per 100,000 of the population in 1954 to 325 nurses per 100,000 people in 1967 (at which time there were 640,000 employed professional nurses), there is a serious gap between the demand for, and the supply of, professional nurses, particularly teachers, supervisors, and administrators.[46] Even the most optimistic estimates of supply suggest that the problem of shortage will not be met entirely by increasing the numbers recruited to professional nursing. New methods of utilization, increases in returns to the nursing profession after absence for family responsibilities, and the development of new kinds of nursing manpower are seen by some as conditions offering the most hopeful approach to reconciling the need-supply discrepancy.

Distribution of Increase. In 1966 there were 41,254 nurses— 18.3 nurses for each 100,000 of the population—employed in public health work, including school nursing. This represents an increase since 1956, at which time there were 27,200 nurses so employed—16 nurses for each 100,000 of the population.[47]

By far the greatest number of these nurses are employed in local health work such as local health departments, visiting nurse associations,

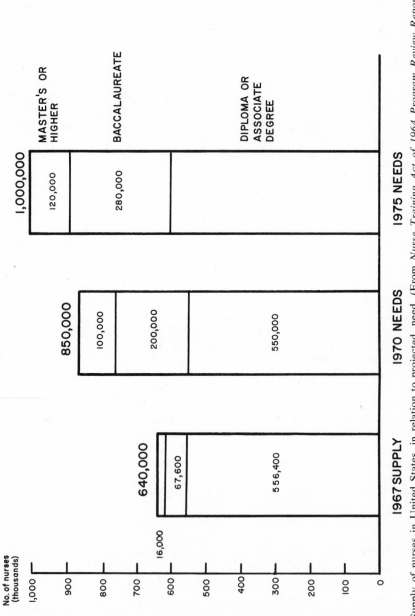

FIGURE 5.   Supply of nurses in United States, in relation to projected need. (From *Nurse Training Act of 1964 Program Review Report*. U.S. Department of Health, Education and Welfare, U.S. Government Printing Office, Washington, D.C., December, 1967, p. 57.)

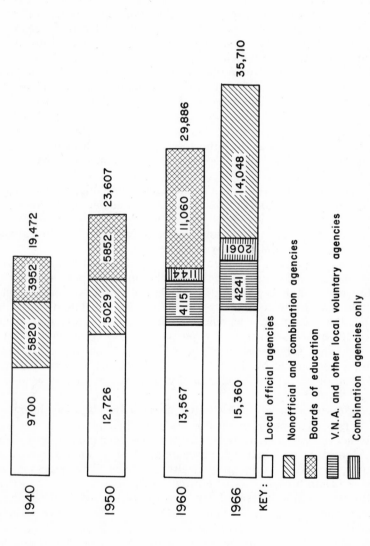

FIGURE 6.   Number of nurses employed by various types of agencies. The number of those employed by boards of education has grown most rapidly. (From *Nurses Employed in Public Health Agencies, 1966.* U.S. Government Printing Office, Washington, D.C., 1966, Table 2, p. 7.)

voluntary agencies; in combination agencies in which government and voluntary services are merged; and in schools. Ninety-five percent of the nurses engaged in public health work in 1966 were in local agencies. The remainder were in state or federal agencies or educational positions.

Greatest Increase in Nurses Employed by Boards of Education. As is shown in Figure 6, nursing under the sponsorship of boards of education has grown more rapidly than has nursing in other types of local employment. Between 1950 and 1960, the number of nurses employed by boards of education increased 89 percent compared to a 15.6 percent increase in local official and combined services during this period. This disparity in growth continued from 1960 to 1966 when the number of nurses employed by boards of education increased by 27 percent, compared to an increase of 15 percent in all other local services. In 1966, boards of education employed 39 percent of all nurses employed for local health work. This is not to imply that schools are overstaffed, but rather that the other community health agencies have made less progress than might be inferred from a cursory look at the figures.

It is interesting that the situation in Canada is quite opposite to that of the United States: the number of school nurses has decreased. In 1966 public health nurses, exclusive of school nurses, numbered 5165, 6.3 percent of all employed nurses; and the number of school nurses was only 505, 0.6 percent of all employed nurses.[48]

The number of persons in public elementary and high schools represents approximately 22 percent of the population. It is apparent that the availability of community nursing in the school setting is considerably greater than that in the community outside the school. The disparity in growth becomes even more significant when one considers that many schools receive nursing services from generalized community health agencies and that school-age children in schools which have full-time school nurses employed by the board of education are frequently cared for in illness, or as part of regular family services, by the nurse in the generalized service agency.

Inadequate Increase.   As noted previously, although the numbers of nurses in community health agencies has increased, the demands for service are increasing at a more accelerated pace. Legislation, such as Medicare and Medicaid, has expanded or created a new consumer group for local community health agencies. The development of intensive health programs directed toward disadvantaged or high-risk population groups has increased the amount of services provided to populations previously inadequately reached. Comprehensive-care programs of various sorts have created new needs for referral and nursing follow-up services in the home. Furthermore, as nursing education has improved and the preparation of nurses employed in community health work has increased, nurses themselves see more opportunities for care; thus the pressure is escalated still further.

To a greater degree, community health agencies are using licensed practical nurses, home health aides, specialized clerical help, and other personnel who can carry out nursing responsibilities not requiring professional-level decisions. Although this does help narrow the gap between demand and supply, it does not decrease the need for a larger complement of professional nurses.

Thus it could be said that the resources for health and medical care, though generous by some countries' standards, appear inadequate to meet the burgeoning demands of this country. Furthermore, the fragmented and uncoordinated system by which health care is provided makes efficient utilization of resources difficult, if not impossible.

HEALTH LEGISLATION

Through legislation, the people of the nation express their commitment to various types of social action. The tempo of introduction and adoption of health legislation has been accelerated in recent years. The 89th Congress has been called the most health oriented Congress in history. It passed 24 health or health-related bills.

The Comprehensive Health Care Planning Act has been discussed earlier as an expression of the public desire for a more rational approach to health planning. A few other representative pieces of legislation will be discussed here.

The Social Security Act

Basic to many of the modern efforts in health is the Social Security Act of 1935, which has been amended many times. It was amended very substantially in 1965 when the Medicare and Medicaid provisions were added. The original statement of principles that guided the development of this legislation express a clear commitment:

1. The national interest requires that all people have sufficient income to maintain a living standard conducive to health and well being.
2. All people should have the opportunity to meet their basic needs for living through their own efforts, with the federal government helping when necessary to make it possible for them to do so.
3. For people who are unable to maintain a minimum standard of health and well being through their own efforts, the federal government should provide grants to states for public assistance and social services.
4. Public programs of assistance and social services should be carried out in such a way as to strengthen family life, since the Nation's welfare is closely linked to the status of its families.[49]

This act provides, through insurance, for certain old age benefits, including (since 1965) provision for a combined compulsory and voluntary health benefit for those 65 years old or over; namely, Medicare. In addition, it provides for grants to states for the following purposes: old age assistance, including medical benefits to the needy aged (Title 1); aid for families with dependent children; aid for the blind; aid for the permanently and totally disabled; care for the aged blind and disabled; and, since 1965, medical assistance for needy or medically needy families (Title 19).

It has been estimated that when the program is in full operation, Titles 18 and 19 (Medicare and Medicaid) will reach over 25 percent of the people.[50]

Regional Medical Programs for Heart Disease, Cancer, and Stroke

As an outgrowth of the report of the President's Commission on Heart Disease, Cancer and Stroke, a bill was passed by the 89th Congress providing for federal aid to establish a system of regional medical programs for this group of diseases (Public Law 89-239). The first grants provided support for planning, and subsequent grants are planned for operational support. The bill requires the coordination of efforts of medical schools and other institutions. It provides for programs that involve research, training, and demonstration services for heart disease, cancer, stroke, and related diseases. A key provision includes the requirement that medical programs be founded on a regional basis and that appropriate geographic boundaries be established for this purpose. This legislation is bound to have an effect on the methods used in planning for general health services as well as on the particular disease entities with which it is primarily concerned.

The Nurse Training Act of 1964

In the spring of 1961, President Kennedy requested the Surgeon General of the Public Health Service to appoint a Consultant Group on Nursing, which, in 1963, published its report "Toward Quality in Nursing: Needs and Goals." This report served as a basis for developing the Nurse Training Act of 1964 (Public Law 88-581). The purpose of this legislation was not only to increase the numbers of nurses but also to improve the quality of the supply. The act provides for a broad program which includes grants for construction, teaching improvement programs, institutional support designed to upgrade and increase educational opportunities, loans to students, and traineeships for graduate nurses preparing for supervisory or teaching positions or clinical specialties.

Prior to the passage of this act, there had been provision beginning in 1957 for some training activities, but this was directed mainly toward increasing the supply of supervisors and teachers. The new legislation is much broader and provides for much greater support. The sum authorized under the Nurse Training Act for the five-year period from fiscal year 1965 through fiscal year 1969 was 283 million dollars.[51] Some idea of the growth in the size of this program may be gained from the fact that in 1957, two million dollars was authorized for nurse traineeships; in 1967, nine million dollars was authorized for this purpose.

The effects of this legislation will be felt not only in the increased numbers of nurses prepared under its various provisions but also in many areas of quality. In the process of reviewing the applications for assistance, both the recipient institution and the responsible government bureau must consider quality factors.

The Economic Opportunity Act of 1964

A health-related Act which has considerable health significance is the Economic Opportunity Act of 1964, amended in 1965. This comprehensive piece of legislation provided the basis for the war on poverty proposed by President Johnson. Its provisions include support for a variety of programs—job corps, work training programs, and work-study programs—designed to fit youth for employment. This act also provides for community action programs. Estimated expenditures for implementation of this legislation in 1966 was 822 million dollars.[52]

Explicit provision is made in this law for the active involvement of aid-recipients in the decisions relating to the implementation of programs. Although much major social legislation requires some "consumer" involvement, to date, those involved have tended to come from the more highly educated and "powerful" segments of the population. The provisions of this law bring to the decision-making table a group that has hitherto had little opportunity to control the social actions that affect it so vitally. It is expected that this involvement will have profound effects on every aspect of the program. Certainly, it will require considerable reassessment of the relationship between those responsible for implementing the health programs and those benefiting from the programs. It will unquestionably change the methods of planning for nursing services to low-income groups.

All of these legislative actions are representative of the broad and forceful stand being taken by the federal government of the United States with respect to health. There are a large number of other pieces of legislation that have significance for nursing. These range from action requiring safety devices to be installed in automobiles to proposals to increase health manpower of all types.

What is taking place in the United States is not unusual with respect to the scope of action and the depth of commitment to health movements, although the approach and the control may differ from those of other countries. Throughout the world this concern with health, as represented in legislative action, represents a major political movement. In most countries, public policy, with respect to extending and improving the health services available, improving the delivery of health-care services in order to equalize their availability, and improving health manpower, is under constant review; and changes tend to occur in the direction of increasing the services required.

Since legislative action is continuous, it is well to keep abreast of changes in health or health-related legislation. Very little of such legislation is without import for community health nursing.

PROSPECTS

Community health nursing is functioning within a large and complex system through which the community is acting to meet its health and health-related problems. The work of the nurse will be conditioned by each and every part of this system. If the nature of the population changes, nursing must change to conform to the new requirements. If the hospitals change the character of their work, community nursing may be called upon to change in order to meet the total needs of the community. If the numbers of physicians in public health expand or contract, this too may be reflected in the nature of the community nursing task. If the people, as represented by their legislators, set new values — whether higher or lower — on health, community nursing must again be responsive and able to expand or contract services.

Equally, the community health nurse has an opportunity to affect this system, since as nursing changes, the other components of the health system must adjust accordingly. As the community health nurse goes to her work with greater preparation, her capacity to influence developments in other fields, as well as in her own, will increase. Her observations, her ability to evaluate and communicate what she has observed, and her ability to make judgments with respect to the ways in which her own work may be used to further the total effort will affect all of her coworkers as well as the community at large.

The excitement and the immense potential for creative and effective work that such a reciprocal relationship affords is a challenge that can only become greater as one's experience increases and as one's sphere of influence broadens.

REFERENCES

1. Gardner, John: Health goals for the great society. New York Medical Quarterly, *10:*224, Spring, 1967.
2. Stewart, William: From an address delivered at the Annual Meeting of the National Academy of Engineering, 1967. Quoted in Public Health Service World, *2:*34, December, 1967.
3. Robson, R. A. H.: Sociological Factors Affecting Recruitment into the Nursing Profession. Royal Commission on Health Services, The Queen's Printer, Ottawa, 1964, p. 11.
4. Dubos, Rene: The Mirage of Health. Harper and Brothers, New York, 1959, p. 13.
5. Pocket Data Book, USA, 1967. U.S. Department of Commerce, Bureau of the Census, U.S. Government Printing Office, Washington, D.C., 1967, pp. 34, 35.
6. Health, Education and Welfare Trends, 1965. U.S. Department of Health, Education and Welfare, U.S. Government Printing Office, Washington, D.C., 1965, p. 3.
7. *Ibid.,* pp. 5-6.
8. *Ibid.,* pp. 5, 6, 10.
9. *Ibid.,* p. S-3.
10. *Ibid.,* p. 32.
11. *Ibid.,* p. 1.
12. The Facts of Life and Death. U.S. Department of Health, Education and Welfare, PHS Publication No. 600, U.S. Government Printing Office, Washington, D.C., 1967, p. 14. (Note: This publication is usually revised annually; see the most recent edition for later figures.)
13. Epidemiological and Vital Statistics Report. World Health Organization, Geneva, *20:*(Nos. 1, 2) 133, 117, 1967.
14. Health, Education and Welfare Trends, *op. cit.,* p. 4.
15. The Facts of Life and Death, *op. cit.,* p. 9.
16. *Ibid.,* p. 27.
17. Health, Education and Welfare Trends, *op. cit.,* p. 11.
18. *Ibid.,* p. S-15.
19. The Facts of Life and Death, *op. cit.,* p. 30.

20. 200 Million Americans. U.S. Department of Commerce, Bureau of the Census, U.S. Government Printing Office, Washington, D.C., 1967, p. 37.
21. Pocket Data Book, *op. cit.*, pp. 279, 286.
22. *Ibid.*, p. 191.
23. 200 Million Americans, *op. cit.*, p. 17.
24. Pakter, Jean, Rosner, Henry J., Jacobziner, Harold, and Greenstein, Frieda: Out-of-wedlock births in New York City. Amer. J. Public Health, Part I, Sociological Aspects, *51:*683, May, 1961; Part II, Medical Aspects, *51:*846, June, 1961.
25. Serum Cholesterol Levels of Adults in the U.S., 1960. U.S. National Center for Health Statistics, PHS Publication 1000, Series 11, No. 22, U.S. Government Printing Office, Washington, D.C., 1967.
26. Gunn, Alexander: Vulnerable groups—12. Life at the top: the health of the business executive. Nurs. Times, *64:*433, March, 1968.
27. Pocket Data Book, *op. cit.*, pp. 191, 186.
28. 200 Million Americans, *op. cit.*, p. 51.
29. Pocket Data Book, *op. cit.*, p. 193.
30. *Ibid.*, p. 190.
31. 200 Million Americans, *op. cit.*, pp. 55-56.
32. Facts About Smoking and Health. U.S. Department of Health, Education and Welfare, PHS Publication No. 1712, U.S. Government Printing Office, Washington, D.C., 1968.
33. Dependence on LSD and other hallucinogenic drugs. J.A.M.A., *202:*141, October, 1967.
34. Health is a Community Affair. National Commission on Community Health Services, Harvard University Press, Cambridge, Mass., 1966, p. 139.
35. McNerney, W.J.: Personal health comprehensive care services—a management challenge to the health professions. Amer. J. Public Health, *57:*1717, October, 1967.
36. Medical Care Financing and Utilization. U.S. Department of Health, Education and Welfare, Health Economics Series 1A, U.S. Government Printing Office, Washington, D.C., 1967, p. 4.
37. *Ibid.*, p. 61.
38. Pocket Data Book, *op. cit.*, p. 141.
39. Medical Care Financing and Utilization, *op. cit.*, p. 141.
40. Pocket Data Book, *op. cit.*, p. 139.
41. Moxley, John H., III: The predicament in health manpower. Amer. J. Nurs., *68:*1486, July, 1968.
42. Family Physician: Meeting the Challenge of Family Practice. American Medical Association *ad hoc* Committee on Education for Family Practice, Council on Medical Education, American Medical Association, Chicago, 1966.
43. Public Health Personnel in Local Health Units. U.S. Department of Health, Education and Welfare, PHS Publication No. 682, U.S. Government Printing Office, Washington, D.C., 1967.
44. Hamlin, Robert: The role of the voluntary agency in meeting the health needs of Americans. *In* Katz, Alfred, and Felton, Jean (eds.): Health and Community. Free Press, New York, 1965, p. 374.
45. Nursing Profession Undergoing Crisis. Pan American Health Organization Release, 1967.
46. Facts About Nursing 1967. American Nurses' Association, New York, 1967, p. 128.
47. Facts About Nursing 1967, *and* Facts About Nursing 1957. American Nurses' Association, New York, 1967 and 1957, pp. 28 *and* 29, respectively.
48. Countdown 1967. Canadian Nurses' Association, Ottawa, Canada, 1968, pp. 13, 14.
49. Public Assistance Under the Social Security Act: Serving People in Need. U.S. Department of Health, Education and Welfare, U.S. Government Printing Office, Washington, D.C., 1966, p. 1.
50. Peterson, Paul: The impact of recent federal legislation on personal health services. Amer. J. Public Health, *57:*1091, July, 1967.
51. Nurse Training Act of 1964, Program Review Report. U.S. Department of Health, Education and Welfare, PHS Publication No. 1740, U.S. Government Printing Office, Washington, D.C., 1967, p. 61.
52. Pocket Data Book, *op. cit.*, p. 94.

SUGGESTED READINGS

Ashenburg, Norman J.: The effects of air pollution on health. Nurs. Outlook, *16:*22, February, 1968.
Baumgartner, Leona: How will we get well and keep healthy? Nurs. Outlook, *16:*40, March, 1968.
Besson, Gerald: The health illness spectrum. Amer. J. Health, *57:*1901, November, 1967.
Conley, Veronica, and Olson, Stanley: Regional medical programs. Amer. J. Nurs., *68:*1916, September, 1968.
Countdown, 1967. Canadian Nurses' Association, Ottawa, 1968.
Dubos, Rene: Man Adapting. Yale University Press, New Haven, 1965.
Dubos, Rene: The Mirage of Health. Doubleday and Company, Inc., Garden City, 1959.
Exploring progress in public health nursing. Papers from Regional Clinical Conference No. 5, American Nurses' Association, New York, 1965.
The Family Physician: Meeting the Challenge of Family Practice. Ad Hoc Committee on Education for Family Health Practice, American Medical Association, Chicago, 1966.
Gordon, John E.: Changing accents in community disease. Amer. J. Public Health, *53:*141, February, 1963.
Health is a Community Affair. National Commission for Community Health Services, Harvard University Press, Cambridge, Mass., 1966.
Kohn, Robert: Emerging Patterns in Health Care. Canadian Royal Commission on Health Services, Queen's Printer, Ottawa, 1966.
Lee, R. V.: Provision of health services—past, present and future. New Eng. J. Med., *277:*682, September, 1967.
Man and his cities. Int. Nurs. Rev., *13:*27, March—April, 1966.
Morris, Robert: The city of the future and planning for health. Amer. J. Public Health, *58:*13, January, 1968.
Moxley, John H. III: Health manpower: the predicament. Amer. J. Nurs., *68:*1486, July, 1968.
Mustard, S., and Stebbins, E. L. (eds.): Introduction to Public Health. 4th ed., The Macmillan Company, New York, 1968, Chapter 1.
Nahm, Helen: Nursing dimensions and realities. Amer. J. Nurs., *65:*96, June, 1965.
Olson, Edith V.: Health manpower: needed—a shake up in the status quo. Amer. J. Nurs., *68:*1491, July, 1968.
Peterson, Paul Q.: The impact of recent federal legislation on personal health services. Amer. J. Public Health, *57:*1091, July, 1967.
Porterfield, John (ed.): Community Health. Basic Books, Inc., Publishers, New York, 1966, Chapter 1.
Position Paper on Educational Preparation for Nurse Practitioners and Assistants to Nurses. American Nurses' Association, New York, 1954.
Roberts, Ida: Health visiting: a view of the future. Nurs. Times, *64:*33, March, 1968.
Roberts, Mary: American Nursing: History and Interpretation. The Macmillan Company, New York, 1954, Chapter 9.
Stainbrook, Edward: Man and his changing environment. *In* Katz, A. H., and Felton, J. S. (eds.): Health and the Community. The Free Press, New York, 1965, 827.
Storck, John: Assessing the community's health in times of change. Public Health Rep., *81:*821, September, 1968.
Terris, Milton: A social policy for health. Amer. J. Public Health, *85:*5, January, 1968.
Toward Quality in Nursing—Needs and Goals. U.S. Department of Health, Education and Welfare. Report of the Surgeon General's Consultant Group on Nursing, P. H. S. Publication No. 992, U.S. Government Printing Office, Washington, D.C., 1963.
World Health Organization Expert Committee on Nursing. Fifth Report. W. H. O. Tech. Rep. Ser. No. 347, Geneva, 1966.

CHAPTER

2

The Nature of Community Health Nursing: Purpose and Goals

Community health nursing is more than nursing in a setting other than the hospital. It is more than the implementation of measures for the protection of public health. It is a unique blend of nursing and public health practice woven into a human service that, properly developed and applied, could have a tremendous impact on human well-being.

THE BASIC PURPOSE: FURTHERANCE OF COMMUNITY HEALTH

The purpose of community health nursing is to further community health through the selective application of nursing and public health measures within the framework of the total community health effort.

It is the nature of this purpose that determines the characteristic attributes of community health nursing. Although the methods through which the purpose is realized and the conditions under which the work of implementation proceeds will greatly vary throughout the world, the essential purpose, and hence the general nature, of community health nursing will remain relatively constant. The areas of responsibility, process, and the areas of interaction in community health nursing are shown graphically in Figure 7.

Community Health Nursing Is Community Focused

Implicit in this definition of purpose is that the focus of community health nursing is the community: the direction and nature of the nursing

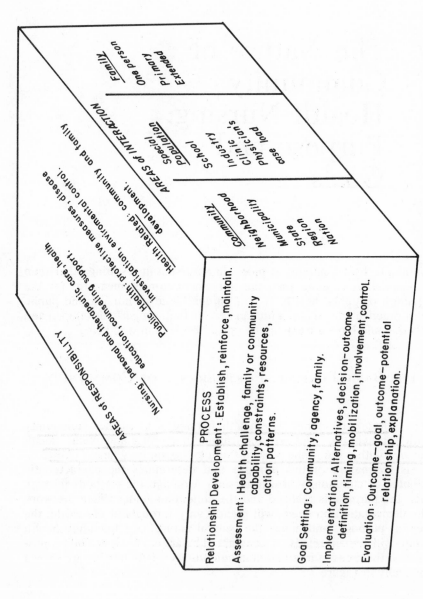

FIGURE 7.   The areas of responsibility, process, and interaction in community health nursing.

program is shaped by the needs of the community as a whole and by the nature of the total community health effort.

The health of the community is as much the product of its physical and social environment, its institutions, and its interactions and interfaces, as it is of the additive health conditions of its population. The interplay between the individual and his environment—whether the micro-environment of family and immediate neighbors or the macro-environment of the city, county, or country—is an essential determinant of family and community health. The betterment of that relationship is one of the major channels for health improvement.

A WIDE RANGE OF PROBLEMS

Whether in Taiwan or New York City, the community nurse cannot limit her attention to the individuals or families in her case load. She must be equally concerned with those who may need care but who have not sought it or who have been unable to find it. It is not enough to give the very best and most complete care possible to a small segment of the population while others are left without any care at all; nor is it possible to limit community health nursing to "patient" care. The community health nurse must be as concerned with the safety implications of a new swimming pool and with the alienating effect of the ghetto psychology as she is with the individual with a diagnosed illness or a defined health problem. She must also be concerned with health-related factors; for instance, the ways in which welfare is administered, since this affects family budgeting and buying habits and consequently the family's ability to remedy nutritional deficits; or the degree to which the school is involved with the community, since this affects the recreational and social behavior of the adolescent population and may therefore have a part to play in the control of venereal disease or pregnancy among unmarried teenage girls.

SPECIAL SKILLS REQUIRED

Just as surgical nursing involves some procedures that are common to both the surgeon and the nurse and just as psychiatric nursing requires some procedures that are common to the psychiatrist and the nurse, so community health nursing involves some procedures, skills, and knowledge that are common to all public health practitioners. The diagnosis of community health problems—the institution of measures designed to evaluate, protect, and advance the health of the population as a whole—requires special competence in epidemiologic methods, in the interpretation of biostatistical reports, and in community organization and planning. None of these skills replaces basic nursing skills, which are at least equally important in the provision of community nursing service. Rather, these special skills are a necessary supplement, especially when the community health nurse is working in a small agency with minimal immediate nursing and public health supervision.

A DEFINED PROCESS

The practice of community health nursing rests on a defined process that has much in common with the process used in many of the "helping" professions. This process is discussed more fully later, but essentially it involves the steps of developing a working relationship, assessment, goal setting, building and implementing a program of action, and evaluating the action taken.

A GENERALIZED APPROACH

Although individuals working in community health agencies may be specialists, community nursing as a whole is, above all, generalized. As will be discussed later, community health nursing may be provided through many different services and under many sponsorships within a given locality. However, the community health nursing effort for the community as a whole must be involved in the entire spectrum of health services, since the object of the service — the community — is made up of people of all ages, afflicted with a variety of diseases, faced with a multitude of genetic, psychological, social, and environmental threats to health, and hampered or helped by all levels of health practice.

Many of those served by the community health nurse will not be sick at all but may need preventive supervision during periods of stress. Vulnerable groups, for instance children in broken homes or suffering from physical or emotional deprivation, may require special protection. Anticipatory guidance, such as preparing a geriatric patient for problems associated with the aging process or readying the family of a hospitalized psychiatric patient for his return, takes an important place in health care. The community health nurse must be concerned with pre-disease manifestations or indications for preventive or supportive medical care that in other settings would be recognized by the physician or picked up in routine medical or laboratory examinations.

At the same time the community health nurse will be increasingly concerned with a variety of illnesses and injuries being cared for outside the hospital. In one and the same day she may serve families in which the main problems are tuberculosis, obstetrics, mental illness, or the supervision of a well school child. Thus the community health nurse is, above all, a generalist.

INDEPENDENT AND INTERDEPENDENT ACTION

Much of the work of community health nursing is done in the home or in small groups. This creates a situation in which it is not always possible to anticipate the problems that will arise and for which the community health nurse will not have immediate access to the advice of a physician or a senior nurse. As a result, to a greater degree than might occur in another setting, she is likely to be called upon to make decisions or to take action on her own initiative. She may be expected to decide whether or not to refer a child to a physician after a school mishap or to advise a family to stop medication pending investigation of symptoms by the physician.

The lines of accountability that characterize work in the community are also somewhat different from those that pertain in the hospital or in other work settings. There may be legislative requirements within which the work must be carried out: health laws or regulations may require periodic vision and hearing tests for school children, or they may specify the procedures to be followed in the care of patients with communicable disease.

In some instances the community nurse will be responsible to more than a single individual for her work. Certain aspects of her work may involve responsibilities to the school authorities, to the family physician responsible for the patient's care or to the medical director of the health unit. Although the nurse supervisor or administrator may be the mediator in the larger agencies, in many instances the nurse may work within a general policy developed by her agency, and her responsibility to another person or agency will be immediate and personal. Care of the individuals and families she serves may be shared by several other agencies or departments with whom she must find ways of relating and coordinating.

Whatever the setting, however, the community health nurse must relate not only to the family as a unit of service but also to many individuals and special groups within the community and to the community as a whole. For example, the nurse in a rural county will collaborate with individual families to provide preventive and curative nursing measures; she will also work with teachers and other groups within the shool to develop the nursing program, and with agricultural extension programs and community action groups to plan health education activities. Even though the distribution of effort and time among these various arenas of interaction will vary in different settings, community health nursing, by its nature, requires such collaboration.

Moreover, the nurse may work with indigenous midwives; she may help plan for the development of better facilities for intrapartum care; or as part of an effort to improve the statistical base for program planning, she may gather information about the outcome of pregnancies. She may also work with community resources for employment, housing, or welfare.

Definitions of Public Health or Community Nursing

The Division of Community Health Nursing Practice of the American Nurses' Association endorses the following definition:

> Community health nursing practice is a field of nursing practice for which there exists a body of knowledge and related skills which is applied in meeting the health needs of communities and of individuals and families in their normal environments such as the home, the school, and the place of work. It is an area of practice which lies primarily outside the therapeutic institution.[1]

A recent statement developed by the Canadian Public Health Association defines the philosophy of public health nursing in the following terms:

> Public health nursing is professional nursing that focuses its attention, through organized community effort, on serving people in their usual environments of home, school and work. As one part of the community's total arrangement for health promotion public health nursing is concerned with well people and with the sick and disabled. It strives to prevent

disease or to retard its progress; to reduce the ill effects of unavoidable disease; to provide skilled nursing care for the non-hospitalized sick and handicapped; to support those facing crisis situations; and to provide information and encouragement to individuals, families, special groups and the community as a whole for the development and practice of habits conducive to health.[2]

Thus community health nursing may be said to represent elements of both nursing and public health practice. It is concerned both with health and the community as an interacting whole and with the entire gamut of health care, which embraces the treatment and prevention of illness and injury and the rehabilitation and promotion of health and vigor. Community health nursing provides an important link between public health and nursing efforts.

THE GOALS OF COMMUNITY HEALTH NURSING

Within this general concept of purpose it is possible to identify the general goals toward which the community health nursing effort appears to be directed. These goals, which apply to the community health nursing effort or movement as a whole, will need to be supplemented by each nurse in her own situation and brought down to more measurable and exact statements.

Goal 1: To increase the capability of families, groups, and communities to cope with health and illness problems.

If this goal is to be realized, several conditions need to be met through whatever program is devised. Although it is fair to say that the community health nurse has a central role, no one of these conditions is the responsibility solely of the community health nurse; yet, no one of these conditions is unaffected by what she does and how she does it.

a. The level of health information held by families and community groups must be adequate to serve as a basis for the health decisions they are expected to make.

b. Families and groups should feel secure in the belief that the services they need and are unable to provide for themselves will be provided by the community. The community in turn should feel secure that the services they are unable to provide will be supplied either by an additional effort of the community itself or by some other level of government.

c. The community and its subgroups should have attitudes toward health care that are consistent with effective health planning and action at the family, group, and community level.

d. Families and groups should have whatever guidance is required to develop general problem-solving ability to enable them to deal with health problems on a rational basis.

e. The potential of families and groups for the direction of, and participation in, action on their own behalf should be fully recognized.

Goal 2: To support and supplement the efforts of other professional

workers or agencies in the control of disease and in the restoration and preservation of health.

Conditions that need to be met for the realization of this goal are likewise the responsibility of many health and health-related workers, but community health nursing again holds an important place in its achievement.

a. A continuing flow of field health intelligence is required for the development of health policy and plans. Reports of the occurrence of reportable or preventable diseases, the presence of health threats such as an apparent increase in the rat population, the results of simple screening tests in the school or community, and the response to offered health services are examples of such data.

b. Nursing support should be given to other members of the health team in the care of families, groups, or the community. Examples include providing information about home conditions and intra-family problems of patients to the family or clinic physician and supporting the sanitarian by reinforcing his instructions regarding the school environment.

Goal 3: To control or counteract as much as possible physical and social environmental conditions that threaten health or decrease the enjoyment of life.

Community nursing should help to effect the following:

a. The environment should be safe from such health threats as unnecessary exposure to accident, communicable disease, inadequate or unsafe water supplies, or indiscriminate access to harmful or habit-forming drugs.

b. The environment should be conducive to self-respect and self-realization. Freedom from discriminatory practices or assaults upon personal dignity is one indication that this condition is being met. Other indications might be adequate affectional interchange between parents and children; attractiveness, as well as safety, in the home; and child rearing practices that provide security and order and allow for individual creativity.

Goal 4: To contribute to the refinement and improvement of nursing practice and of public health practice and service.

Again, several important conditions may be identified as basic to the achievement of this goal:

a. Relevant research questions must be generated by those in practice as well as by those in research.

b. Continuing systematic study and appraisal must be an integral part of all professional practice.

c. New entrants to the field must be oriented and trained.

d. Multiprofessional research efforts must be supported by each of the disciplines involved at the planning, interpretative, and data collection phases of the investigation.

With no one of these goals is it possible for the nurse to carry the full responsibility. Nor is it possible for the nurse in community health practice to divorce herself from any of them. Within this goal context, the opportunity for creative, independent, and rewarding practice is limited only by personal inclination or by the failure to consistently and continually expand one's professional competence.*

REFERENCES

1. American Nurses' Association, Division of Community Health Nursing Practice. New York, April, 1967 (mimeo.).
2. A Statement of Functions and Qualifications for the Practice of Public Health Nursing in Canada. Canadian Public Health Association, Ontario, 1966, p. 1.

*The Suggested Readings for Chapter 2 are combined with those for Chapter 3 on p. 48.

3

Roles and Functions of the Community Health Nurse

What the community nurse actually does in a given situation will depend in part upon the concept she and others have of her role (that is, what is expected of her as a community health nurse) and in part on the functions that the professional organizations deem appropriate for the position of community health nurse.

ROLES

A consideration of some current perceptions of the role of the community health nurse helps to explain a few of the seeming inconsistencies (and sometimes, absurdities) that creep into the program planning in this field.

Provider of Personal Care to the Sick, Especially the Poor

Despite the facts that much of health care is not involved with illness and that even when illness is present, relatively little personal care is likely to be required, the community health nurse is still seen, particularly by the recipients of her aid, as one who cares for the sick. This image persists, rooted perhaps in the tradition of selfless service engendered by the Roman widows and reiterated in a different context by the Nightingale nurses; or possibly in the fact that many come to know the nurse first in the hospital setting where she may be the first source of help and the only one there day and night.

This perception is at once a blessing and a handicap. On the one hand, it creates a high degree of acceptance and trust on the part of the patient, since the nurse is an appreciated and tangible form of help. On the other hand, it may create a very limited view of the nursing potential for other types of care such as health teaching or the provision of emotional support.

Moreover, in many communities, especially in large urban areas, the community health nurse may be seen as one who "helps the poor." It is true that the case loads of community nursing services are usually heavily weighted with families from lower income groups; this is partly because the low-income groups tend to have a proportionately greater amount of illness and more health problems than the more fortunate groups. In many instances, however, this preconception, a hangover from a previous era, results in the neglect of middle and upper income groups who may have very pressing health problems, even though these problems are not as numerous. Drug abuse by high school students, for example, is by no means limited to the ghetto.

Willing Advocate

With the advent of specialization in medical practice and the consequent great fractionation of health and other human services, the community health nurse is often seen as an advocate of those being served. She is a kind of ombudsman in the home: one who will try to explain to the doctor the difficulties of following a prescribed treatment regime, expedite welfare action for the Medicaid patient, arrange for the sanitarian to visit the rural school, or talk to the school authorities when a student is constantly kept home to help with family work or to care for the home when someone is ill. She is seen as one who can stand between the family and the frustration, delay, and confusion imposed by fragmented and depersonalized health services.

Approachable and Concerned Adviser

From the standpoint of the recipient of community health nursing, perhaps the most significant role attributed to her is what Gerald Caplan has called that of a "wise older sister." This implies a commitment to the individuals being served that goes beyond casual interest or an impersonal provision of goods and services. It involves a certain amount of identification with the problems that are of concern to the patient and his family. It implies, also, a kind of claim on the part of the family for the nurse's concern, interest, and intervention on their behalf, since the relationship is not entirely one of equal exchange because of the nurse's professional preparation. The nurse's role is somewhere between that of teacher and collaborator, between that of counselor and friend.

This relationship can be observed when one looks at the differences in the ways patients use the physician and the nurse: in the types of problems they bring to the one or to the other, in the degree of freedom they feel in revealing themselves and their concerns, and in their willingness to identify and discuss those problems with the nurse which they feel are "too silly" to bring to the physician.

Patients and families, however, see the nurse as an adviser largely in practical and urgent matters. They may appreciate her willingness to listen, but they will not relate these less tangible acts to her role as a nurse and practical adviser.

Coworkers, too, see the nurse as an adviser. For instance, the health director may see her as a source of information about planning aspects of an immunization program; the school principal considers her as someone knowledgeable about the detection of disease among school children, or the industrial physician sees her as one who can anticipate the problems in securing employee compliance in a cancer screening program among women workers.

Sensitized Observer

For other members of the health team, particularly the medical care team, the community health nurse's role as a sensitized observer has an important place. The physician expects that the nurse will be alert to any deviation from expected behavior with respect to illness, growth and development, response to drugs, and general well-being. He is also dependent upon the nurse to be sensitive to, and to report, environmental conditions which are of importance in case management. He expects that she will be able to sort out and transmit to him those observations which are relevant to the situation.

The nurse's observations are especially needed in the home situation where the physician's contacts with the patient and the patient's family may be brief and infrequent. For example, the pediatrician may rely on the nurse to estimate and report the degree to which the father in a family is supporting the preventive care recommended for the children, the capacity of the family to carry through medical recommendations that are made, and the confidence or lack of confidence the family has in the treatment he has recommended. Families, too, share this expectation. Frequently they will say of the nurse, "I'm glad she came; she'd know if anything was wrong."

This role of sensitized observer extends to the community as well as the family. It is assumed that the community health nurse will be aware of and will report any unusual occurrence of disease symptoms; environmental threats; or unusual family or community stresses that may indicate a need for further epidemiologic, social, or environmental study.

One Who Influences Decisions and Produces Change

The community health nurse, by virtue of her expertise in public health practice, as well as in nursing, is expected to influence decisions at the individual, family, and community level and to manage change in the direction of more effective health care.

In the developmental period of rural health services, the public health nurse was frequently the only representative of community health services. The employment of a public health nurse usually increased the likelihood of a more comprehensive health organization and led to greater use of medical supervision, prenatal care, and immunization.

Currently, as health care becomes more and more dependent upon the willing and knowing action of the public, the role of the community nurse assumes a still more central position in enabling the individual, family, or group to make good decisions about health, to take appropriate and prompt action, and to deal constructively with inescapable illness and death. Lundberg describes this role as a "potentiator": someone who serves as a catalyst; one who is able to make others more effective.[2]

The community health nurse is expected to increase the family and community capacity to cope with their health problems as well as to provide care herself; to help school children utilize the educational facilities of the school more effectively; to bring the accident control program into the homes, schools, and industries of the community; and to encourage support and participation in the total health program. Whether the barrier to action is logistical, such as poor scheduling of a crippled children's clinic, or attitudinal, such as distrust of any authoritative figure on the part of a low-income family, the nurse is generally expected to "do something about it." She is counted upon to try to overcome whatever stands in the way of forward movement.

It is also expected that the nurse's efforts on behalf of change will extend to promoting action on more general fronts as she sees, interprets, and urges action with respect to unmet human needs or incongruous community responses to health-care requirements.

Organizer and Manager

Whether in family care or in carrying out agency responsibilities in homes, schools, and places of employment, the community health nurse is often seen as an organizer who welds the many aspects of service into some kind of suitable pattern.

She may be thought of as the one who keeps the clinic running smoothly, who gathers together all of the many strands of care being provided to a particular family, and who organizes and supervises auxiliary workers. She may be expected to identify, interpret, and maintain the linkages between hospital and community nursing services and between developments in professional nursing practice and the health agency program. The nurse may be seen as the one who keeps things "under control."

Knowing Participant in Community Planning and Action

In deliberative groups in the agency and in the community, there is almost always provision for "a representative of nursing," or for someone who can provide the "nursing point of view."

The special ingredient provided by the community health nurse is considered important in molding decisions not only about nursing but also about community health and about health and health-related facets of education and welfare programs. Whether seen as someone who provides the essential information on which decisions are made or as an active member of a deliberative action group, a representative of community nursing interests is rarely absent from decisional activities in areas where community health and nursing are involved.

Decisions relating to the timing of a particular program, the methods of approach that might be used in securing community participation and support, and the people who might be appropriately involved in carrying through community action programs are areas in which nursing knowledge and nursing know-how carry a great deal of weight. However, it must be added that the nurse's role as a decision maker is sometimes clearer to the nursing profession than it is to others involved in the decisions!

Provider of personal care, advocate, teacher and counselor, observer, potentiator, organizer, and decision maker: in different ways and in varying degrees, the community nurse is expected to fill all of these roles. The nature and the scope of these expectations has a strong effect on what the community health nurse is able to do. The degree to which the expectations of others are congruent with those of the nurse herself will have much to do with the satisfaction she derives from her work.

FUNCTIONS

The functions of community health nursing represent those broad areas of responsibility that the community health nurse is expected to assume. Functions of any professional group are generally defined by the professional group itself. In the case of community health nursing, both the American Nurses' Association and the American Public Health Association have provided official statements, as has the Canadian Public Health Association.[2-4] On an international level, the World Health Organization has described public health nursing in an official technical bulletin.[5]

The official statement of functions, emanating in most instances from the appropriate professional association, is based on the judgment and the will of the practitioners in that field. However, this statement is also influenced by many factors of the environment. The numbers, preparation, and distribution of medical practitioners, the types of health institutions, the social position of women, the acceptability of male nurses, the state of health science, and public policy and commitment to health care all have a bearing on the final definition of functions. Since these conditions are always in a process of change, changes may also be expected in the functions of any professional worker. For this reason, every community health nurse, and all others involved with the provision of community nursing service, should not only be aware of current official statements but should also be alert to the indications that may presage change.

The following statement of functions differs from the official statements previously noted, but it is not inconsistent with them.

Function 1. The community health nurse provides and promotes comprehensive nursing service to families. These services include personal and therapeutic care to the unhospitalized sick; preventive tests and procedures that are within nursing competence; anticipatory, crisis, or continuing health guidance and support; and health counseling. The provision of comprehensive nursing care by or under the direct supervision of a nurse to everyone who is sick, likely to be sick, disabled, in need of preventive care or preparation for a predictable crisis, or whose health practices constitute a threat to health is obviously far beyond present or anticipated nurse manpower capability. Therefore, the accomplishment of this function requires a variety of approaches, which includes:

a. Assuming direct responsibility for providing care or for supervising and directing others who provide care, for those families or groups to whom the agency has a specific commitment (such as Medicare patients) and for others within the limits of agency policy.

b. Teaching others, or arranging for the teaching of others, to give such care as is required. For example, the nurse may teach family members or groups to give care to longterm patients at home, she may arrange for the American Red Cross to develop classes in home nursing or child care, or she may organize volunteers or the regular staff to teach home nursing in the secondary school. This approach permits reaching a much wider group than is possible with the procedures noted under *a.*

c. Referring to other sources for care. For example, the nurse in the local department of health may refer a family to the Visiting Nurse Association, suggest that the nurse in the industrial plant would be willing to help with dressing a small wound, or recommend that the nurse in the diabetic clinic might be able to help with injections of insulin.

Often a combination of two or more approaches will be used. For example, the nurse might teach a family member to provide personal care for a geriatric patient, but she herself would continue to provide guidance and support to the family as they anticipate and prepare for changes with advancing age of the patient.

Function 2. The community health nurse uses nursing as a channel for strengthening family life and for promoting personal or family development and self-realization. Even though in many ways this is a "bonus function" and is achieved largely in the course of fulfilling other functions, it is an essential and powerful ingredient of community health nursing. Thus, deliberately and progressively engaging socially alienated families in decisions regarding their own care may engender a degree of self-confidence and skill in handling other family problems; engaging the rebellious "way out" adolescent in the care of others offers him a channel for expressing social concern and may perhaps be a first step toward meaningful social action. Such general skills are inextricably interwoven with the social and emotional health of the individual and with the development of the favorable home environment so essential for nurturing the growing child.

Function 3. The community health nurse participates in disease control activities through general preventive measures, early identification of disease, provision of care, and supervision to reduce the effects of disease. Examples of ways in which the nurse might implement this function are:

a. Using a variety of channels to alert parents, teachers, possible patients, vulnerable groups, or the general public to symptoms that merit further investigation or preventive intervention.

b. Using the family and patient history as a tool for eliciting symptoms of undiagnosed disease, impairment, or health risk. For example, a 45-year-old woman who has requested care for an acute illness might be observed and queried as to symptoms of disease or health conditions likely to be found in that age group.

c. Participating in epidemiologic alerts and investigations. For example, the nurse might alert an individual reporting a gastrointestinal upset to watch for and report others with similar symptoms, alert school personnel to the existence and probable curve of an outbreak of influenza, or help carry out an epidemiologic survey or investigation.

d. Participating in screening and mass preventive procedures. The nurse could recruit participants, assist with the screening or immunization programs, interpret the program, and assist those needing further study or care.

Function 4. The community health nurse works with appropriate personnel in special settings, such as schools and places of employment, to plan and implement the nursing phases of their health programs. The following are representative measures for carrying out this function:

a. Reviewing and interpreting data—such as absence records, service reports, or teacher-nurse conference notes—relevant to health needs of these special population groups.

b. Arranging with appropriate administrative personnel for schedules and procedures for reporting and evaluating ongoing and special health activities. This may include such activities as scheduling visits to schools or nursing homes or setting up plans for medical examinations of a migrant labor crew.

    c. Serving as a member of committees for health planning and action.

Function 5. The community health nurse plans and evaluates the nursing services for the population group under her care to maximize the benefits of nursing care and to bring the nursing effort into proper relationship with that of other health workers serving the same population. Examples of ways in which this function is accomplished include:

    a. Identifying service developments and demographic and vital statistics trends that might have relevance for nursing, such as changes in the age distribution in the population, trends in incidence of tuberculosis, and plans for glaucoma screening or increased home care for psychiatric patients.

    b. Setting goals and clearly defined outcomes for the nursing service and establishing a systematic method for checking progress.

    c. Conferring and planning with other health workers for the care of families or groups such as discharged tuberculosis patients or those participating in a screening program.

    d. Working with the nursing supervisor or administrator to evaluate nursing accomplishments and to plan for improvement.

Function 6. The community health nurse contributes to decision and policy setting in the agency and community. This function may be realized through such activities as:

    a. Sending reports or suggestions, based on field observations or other personal experience, to appropriate individuals involved in policy setting within the agency.

    b. Accepting (or when appropriate, prompting) membership on agency or community planning committees concerned with making recommendations regarding agency program and policy.

Function 7. The community health nurse contributes to the extension of knowledge in nursing and health care by engaging in surveys, studies, or research. This may be done through:

    a. Proposing problems that need systematic study for their resolution.

    b. Planning and carrying out simple studies as part of the continuing service effort. One typical inquiry would be the postnatal examination return rate of those who had received prenatal nursing supervision in groups, as compared to those whose care was provided on an individual basis.

    c. Participating in research done by others when it is appropriate. In general, "appropriate tasks" include those that require nursing skill, that provide experience which will increase the nurse's capacity for later independent research, that contribute to the nurse's research competence, and that can be undertaken without detriment to ongoing service commitments.

Expanding Responsibilities of the Nurse

Recently there has been considerable attention given to the expansion of the responsibility of the nurse, particularly as related to her assumption of some activities and some decisions that have customarily fallen within the realm of medicine. The increasing production and use of the clinical specialist in the hospital has been accompanied by the use of the community health nurse in an expanded role in the community setting.

Siegel and Bryson, for example, suggest that the role of the nurse in child health supervision might be considerably expanded in view of the nature of the problems presented. They suggest that the nurse see the child before the physician and that in many instances the family could be seen only by the nurse.[6]

In Colorado, a "pediatric nurse practitioner" has assumed expanded responsibilities in pediatric care. Fortified by special training and a close association with the pediatrician, she is equipped to furnish comprehensive well-child care to children of all ages. This care includes the assessment of physical and psychosocial development, immunization, and counseling on child rearing problems. She is also prepared to render emergency services when indicated and to identify and refer acute and chronic conditions that require medical care.[7] Lewis and Resnick report expanded responsibilities of a community health nurse who functions in a special "nurse clinic" for selected patients in which there is a wide latitude for independent action and decision.[8] Miner reported that in the year 1960-61, nurses in the Saskatchewan Health Region and Northern Health District gave over 434,000 immunizations.[9]

This enlargement and transfer of functions is understandable. First of all, such shifts have characterized the physician-nurse relationship for many years. At one time, taking a patient's temperature was strictly a medical function! In addition, the nature of health care has changed so that much of the care required is not primarily medical in nature but rather observational, educational, or supportive and thus properly a nursing practice area. Also, the increasingly professional character of basic nursing education and the expanding opportunities for preparation in specialty areas is creating an able and highly independent group of nurses who respond enthusiastically to the challenge such extended responsibilities offer. There is every likelihood that this extension will continue to spread.

The functions of community health nursing are at once broad and susceptible to the use of specific measures for their realization. Their accomplishment must be based upon both nursing and public health skills and knowledge. Most of all, their appropriate application demands judgment in a high degree. Distortion or inappropriate application of these various aspects of practice in a particular setting may make even "good" nursing unproductive in its outcomes.

REFERENCES

1. Lundberg, Helen G.: A community health potentiator. Nurs. Outlook, *14:*43, September, 1966.
2. Functions and Qualifications in the Practice of Public Health Nursing. American Nurses' Association, New York, 1964.
3. Educational Qualifications of Public Health Nurses. American Public Health Association, Committee on Professional Education, Amer. J. Public Health, *52:*501, March, 1962.
4. A Statement of Functions and Qualifications for the Practice of Public Health Nursing in Canada. Canadian Public Health Association, Toronto, 1967.
5. Public Health Nursing. World Health Organization, Technical Report Series 167, Fourth Report of the Expert Committee on Nursing, Geneva, 1959.
6. Siegel, E., and Bryson, S.: A redefinition of the role of the nurse in child health supervision. Amer. J. Public Health, *53:*1015, July, 1963.
7. Silver, H. K., Ford, Loretta, and Stearly, Susan: A program to increase health care for children: the pediatric nurse practitioner program. Pediatric Nursing Currents, Ross Laboratories, Columbus, Ohio, Vol. 14, No. 4, July, 1967.
8. Lewis, C. E., and Resnick, B. A.: Nurse clinics and progressive ambulatory care. New Eng. J. Med. *277:*1236, December, 1967.
9. Miner, E. L.: The public health nurse in diagnosis and treatment. Canad. J. Public Health, *54:*378, August, 1963.

SUGGESTED READINGS (CHAPTERS 2 AND 3)

Abrams, Rhoda: Patterns in public health nursing home visits. Amer. J. Nurs., *63:*102, March, 1963.
Asplund, Brita: The nurse's role tomorrow. Int. Nurs. Rev., *13:*25, November–December, 1966.
Baldridge, Patricia: The nurse in triage. Nurs. Outlook, *14:*46, November, 1966.
Bauer, Herbert: Public health: a medical specialty? Amer. J. Public Health (Letters to the Editor), *58:*1581, September, 1968.
Bergman, Rebecca Lyons: Public health nursing functions: assisting, complementing, initiating. Nurs. Outlook, *14:*42, July, 1966.
Bryant, Zella: The public health nurse's expanding responsibilities. *In* Stewart, D. M., and Vincent, P. A. (eds.): Public Health Nursing. William C. Brown Company, Publishers, Dubuque, Iowa, 1968, p. 3.
Bulbulyan, Ann, Davidites, R. M., and Williams, Florence: Nurses in a community mental health center. Amer. J. Nurs., *69:*328, February, 1969.
Coffey, Kenneth J.: Nurses and the Peace Corps. Amer. J. Nurs., *62:*50, July, 1962.
Cotter, Sister Mary D.: The public health nurse and community mental health. Nurs. Outlook, *16:*59, April, 1968.
DeYoung, Carol D.: Nursing's contribution to family crisis treatment. Nurs. Outlook, *16:*60, February, 1968.
Educational Qualifications of Public Health Nurses. Amer. J. Public Health, *52:*501, March, 1962.
Field, W. E. Jr., Patterson, E. Gene, and Dayton, Mildred: The senses taker. Amer. J. Nurs., *66:*2654, December, 1966.
Ford, Patricia A., Seacat, Milvoy S., and Silver, George A.: The relative roles of the public health nurse and the physician in prenatal and infant supervision. Amer. J. Public Health, *56:*1097, July, 1966.
Freeman, Ruth B.: The criterion of relevance. Amer. J. Public Health, *57:*1522, September, 1967.
Functions and Qualifications in the Practice of Public Health Nursing. The American Nurses' Association, New York, 1964.
Glidewell, John C.: The role of epidemiologic research in local health departments, Part I. Nurs. Outlook, *10:*733, November, 1962.
Ibid., Part 2. Nurs. Outlook, *10:*804, December, 1962.
Hale, Rosemary, Loveland, Marion, and Owen, Grace: The Principles and Practice of Health Visiting. Pergamon Press, Inc., London, 1968, p. 17.

Hammerly, Aloha B.: The army's public health nurses. Amer. J. Nurs., 66:765, April, 1966.
Hanlon, John: Principles of Public Health. 5th ed., The C. V. Mosby Co., St. Louis, 1969, p. 585.
Hansen, Ann, and Levy, Judith M.: What is a public health nurse? Nurs. Res., 10:100, Spring, 1961.
Haugen, Idunn: Changing role and functions of a nurse in the community. International Journal of Nursing Studies, 3:111, September, 1966.
Helvie, Carl O., Hill, Ann, and Bambino, Charlotte: The setting and nursing practice. Part I. Nurs. Outlook, 16:27, August, 1968. Ibid., Part II. Nurs. Outlook, 16:35, September, 1968.
Henderson, Virginia: The Nature of Nursing: A Definition and Its Implications for Practice, Research and Education. The Macmillan Company, New York, 1966.
Holliday, Jane: Public Health Nursing Care of the Sick at Home: A Descriptive Study. Visiting Nurse Association of New York, New York, 1967.
Leone, Lucille: Center for creative nursing. Public Health Rep., 78:347, April, 1963.
Lewis, C. E., and Resnick, B. A.: Nurse clinics and progressive ambulatory care. New Eng. J. Med., 277:1236, December, 1967.
Lundberg, Helen G.: A community health potentiator. Nurs. Outlook, 14:43, September, 1966.
Mauksch, Hans O.: The nurse: coordinator of nursing care. In Skipper, J. K., and Leonard, R. C. (eds.): Social Interaction and Patient Care. J. B. Lippincott Co., Philadelphia, 1965, p. 251.
May, L. K.: Changing trends in health visiting. International Journal of Nursing Studies, 3:27, May, 1966.
Miner, E. L.: The public health nurse in diagnosis and treatment. Canad. J. Public Health, 54:378, August, 1963.
Mitch, Anna D., and Kaczala, Sophie: The public health nurse coordinator in a general hospital. Nurs. Outlook, 16:34, February, 1968.
Murphy, Marion: Why a master's prepared practitioner in public health nursing? Part I. Nurs. Outlook, 15:33, March, 1967. Ibid. Part II. Nurs. Outlook, 15:56, April, 1967.
Mussalem, Helen: The changing role of the nurse. Amer. J. Nurs., 69:514, March, 1969.
Public Health Nursing. Fourth Report of the Expert Committee on Nursing. World Health Organization, Technical Report Series No. 167, Geneva, 1959.
Reese, Eva M.: Public health nursing and comprehensive health care. Nurs. Outlook, 16:48, January, 1968.
Schulman, Diane, and Schulman, Sam: The nurse as catalyst. Amer. J. Nurs., 68:1890, September, 1968.
Schulman, Sam: Basic functional roles in nursing: mother surrogate and healer. In Jaco, Gartly E. (ed.): Patients, Physicians and Illness. The Free Press, Glencoe, Ill., 1958, p. 528.
Sheps, Cecil G., and Bachar, Miriam: Nursing and medicine — emerging patterns of practice. Amer. J. Nurs., 64:107, September, 1964.
Siegel, E., Dillehay, R., and Fitzgerald, C.: Role changes within the child health conference: attitudes and professional preparedness of public health nurses and physicians. Amer. J. Public Health, 55:832, June, 1965.
Silver, George: Family Medical Care. Harvard University Press, Cambridge, Mass., 1963, Chapter 5.
A Statement of Functions and Qualifications for the Practice of Public Health Nursing in Canada. Canadian Public Health Association, Toronto (1255 Yonge St.), Ontario, 1966.
Staub, Mary and Parker, Kitty (eds.): Continuity of Patient Care: The Role of Nursing. Proceedings of a Workshop. Catholic University of America Press, Washington, D.C., 1966.
Wald, Florence S.: Emerging nursing practice. Amer. J. Public Health, 56:1252, August, 1966.
Wiedenbach, Ernestine: The helping art of nursing. Amer. J. Nurs., 63:54, November, 1963.

Community Health Nursing: The Process

Community health purposes and goals are realized through the application of a process: an orderly series of steps which, if taken, are expected to lead to a desired result. The process is similar to that of problem-solving itself, and predictably the steps will have much in common with those of the other helping professions such as medicine and social work. The uniqueness of the process as used in community health nursing will depend both on the nature of the end, which is the best possible application of nursing to the community's health problems, and on the nature of the means, which is a synthesis of nursing and public health skills.

Five major steps may be identified in the process through which community health nursing is effected:
1. Establishing, reinforcing, or maintaining a working relationship.
2. Assessing the health and nursing situations.
3. Establishing the goals for health and nursing care.
4. Constructing and implementing a program of action (which includes choosing among alternative actions).
5. Validating or evaluating the action taken.

PROBLEMS CHANGE, BUT THE PROCESS FOR MEETING THEM REMAINS CONSTANT

Even though the problems with which the nurse is faced will vary considerably, the process by which she moves to deal with them should remain constant. Whether working with an individual being treated in a venereal disease clinic or with a community organizing to prevent accidental injuries on the highway, the same steps will be required to move toward a solution.

THE PROCESS SYNTHESIZES THE DECISIONS OF MANY

The process by which an effective community health nursing program is established involves the integration of the decisions of the many workers, both professional and nonprofessional, who are involved. The decisions of the client, be it a family, a fellow health professional, or a community committee, must be developed and reconciled with those of the nurse in a way that makes the final action satisfactory to both.

The family, as well as the nurse, decides the kind of relationship or interchange that will be acceptable as a "working" relationship; the community planning committee, as well as the nurse, will define the goals that should govern the action to be taken; the medical health director, as well as the nurse, will be involved in determining the effectiveness of the nursing services provided.

ESTABLISHING A WORKING RELATIONSHIP

The health problems that are handled by the community nurse and by those she serves are not simple. Their solution often depends upon the willingness of individuals, families, and community groups to make careful decisions, to persist in a long course of action, or to change fundamental patterns of living. The support of the care recipients in achieving this end requires that the nurse, through the use of interpersonal and other therapeutic measures, draw out and clarify the attitudes and feelings that are apt to influence their evaluation of the problem. To achieve the desired ends, the nurse and the family, agency, or community group must establish a relationship that permits them to work together in such a way that the best efforts of both can be fused into action for improving the situation. This relationship may best be described as a "working" relationship, one which, in itself, constitutes a positive force in achieving the goals of the community health nursing service. It is a relationship that works. It is a relationship that is consistent with the demands of a particular situation and that creates a climate which fosters the required action, whether the action is to help the family or to protect the community. The development of such a working relationship becomes the foundation for all subsequent nursing action.

Characteristics of a Working Relationship

PRODUCTIVE

The primary criterion for a working relationship is that, in the long run, it produces the intended results. Thus, in an emergency situation that requires an individual to be hospitalized immediately and the patient and family are too distraught to think clearly, an authoritarian or "hard sell" persuasive relationship may be entirely appropriate. However, if nursing home care is required for a geriatric patient whose presence in the home is threatening the well-being of other family members, an authoritarian relationship may be totally inappropriate. The hard sell may produce immediate results in terms of initiating nursing-home care, but the decision has not been made by the family; moreover all of the possible factors have not been discussed and evaluated in advance. In consequence, the longterm result may be either the return of the patient to the home or the development of emotional problems among guilt-ridden family members, the latter resulting from a lack of confidence in the decision that has been made. The situation may thus be worsened, not improved.

TWO-WAY COMMUNICATION

A working relationship is characterized by free two-way communication; that is, each party communicates his feelings, his ideas, his concerns to the other. This openness is a critical factor in assessing nursing needs and in determining what action may be appropriate. Three conditions — trust, empathy, and "outreach" — are essential for the development of a communicating relationship.

Trust.   Trust is the *sine qua non* of any truly joint endeavor. If the family sees the nurse as a representative of the authorities who have the power to cut off welfare aid or as someone too well-off, too young, or too protected to accept them as they are and to appreciate real-life problems, they are unlikely to trust her sufficiently to reveal their true feelings. If the nurse expects her clients to be lazy and unwilling or unable to do what is expected of them, she too will find it hard to deal openly and objectively with the problems at hand. Both the nurse and the client must be confident of the other's basic integrity. Even though cultural or educational background may create differences in value concepts and in behavioral patterns, the achievement of mutual respect is not only possible, it is imperative.

To work together effectively, the recipient of care must feel that the nurse's primary concern is the good of the family (or the agency or the community) and that her primary objective is to help. The nurse, in turn, must feel that those with whom she is working sincerely desire to improve the situation and that each individual with whom she deals is a person of worth and consequence.

Empathy.   Empathy has received growing emphasis as an essential to any helping relationship. Appreciation of the importance of general attitudes and feelings in determining health action has reinforced the notion that, as a basis for planning specific health care, it is necessary to see another's problem and to understand how he feels. At the same time a growing reliance on the family (or community) in decision making and in action for health care has produced new problems of interaction. The professional health worker who is trying to merge his own decisional abilities with those of recipient groups must have an undistorted picture of how his partners in planning feel about various facets of their health problems and about the health-care system. This kind of understanding rests for the most part on the ability to sense the feelings of others; to accept, rather than to judge, the ways in which people relate to their world. For the health professional, it is essential that there be the capacity not only to enter into another's feeling world, but also, when the occasion demands, to step back out of it and become an objective observer and planner.

Outreach. Outreach, taking the initiative in introducing discussion of a problem or in offering assistance, has assumed greater importance than it has held previously. Recent studies of failure of community services to reach certain segments of the population suggest that many families and groups, especially those living in poverty, take a passive role with respect to the community services afforded them. This may arise from a failure to recognize that a problem exists, from a feeling that they are expected to be grateful and not demanding, or from an inability to express their needs because of poor communication skills. In such cases, the service personnel must take the initiative rather than wait for the topic to come up in the course of the visit. The nurse may need to raise the issue of birth control or to propose that the father of the family might be more involved in a particular health situation.

CONFIDENT

A working relationship must be based on the assumption that the relationship is worthwhile, that something will come of it. Both the nurse and those with whom she works must be convinced that the nursing input — that is, what the nurse does — has relevance and is likely to help. The family must feel that the nurse's advice regarding prenatal medical supervision is truly germane to their well-being; the public health physician consulting with the nurse must feel that the suggestions she offers are practically related to the problems of the program as a whole.

On the other hand, the nurse, too, must have confidence in those she serves. She must accept the validity of a parent's estimate of the probable behavior of his offspring. She must accept the existence of motivations that create behavior different from that which the nurse herself would find natural — for example, the over-striving of the suburban middle class parent or the all-or-nothing orientation of an adolescent — without letting this difference undermine or distort her belief in the basic competence of most people to make wise decisions or to consider the alternatives.

SPECIFIC AND GENERAL DEVELOPMENT
FOSTERED

A working relationship is one in which those involved build upon one another's abilities so that each participant grows through encounter with the other. The ego-damaged parent living in a low-income area may gain strength and self-confidence through the way in which the community health nurse provides help. The parent, in turn, because of the nurse's willingness to expose her thoughts and her feelings, increases the nurse's understanding of, and competence in dealing with, these kinds of situations.

Moreover, a building relationship is concerned with general, as well as specific, development. The abilities to solve problems, to deal with one's daily tasks more effectively, and to gain a little insight into problems in wider spheres of action are as important in building health competence as they are satisfying as measures of personal development.

A Working Relationship Is Developed, Not Discovered

It is likely that few practitioners develop their capacity for using interpersonal relationships to the fullest potential. Certainly the capacity to develop and to use one's relationship with others as a means of achieving service goals should be expected to grow with professional maturity and experience. However, it cannot be assumed that experience alone will assure this growth. There is need for a firm conviction that such relationships are an integral part of successful practice and that a persistent effort toward improvement of interpersonal skills is both necessary and rewarding.

GET TO KNOW THE PATIENT AND ENVIRONMENT

To understand and appreciate another person usually requires knowing something about him. To know how a father who is not the family wage earner feels about his condition and how he sees himself as a father helps to explain his attitudes and behavior with respect to child rearing and the use of medical resources. The nurse can "put herself in his shoes" as he faces the combination of pressures with which he must live. To know of the frustrating and ego-damaging experiences apt to be encountered by a young unmarried mother in her use of health facilities may make it easier to feel with her the great courage it may take to try again.

Observation.   Learning about diseases is relatively easy; learning about people is considerably less easy. However, much will be learned by observation, for example, of the way a mother holds her infant, of the pride or exasperation in the voice of a patient telling about the members of her family during the taking of the family history, or of the way in which an elderly patient explains for the ninth time how lonely it is with everyone away during the day. But observation alone is not enough; there is also need for a kind of relaxed "sopping up" attitude on the part of the nurse. That is, she must put aside, for a while, all of the pressures in her own work in order to "tune in" on the family or group and to understand what they are trying to communicate often without words or in words that express something quite different from their literal meaning.

In any interpersonal exchange there are clues to meaning that are essential guides. Hodgins talks about the silent patient who may be saying by his silence that he thinks no one wants to help; that no one can help; or that should he raise a question, it will not be answered honestly. The family member who agrees too quickly to suggestions that are bound to be hard to carry through, the family physician who talks about the "wonderful girls in the VNA" but who seldom refers a patient, the adolescent who appears overly unconcerned about the possibility that he has contracted gonorrhea: all are saying things of importance, and by the way they select what they say or do not say, they are expressing the quality of the relationship that has been developed.[1] The virtue of quiet repose, listening without talking, cannot be overestimated as an investigative method.

In community health nursing, getting to know the patient implies becoming acquainted not only with the patient but also with the environment which has produced him. A patient divorced from his environment cannot be fairly evaluated. Nor, for that matter, should a particular social climate be condemned on one's first impression. An environment which, to the nurse, seems grossly inadequate for the needs of the community may in fact be the lesser among the available evils. Peripheral attractions, such as a high level of interchange among neighbors or the excitement of a continually changing scene, may blind residents to those faults their area shares with the rest of the poverty region. How the environment affects the nurse is not germane; how it affects her patients is.

Records.   Other sources of information about a particular individual or group include service records and conferences with other workers who have known the family. Reading about cultural patterns that prevail in subgroups of the population will also help in understanding the families with which the nurse works, thereby making it easier to build bridges between her own experiences and values and theirs.

DECLARE IN EXPLICIT WAYS THE INTENTION TO HELP

There are many ways of declaring oneself as committed to helping. Some of these are verbal. No one would underestimate the importance of the right word at the right time: the words of respect and appreciation for the harassed mother who still finds time to give her children warm and loving support, or the assurance to the clinic patient that his history is indeed a confidential document.

However, there is also great force in nonverbal expression. Johnson points up the significance of touch in nursing practice.[2] Similarly, it would appear that the nurse's facial expression, such as an expression that mirrors shock or disapproval; her manner of wearing a uniform; her manner of dress when a uniform is not required; or her bodily posture, such as posture that suggests a readiness for flight, may serve to alienate the family from the practitioner.

When there are obvious differences in the backgrounds of the nurse and those with whom she is working, the identification of shared interests, like the baby, cooking, or growing plants, may diminish strangeness and declare the nurse's intention to establish some common bonds.

Doing something tangible to help is one of the most effective means of developing a relationship that works. Whenever possible, nursing service patterns should be geared to provide immediate and responsive action. For example, it may be possible to provide help with a new problem right now instead of putting it off for another visit, or to provide treatments in the home rather than in a clinic that would require a long, tedious trip across town. In the latter case, agency policies may not foster this kind of action, but if it appears to be a helpful approach, the field nurse may suggest, through her superiors, that policies be revised to allow such adaptation.

STUDY TO IMPROVE

The improvement of interpersonal skill depends upon repeated analyses of the effectiveness of the nurse-patient relationship. The primary questions should be: *How well does the relationship work?* Does this nurse-family or nurse-group relationship make it easy for us to work together on the problem, or are there aspects of the relationship that get in the way? Is my relationship with a family that does well different from that with a family which does not deal effectively with its health problems? If so, is it possible to tell just what aspects of the relationship are different?

GO THE SECOND MILE

The late Harry Emerson Fosdick once wrote a short essay on the theme "should a man ask you to walk a mile with him, go with him the second mile as well." For the professional health worker, the development of a relationship with others may require that she go more than the distance, more than the halfway, that might be expected. This second mile may be the willingness to take the initiative in offering help; the willingness to wait for another to reach the point of being able to engage fully in an interchange; or the willingness to offer help over and over again in different forms and ways, if there is evidence of need for such help and the possibility of making it acceptable to the recipient.

In most cases what is desired is the expansion of the recipient's ability to use the services available to him, which is tantamount to guiding his capacities toward management of his own health problems. If this self-sufficiency is indeed the outcome desired, it becomes immediately apparent that the relationship must be one that expands, rather than diminishes, the patient. Interpersonal behavior should therefore be analyzed as to the degree to which it contributes to or hinders the realization of that outcome. Hodgins points out, for example, that the unwillingness of a professional to share what he knows with the stroke patient while engaging in exclusive medical discussion about the patient at the bedside tends to "diminish" the sufferer and thus makes him less able to deal with his already severe problems of adjustment.[1] Failure to listen to the family's plan for treatment before proposing action or failure to view family health care as a concern of the father, as well as of the mother, may be equally "diminishing" and hence moves one away from, rather than toward, the goal.

The Working Relationship Is Rarely Coercive

The community health nurse may on rare occasions face a situation in which the behavior that the family considers desirable or is willing to accept conflicts with the safety and well-being of the community as a whole. The nurse of a local health department, for example, may know that the frankly psychotic patient must take the required treatment if he is to avoid the possibility of harming others. The family may refuse to comply with the prescribed regimen for tuberculosis at home or to accept hospitalization when it appears necessary. In such an instance the nurse is not free to let the family decide; the constraints of agency and public policy make this alternative impossible.

When agreement on action that is required to meet both community and family needs seems hopeless, the staff nurse must be sure she has exhausted all possible noncoercive methods before resorting to the use of authority to demand compliance. Securing advice from her supervisor or medical director, pooling her ideas with those of others in a case conference, or sometimes letting another nurse try may produce at least minimal acceptance. It may be necessary to confront the family with their responsibility as citizens, or with the legal and social implications of their failure to comply with the medical recommendations. The errant family may end up heartily disliking the nurse, but although unpopular, the nurse's decision would be reasonable and just. Granted that these occasions are infrequent, they do occur.

The Nurse Must Teach Others How To Establish and Maintain Working Relationships

A relationship is something that can't be done by one. Parents must develop a working relationship with their children: they must earn trust, learn to communicate, and learn the importance of interpersonal relationships in the development of children. The nurse's aide or home nurse must learn to use her relationship with the patient in a knowing way and learn to balance her own need to be appreciated and liked as one who helps against the need of the patient to develop self-reliance. For these reasons it is important that the nurse know the reasons why certain relationships develop: growth, recognition, and belonging are of importance to every individual. She must appreciate the force of cultural conditioning and the essential nature of the process of communication. As she recognizes and uses the social and behavioral principles that are basic to the creation of an effective relationship, she is better able to teach others in a consistent and sound manner, and through teaching, to reinforce her own interpersonal skills.

THE NATURE OF THE ASSESSMENT PROCESS

Assessment—defining the nature and the essential particulars of the problem complex to be dealt with—determines the conditions for nursing intervention. Precision in selecting the amounts and types of nursing intervention to be employed, efficient definition of the nurse's case load and priorities, and a valid evaluation of the outcomes of service are all dependent on this first critical step. Future chapters will consider the assessment of family and community health in detail; the purpose here is to discuss the nature of the assessment process itself.

A TOOL FOR ACTION

The purposes of nursing assessment are first, to provide an estimate of the degree to which a family, group, or community is achieving the level of health possible for them; second, to identify specific health deficits or guidance needs; and third, to estimate the probable effect of nursing intervention on these conditions. In other words, the overall purpose is to evaluate the extent to which a community health nursing effort may be expected to close the gap between present and potential levels of health or between health behavior and health understanding.

MORE THAN A COLLECTION OF MEDICAL DIAGNOSES

Participation in the management of disease and disability is one important aspect of the work of the community health nurse. The nature and extent of illness and disability in a family, group, or community is an important determinant of nursing need and therefore represent data essential to the nursing assessment. But the focus of the nursing diagnosis is as much on the relationship between the demands imposed by the disease and the willingness and the capability of the family to deal with these needs (*i.e.,* their ability to cope with the problem) as it is on medical management. In fact, many of the situations with which the community health nurse will be concerned are not characterized by the presence of illness or disability at all. Reducing smoking among school children, offering health guidance to expectant parents, promoting a screening program in a presumably healthy population group, and improving intergenerational relationships in three-generation families are all examples of situations where the emphasis is on prevention or on improvement of the quality of health rather than on the care of illness or disability.

A COMBINATION OF FACT GATHERING AND INTERPRETATION

Assessment may be considered in terms of seven components, here formulated as questions, each of which demands for its solution a combination of fact gathering and interpretation.

What Health Threats, Deficits, or Foreseeable Crises or Stress Points Exist?   *Health threats* are conditions that are conducive to disease, accident, or failure to realize one's health potential. These include such conditions as inadequate immunization status among adults and school-age children who may have been immunized in infancy or early childhood; unsafe equipment or lack of supervision of children during play periods; poverty accompanied by hopelessness, hostility, or feelings of inadequacy; overweight in members of a family in which there is a familial history of diabetes; or unrealistic and stressful striving in an upwardly mobile family.

Health deficits may be defined as instances of failure in health maintenance, such as untimely death, illness, or disability; failure to thrive or to grow and develop at the expected rate; or failure to adapt to the realities of life with reasonable emotional control and stability. These represent, in effect, the health breakdowns.

Foreseeable crises or stress points are anticipated periods of unusual demand on the family or community; pregnancy, retirement from work, adolescence, and resettlement in new community housing are examples.

What Problems Does the Family, Group, or Community Face in Dealing with These Conditions? The health-care problems with which a community or family are faced may range from a critical and urgent need for medical care to a lack of appreciation of the importance of stimulating young children, a task necessary to optimize their social and intellectual development. In nursing assessment it is important to focus on the nursing problem of the family or community rather than on the underlying condition that may precipitate, but not be, the problem. For example, pregnancy among young unmarried mothers is not a problem in the nursing or medical sense if "problem" is defined in operational terms. It is a condition which may or may not produce problems of alienation within the family, increased social dependency, and additional or unusual requirements for health and medical supervision. Thus, in this instance the nursing problem is one of enabling the family to deal with problems of family life and utilization of health services rather than the illegitimacy *per se.*

A typology developed by the nursing staff of the Richmond Community Nursing Service suggests that family problems in nursing-care management may be considered generically within a nine-category system independent of the medical or developmental diagnosis.[3] These problem categories are shown in Figure 8, the Family Coping Estimate. In practice, this breakdown offers a useful approach to delineating the specific difficulties families face in managing their health problems and thereby serves as a guide for nursing intervention.

How Successful Is the Family in Dealing with These Conditions? The capacity of the family or community to cope with its problems and the delineation of the specific areas in which difficulty occurs comprise the next concern. In many instances, families or communities with rather substantial health problems may manage exceedingly well without assistance. The diabetic patient or his family may be fully capable of providing the required care at home; he may know how to use the family or clinic physician wisely; and he may have adapted to this condition intelligently and serenely.

Could the Family, with Nursing Help, Deal with Their Problems More Effectively or More Economically? With nursing assistance, the management of some aspects of health care could be improved for the great majority of families and communities. However, there will also be situations or aspects of care which, because of the nature of the problem or the unavailability of nursing or health resources, no amount of professional health service could change. For example, the senile and slightly disoriented woman living alone, even with the plentiful help of responsible and warm neighbors, may have badly kept living quarters, a poor diet, and inadequate general supervision. However, if the patient values her "independence" above all else, if habits of hoarding "my things" and eating erratically are deeply rooted, and if the community has grossly inadequate care facilities, there is little likelihood that the nurse will be able to help with these matters.

What Conditions Are Inherent in the Problem Situation that Might Help or Hinder the Achievement of a Satisfactory Coping Level? This question seeks out the barriers and the strengths, whether internal or external, that interfere with or invite achievement of satisfactory

FAMILY COPING ESTIMATE		
Family_____	Nurse_____	Date_____
Initial_____	Periodic_____	Discharge_____

Coping Area	Rating x-status 0-est. change Poor...................Exc.	Justification
Physical Independence	1 2 3 4 5 Not Applicable ☐	
Therapeutic Independence	1 2 3 4 5 Not Applicable ☐	
Knowledge of Condition	1 2 3 4 5 Not Applicable ☐	
Application of Principles of Personal Hygiene	1 2 3 4 5 Not Applicable ☐	
Attitude Toward Health Care	1 2 3 4 5 Not Applicable ☐	
Emotional Competence	1 2 3 4 5 Not Applicable ☐	
Family Living Patterns	1 2 3 4 5 Not Applicable ☐	
Physical Environment	1 2 3 4 5 Not Applicable ☐	
Use of Community Resources	1 2 3 4 5 Not Applicable ☐	
Comments		

FIGURE 8.   Reverse side is used for nursing care plan. (Developed jointly by the Richmond IVNA City Nursing Service and the Johns Hopkins School of Hygiene and Public Health, 1964.)

health action. Such barriers may be physical, social, economic, or perceptual; and they may exist in either the recipient or the provider of the care.

To What Degree Are the Barriers to Adequate Management of the Health Situation Subject to Change, and to What Degree Can the Positive Forces Be Strengthened and Utilized?

What Are the Implications of the Six Preceding Considerations for Community Health Nursing?   It is at this point that the nurse looks realistically at what she can offer and the probable effect of such nursing intervention on the situation confronting her. The question is not what kinds of nursing action are *possible* in this problem category, but rather what kinds of nursing intervention are *likely to be effective* in this particular situation, at this particular time, with this particular kind of nursing resource.

The diagnosis of many of these problems—such as the existence of pregnancy, the child already known to the courts as unruly, or the specific medical diagnosis—involves data that are essentially objective or previously defined. However, diagnosis may also involve data that are more subjective, more subtle and hazy. There is no statistical measure of how deeply the family feels about a particular problem, how far they are willing to go in self-help, or whether the "health establishment" recommendation is really relevant to them when all factors in the situation are considered.

Thus, the process of assessment in community health nursing includes not only intensive fact finding, but also the application of professional judgment in the estimation of (1) the meaning and importance of these facts to the family and community, (2) the possible avenues of nursing service, and (3) the degree of change which nursing intervention can be expected to effect.

ESTABLISHING GOALS FOR HEALTH AND NURSING CARE

Goal setting has been increasingly recognized as a highly important component in planning for any program of social action. Whether dealing with a family, a group, a community, or a nation, the development of clear-cut, specific, and acceptable goals in nursing matters is crucial. To the extent that the desired ends of nursing service are defined and accepted as valid by all involved, the resultant action is likely to be sustained and relevant.

Goals Exist in a Multilevel System

Goals exist at all levels—from the broad statement of the purposes of a program to the most explicit statement of desired outcomes for an immediate and specific action. Sometimes there is an unfortunate tendency to concentrate on defining immediate and measurable outcomes in order to "get on with the job" without clarifying the more general goals, which are sometimes described as academic. However, it is usually true that specific goals have meaning only in the context of the more general goals.

For example, the goal of getting an individual under care for gonorrhea may be a response to the immediate task that has been assigned: getting the patient registered for treatment by whatever means possible. However, broader goals of the program, such as those concerned with the preservation of the family and the enhancement of individual potential, impose new responsibilities and constraints upon the nurse's means. Nursing care must, of course, be directed toward assuring that the individual gets the necessary treatment and ensuring that the spread of infection is prevented by identifying and treating those of his contacts who may also need care. However, if the more comprehensive goal is accepted, the nurse's concerns extend to more general problems related to the illness, such as its effect on his self-image, its effect on his family relationships, and the need of his family and contacts for support and understanding. It would involve trying to understand the situation more deeply: whether the infection is incidental or whether it is the symptom of more fundamental emotional problems—for example, promiscuity growing out of a sense of frustration and isolation that, in turn, has been engendered by lack of job training and job opportunity. Thus the task of the nurse might involve support to the family, helping the patient to express his concerns, or referral of the patient to a community agency for job training, social work, or psychiatric help.

Goals for health care will represent only one area of aspiration. Because the nurse wants to live as an individual, apart from her work, she will have goals relating to her personal or family life that may on occasion compete with the goals that are rooted in her professional commitment. A family may be committed to unusual responsibility for older dependent family members and yet want a college education for the children. The agency wants a broad spectrum of health services of which nursing constitutes only one part. The community wants roads and schools and welfare as well as health programs. Thus the problem of goal formulation involves an understanding of the broader goal system in which the nursing-care goals must fit and also an appreciation of the relative pull of these various goals.

Two Kinds of Goals

In community health nursing there are usually two sets of goals operating: the goals of the professional care provider and the goals of the patient (*i.e.,* individual, family group, or community). Sometimes these are in harmony; for example, there is little opposition from either group to the goal of assuring a safe birth for every child. However, in many instances there will not be such complete agreement. A health agency may feel that the interests of the public can be promoted through the assurance of a continuing supply of well-prepared nurses, and to that end the agency proposes that there be considerably greater support to baccalaureate nursing education. The patient, in this case the local public, might feel that the preservation of nursing at its present level is a better goal and that there is no need to raise the level of training. Unless these goals are reconciled, there is little hope of securing the necessary support for any program to expand the supply of nurses.

Nursing Goals Must Be Reconciled Three Ways

In establishing goals for nursing service, the community health nurse has the problem of a three-way reconciliation. First, her own goals (which are largely determined by her professional preparation and, to a lesser extent, by her own personal values) must be reconciled with those of the recipient of her services, who will in the long run decide what he is willing to do. Community health nursing, by definition, involves interaction, and the desired health action can seldom be achieved by the nurse alone. For this reason, prior to the initiation of the action process, all parties involved need to have an understanding of why the action is being taken and a sense of personal commitment to it. In other words, the goals of the nurse and those of the recipient of her services must become fused to the point that the action undertaken can be clearly focused on the problem and its resolution.

Because the professional health worker has greater access to health knowledge, particularly knowledge of a comparative or predictive character, he may in some instances hold goals for health care that the family or the community is not yet ready to understand and to share. The nurse may see the need for an elderly disabled woman to become more independent, even though the achievement of this independence will cost much effort or pain. Her goal is maximization of the patient's potential for self-help. The family may feel the goal should be to do everything humanly possible for a beloved parent, relieving her of effort or pain whenever possible. The goal acceptable to both at this point in time may be to prevent damage, a goal that both can share and on which plans for care can be based. The nurse's goal of making the patient more independent and perhaps freeing the family from undue burden may have to go into cold storage for awhile, not forgotten, but not brought into this phase of the transaction between nurse and family. With more experience, the family's appreciation of the patient's needs may be broadened, and the self-care goal can be resurrected and made operative. To proceed on the basis of goals that are not understood and accepted by the recipient of care is likely to be a wasteful tactic, inasmuch as it encourages unknowing response with little carry-over value. Furthermore, it must be recognized that the professional worker, despite his training, *can* be wrong.

A distinction must also be made between setting goals and then securing the compliance of others, and truly mutual goal setting. In the latter, the competences and the commitment of the nurse and of the recipient are truly merged to produce a viable objective.

Secondly, nursing goals must be reconciled with the goals of the nursing profession; that is, they must be consistent with the ethical and expert characteristics that are expected of the professional. Finally, goals must be reconciled with the overall goals of the agency.

The Goals of Others Must Be Elicited

If nursing goals are to be reconciled with the goals of others, it is important that the nurse be clear as to what these latter goals are. Often families will be unable to explain, or even to think through, goals which do not exist full-blown. Administrators, too, may not be in the habit of verbalizing or writing out goals, even though they may be quite clear in their own minds about what is needed. The nurse may patiently have to uncover the health and health-related goals of others that are pertinent to the formulation of her nursing-care aim.

Specific Commitments Must Be Declared

The efficacy of goal setting as a means of facilitating and directing health action is largely dependent on the degree to which the commitment implied by the goal is explicit and declared. A vague idea that nursing should improve the quality of family health is not sufficient as a guide to action. It must be further delineated into objectives that are tangible, time-related, and measurable. The establishment of time limits accomplishes two purposes: first, it provides a timing mechanism for the activity; and second, it sets an evaluation checkpoint, which helps make it possible to modify goals when necessary. Thus in working with a family, the nurse might establish as one goal the improvement of the mother's ability to relate positively to her infant; she will want to set a time tag of perhaps a year for the accomplishment of this objective. A second example: one objective in neighborhood nursing care might be to increase the participation of the general public in its own health care through the creation of a representative advisory committee; again a time target would be indicated. For the nurse, the integration of goal setting into the nursing process usually includes putting goals in writing and including them as an integral part of her record.

The Reality of the Goals Must Be Tested

Unrealistic goals exert a negative effect in the long run because they lead to disappointment, frustration, and a loss of confidence. In nursing care today, it is important that what is "reasonable" or "possible" is not confused with what is possible *under the present level and type of nursing intervention*. There is sometimes danger of underestimating, as well as overestimating, the capacity of a family or group for self-help or for decision making, particularly if the family has gotten out of the habit of self-reliance or if the nurse has adopted an over-helping stance that inhibits family initiative. Constant testing is required to check not only whether or not the goals really can be achieved, but also if the goals are challenging enough to stretch the capabilities of those involved. The objective of goal setting in health care is to secure internalization and commitment to a clearly defined, desired outcome that is compatible with the life goals of the recipients of care and with the reality of the situation.

Constructing and Implementing a Program of Action

The implementation phase of the community nursing process is concerned with:

1. Choosing among alternative courses of action.
2. Selecting appropriate types of nursing intervention.
3. Mobilizing available resources for care.
4. Developing an operational plan.

Choosing Among Courses of Action

In most instances there will be more than one possible course of action that appears suitable to the problem. For example, five alternative plans for providing personal care to the incapacitated arthritic patient could be considered. Care could be furnished by the nurse herself, by a home health aide supervised by the community nurse, by a registered nurse who would provide care without the supervision of the community nurse, by the daughter in the home, or by some combination of the four alternatives. No nursing action is, of course, also an alternative. The selection of one course of action over another, in this case, would depend upon many corollary factors such as the acceptability of a specific plan to the family; judgment levels required in care and the seriousness of possible error; expectations of the community; availability of community nursing resources; sources of payment for nursing care; and the stamina and commitment of the daughter. Too narrow a concept of the range of possible alternatives in nursing action may result in stereotyped or ritualistic practice, which tends to diminish the relevance and impact of the action taken.

For most actions there are negative, as well as positive, consequences. For instance, the elderly patient who is being pushed into greater self-help may feel deserted or rejected, the decision to keep a patient at home may place additional burdens on an already over-burdened wage earner or homemaker, permissive approaches to child rearing may produce in-law problems, or home psychiatric care may lessen the stress for the patient but may increase the stress within his family.

The positive outcomes anticipated must be seen against these possible negative responses. Selection among alternatives involves weighing the plus and minus values of each and attempting to identify the "best buy." For example, having the daughter provide care may be most economical of scarce nursing time, but it may have a negative effect on the daughter's emotional health. The provision of care by the nurse herself might be most satisfying to the family, especially if they have known her in other situations, but this responsibility may take the nurse away from other higher priority concerns. The use of a home health aide may not be acceptable to the family, particularly at first, but this plan would be most economical of nursing time if the aide is capable of meeting the care needs of the patient satisfactorily. In the community, a "comprehensive nursing-care" approach may meet the needs of a particular family, but it would reach only a fraction of those who need help. The essential relationship is that between the *cost* of a given course of action in terms of effort or money and the *benefits* in terms of the improvement which that action is expected to produce.

Sometimes such benefits are "spillover" benefits. For instance, when the family is encouraged to take the responsibility for selecting a given course of action, the action selected may in fact be less productive than one the nurse would have chosen; but the value of improving the ability of the family to solve its own problems and make decisions in health matters may outweigh the "efficiency" advantage of the nurse's method.

Selecting Appropriate Types of Nursing Intervention

Nursing intervention may be of three types: supplemental, facilitative or developmental.

Supplemental intervention means doing things that the family, group, or community cannot do for itself. It may take the form of providing personal or therapeutic care for the sick, planning a community program when the community is not organized to participate through its own representatives, or making decisions when the head of a household is immobilized in the face of a crisis.

Facilitative intervention is concerned with removing barriers to care, whether these barriers are economic, such as lack of car fare to get to the source of medical care; social, such as culture-linked resistance to necessary change; or behavioral, such as a lack of information or motivation on the part of those who are expected to take the necessary action. This type of intervention involves a careful delineation of the barriers and a realistic program for neutralizing the situation's negative factors and for reinforcing the situation's positive factors in order to expedite achievement of desired action.

Developmental intervention is based on improving the capacity of the recipient to act on his own behalf. Teaching families and groups to make responsible health decisions, supporting them in developing a sense of identity and worth, and guiding them in dealing with predictable crises or points of stress are examples of developmental intervention.

Most nursing service will, of course, involve elements of all three types of intervention. It is important, however, to be sure the intervention used is indeed suitable to the situation. A prolonged use of supplemental intervention, for example, may militate against progress toward independence, whereas trying to encourage self-help by withdrawing supplemental assistance too early may create negative responses in the recipient, which will interfere with future utilization of needed nursing services.

Mobilizing Available Resources for Care

In additon to the nurse and other members of the nursing team, there will be many other individuals, agencies, or groups involved in accomplishing health objectives. Most central are the recipients of care—the patient, his family, the neighborhood, the school, the industrial population—who are called upon to make relatively sophisticated judgments and to take responsible action on their own behalf.

In addition, the whole medical care system—the hospitals, health departments, clinics, private and group practitioners of medicine, and the health units of welfare departments, voluntary health agencies, and health-related agencies—serves as a resource that must be selectively used and activated.

A third group of resources are the nonhealth facilities that are essential to the well-being of the population; namely, the social case work, educational, and counseling services.

MOTIVATION MUST BE PRESENT

Mobilization implies, among other things, motivating others to the action required for the improvement of a problem situation. Thus, a discouraged mother must be helped to see that it really is worth the effort to play with and talk to her small child and a neighborhood group must be persuaded that it is possible to do something about the rat population with the help available. This process is one of clarifying the required health action in terms of the other life goals of the recipient; only if these two facets are incorporated will the remedial action be worthwhile.

Frequently the required action involves change, such as a change in living habits, in ideas, or in attitudes. Change itself is not necessarily distasteful. What threatens a patient is activity in areas in which he feels insecure, the feeling that he is not prepared to make the change that is required. Also, he may feel that the change proposed by health authorities is not necessary.

There are three prerequisites to effecting change. First, it must be made desirable; second, it must be made possible; and third, it must be made rewarding. Part of the process of facilitation is to take whatever steps are necessary to meet these three conditions. It can be done by building bridges between a patient's present knowledge or practice and that which will be required of him in the new behavior pattern.

FUNCTIONAL ORGANIZATION MUST BE ESTABLISHED

Mobilization also includes the functional organization of those involved in the action; that is, a clarification of the relative roles of each of the participants. Thus, the family must understand what help may be expected, and not expected, from the social worker or job counselor. The nurse must see the developmental role of the very young mother who will need time to grow into the responsibility society expects of parents. The physician must understand the limits of community nursing service and at the same time realize that nursing service may provide care other than that related to the immediate illness situation that is his main concern. As each participant understands the other's role and limits, the stage is set for coordinated effort.

Developing an Operational Plan

These several components of the plan for implementing nursing care need to be drawn together into some sort of organized schedule for action. This procedure will involve the establishment of priorities and the phasing and coordination of activities.

Priorities are established by ordering the various aspects of care in terms of urgency or impact in order to define those that warrant the earliest and most inclusive attention. The relative importance attached to a particular problem depends upon the degree to which it actually threatens health, or sometimes it may depend upon the public perception of the danger it raises. Thus with the family in which a member has active tuberculosis, the highest priority would certainly go to implementing those phases of care that have to do with maintaining an adequate drug regime. In a country with a very low productivity, first priority might be assigned to improving the health of those in the producing age groups—the young and middle-aged adults who are most involved in the production of food and goods—in order to provide an adequate base for maintaining life and health in the rest of the population. In a neighborhood where sanitation is at a very low level, the control of rats may assume such importance that all other measures must take a second place.

Phasing the various aspects of the nursing action selected is a threefold process. It first involves breaking multifaceted problems into manageable units for attack. It is, second, putting these units of attack into a reasonable sequence in which each phase of action is dependent upon that which precedes it. Finally, phasing involves the establishment of checkpoints that permit periodic evaluation and replanning. Thus in the school nursing program, meeting with new teachers to acquaint them with the services afforded by the school nurse must precede joint conferences on the health of a specific class. The school nursing program would therefore be phased so as to allow for a teacher-nurse meeting early in the year and for classroom conferences later.

Phasing may also involve postponement of some phases of care in order to keep the problem manageable from the family's point of view. In the multiproblem family it is often wise to take one problem at a time, deferring consideration of others that may seem equally important.

Coordination assumes an important place in planning for community health nursing. In many localities the extreme fragmentation of health care creates a multitude of incursions on the family and community, each demanding some sort of response. All too often there is no place the patient or family can go to be put together again. The community may have no way of preventing or regulating the wasteful proliferation of basically worthy, but scattered and incomplete, health-care services. The community nurse is in a key position to keep the many and varied forces in some sort of relationship. Through observation, consultation, and report systems the nurse picks up inconsistencies or inadequacies in the health care provided, and she reports such failings to appropriate groups. She may, for example, interpret to the hospital and to the medical practitioner the implications for the family of new hospital admission and discharge procedures and inform the hospital personnel of home conditions that may affect their patient-care decisions.

EVALUATING THE ACTION TAKEN

There are two major approaches to the evaluation of community nursing services: the first is based on evidence of effectiveness of the service provided, and the second is based on evidences of excellence of professional practice.

Effectiveness of Service

Health and health-related changes occurring in the recipient of nursing services are without doubt the most relevant measures of the effectiveness of nursing care. At the same time, it is one of the most frustrating of measures to apply: first, because of the difficulties of establishing objective indices of outcomes; and second, because of the many factors other than nursing that may effect the changes that occur.

Despite these difficulties, changes that occur in recipients or recipient groups in the course of nursing service may be a valuable source of evaluation data. Roberts and Hudson have developed a method of measuring patient progress that is based on the reduction of nursing needs in the course of care.[4] By measuring changes in the nursing needs of patients as reflected by differences in health conditions or health behavior, it is possible to document the changes and to locate areas where changes are most likely to occur. However, certain safeguards must be established if evaluation rests on patient, family, or community change:

1. The change to be measured should be one that is largely dependent on nursing intervention. For example, the nurse might be very influential in changing patient and family behavior with respect to following a prescribed medical regime for tuberculosis; moreover, changes involving regularity of taking drugs or reporting to clinic might constitute a legitimate measure of nursing effectiveness. However, nursing care would not be expected to influence directly the actual progress of the disease; this is much more a factor of the drug prescribed and the basic condition of the patient. Thus, to evaluate nursing care by the degree to which the patient's physical condition improves may not be appropriate. The measurement of changes affected by nursing inputs may include changes in behavior that are related to health.

2. When changes are observed over a period of time, it is important to develop baseline data at the point when nursing service is initiated. Only by knowing what the situation is at the start of service is it possible to document and interpret the extent and direction of the changes that occur.

3. In relating changes in the family or community to nursing, it is also important to take account of other care inputs that may be operating concurrently. For example, the patient-physician relationship may produce strongly positive or strongly negative reactions to the care prescribed. The support or nonsupport of the family may facilitate or impede conformity to recommended health practice. Economic constraints may interfere with proper nutritional practices. Sometimes these other forces are so strong that they outweigh any effect community health nursing might be expected to produce.

4. The reliability of information relating to change should also be

considered. The two most frequent sources of data about change are the nurse herself and the family or the representatives of the community being served. Both sources are obviously subject to bias in reporting: the nurse, since she is involved and may see what she hopes to see rather than what is actually there; and the family because they may not be able to recall the information accurately or to make the observations required with sufficient judgment or skill.

Quality of Professional Service

Evaluation of the quality of nursing input is frequently used as a criterion in evaluation. In this approach, the nurse's performance is compared to the performance that, in the judgment of the public health and nursing profession, would exemplify "good community health nursing practice." The characteristics of good practice appear in official statements of professional organizations, professional literature, agency and service manuals, or policies.

One characteristic of good practice may be the fullest possible involvement of the client in his own care; another may be the use of a "comprehensive" approach in rendering service. One could first seek out evidence of these measures of excellence by analyzing what happens in family care or by reviewing service records and then arrive at a judgment as to the degree to which the nurse's practice exemplifies this professional ideal. For example, indications of identifying and dealing with family problems other than the one that occasioned the request for service may be evidence of a "comprehensive" approach; systematic inclusion in the service record of the family's perception of and plan for dealing with their health problems may be evidence of involving the client in his own care.

The usefulness of this type of measure is currently limited by the paucity of evidence that the officially approved methods of approach are significantly operative in the degree of change that occurs in a family. However, professional standards are widely used in all fields as criteria of quality because they are likely to be based on logical theoretical considerations and are therefore believed, by the profession, to have a desirable effect on outcomes of care.

The quality of nursing input can also be measured in some instances by direct or indirect evidence of consumer satisfaction. Families or representative community groups may be asked to express their opinions about the quality and relevance of the community nursing care they receive and the degree to which it meets their expectations of care. A less direct evidence of the degree of consumer satisfaction and acceptance of services is the study of patterns of utilization of care or of the nurse-family interaction. The weakness of both measures is that the patient is often unfamiliar with the technical aspects of "good care." Conversely, both measures have great potential for identifying the degree to which the recipient of care *feels* the service is relevant to the needs of his family or of his community.

Those who find the attempts to analyze health improvement or quality of nursing input too imprecise may estimate the amount of nursing care that is afforded to a particular family or to groups having a particular type of medical problem. They thereby define in quantitative, rather than in qualitative, terms the way in which nursing care is distributed throughout the community. Thus the achievement of a higher nurse-population ratio (moving, say, from a ratio of one community health nurse to each 5000 of the population to a ratio of one community health nurse for each 3000 of the population) might be considered as a measure of achievement.

However, the distribution, as well as the amount, of service provided is crucial to community health nursing, inasmuch as the community health nurse's obligation is to the community as a whole. For example, the number of nurse-family contacts during the maternity cycle might be increased from three to six for those families known to the nursing service, whereas at the same time care is being provided to only about 25 percent of those estimated to need it. In this instance the increased visit ratio might be a good measure of change in the care of this particular segment of the population, but it would be a poor measure of the nursing care provided to the population as a whole.

There are obvious limits to this quantitative approach to evaluation because the impact of nursing care will depend upon qualitative, as well as quantitative, factors. However, agency or community goals are sometimes set in terms of increasing the availability of specified services to the population, in which case quantitative measures are indeed appropriate.

THE PROCESS—A NEED FOR GREATER PRECISION

This, then, is the process involved in community health nursing practice: relating, assessing, goal setting, implementing, and evaluating. Each step is essential for the accomplishment of the others; each step is related to all of the others.

Although the explanation given here may seem lengthy and involved, it is important to understand the process as basic to community health practice. With experience, the sensitive nurse comes to apply some parts of it more and more intuitively and to recognize and respond to complex situations in a synoptic fashion.

Intuitive response, however, is reliable only as it is firmly rooted both in the mastery of the scientific and the behavioral content basic to nursing and to public health practice and in the knowledge of the nature of the process by which this content is transformed into the professional practice of community health nursing.

Undeniably, there is need for much more precision in evaluating aspects of community health. Achieving greater exactness will, however, rest on the acquisition of much more detailed knowledge of the nature of nursing input, a more precise definition of the changes that may be classified as measures of nursing achievement, and the application of comparative "cost" and "benefit" estimates as they apply to the realization of stated goals for community nursing care.

REFERENCES

1. Hodgins, Eric: Listen: the patient. New Eng. J. Med., *274:*657, March, 1966.
2. Johnson, Betty Sue: The meaning of touch in nursing. *In* Stewart, Dorothy, and Vincent, Pauline (eds.): Public Health Nursing. William C. Brown Company, Publishers, Dubuque, 1968, p. 59.
3. Freeman, Ruth B., and Lowe, Marie: A method for appraising public health nursing needs. Amer. J. Public Health, *53:*47, January, 1963.
4. Roberts, Doris, and Hudson, Helen: How to Study Patient Progress. PHS Publication No. 1169, U.S. Government Printing Office, Washington, D.C., 1964, p. 1.

SUGGESTED READINGS

Apple, Dorian: How laymen define illness. J. Health Hum. Behav., *1:*219, Fall, 1960.
Aring, Charles D.: Sympathy and empathy. J.A.M.A., *167:*448, 1958.
Baumann, Barbara.: Diversities in conceptions of health and physical fitness. *In* Skipper, J. K., and Leonard, R. C. (eds.): Social Interaction and Patient Care. J. B. Lippincott Co., Philadelphia, 1965.
Berggren, Helen, and Zagowick, A. D.: Teaching nursing process to beginning students. Nurs. Outlook, *16:*32, July, 1968.
Brunclik, Helen, Thurston, John R., and Fedlhauser, John: The empathy inventory. Nurs. Outlook, *15:*42, June, 1967.
Burton, Genevieve: Personal, Impersonal and Interpersonal Relations. 2nd ed., Springer-Verlag New York Inc., New York, 1964.
Collins, R. D.: Problem solving: a tool for patients, too. Amer. J. Nurs., *68:*1483, July, 1968.
Conant, Lucy H: Give and take in home visits. *In* Stewart, Dorothy and Vincent, Pauline (eds.): Public Health Nursing. William C. Brown Company, Publishers, Dubuque, 1968, Chapter 6.
Dilworth, Sarah E.: Identification of selected nursing needs of post partum patients as recorded by public health nurses. *In* Exploring Progress in Public Health Nursing Practice. American Nurses' Association Regional Clinical Conferences, vol. 5, 1965, American Nurses' Association, New York, 1966.
Elder, Ruth: What is the patient saying? *In* Skipper, J. K., and Leonard, R. C. (eds.): Social Interaction and Patient Care. J. B. Lippincott Co., Philadelphia, 1965, pp. 102.
Friedson, Elliott: Patient's Views of Medical Practice. Russell Sage Foundation, New York, 1961.
Gregg, Dorothy: Reassurance. *In* Skipper, J. K., and Leonard, R. C. (eds.): Social Interaction and Patient Care. J. B. Lippincott Co., Philadelphia, 1965, pp. 127.
Hay, Stella I., and Anderson, Helen: Are nurses meeting patients' needs? Amer. J. Nurs., *63:*96, December, 1963.
Henderson, Virginia: The Nature of Nursing: a Definition and Its Implications for Practice. The Macmillan Company, New York, 1966.
Hodgins, Eric: Listen: the patient. New Eng. J. Med., *274:*657, March, 1966.
Jacobson, Gerald F., Strickler, Martin, and Morley, Wilbar: Generic and individual approaches to crisis intervention. Amer. J. Public Health, *58:*338, February, 1968.
Johnson, Betty Sue: The meaning of touch in nursing. *In* Stewart, Dorothy, and Vincent, Pauline (eds.): Public Health Nursing. William C. Brown Company, Publishers, Dubuque, 1968, Chapter 7.
Johnson, J., Dumas, R., and Johnson, B.: Interpersonal relations: the essence of nursing care. Nurs. Forum, *6:*324, 1967.
King, Imogene: A conceptual frame of reference for nursing. Nurs. Res., *17:*27, January-February, 1968.
Komorita, Nori I.: Nursing diagnosis. Amer. J. Nurs., *63:*83, December, 1963.
Lindeman, Ruth S.: Empathy: a component of therapeutic nursing. Nurs. Forum, *7:*275, 1968.
MacGregor, F. C.: Social Science in Nursing. Russell Sage Foundation, New York, 1960.
Measurement of Levels of Health: Report of a Study Group. Technical Report Series 137, World Health Organization, Geneva, 1957.

Mendelsohn, Harold: What shall it be: mass education or mass persuasion for health? Amer. J. Public Health, *58:*131, January, 1968.

Murray, Jeanne B.: Self knowledge and the nursing interview. Nurs. Forum, *2:*67, 1963.

Orlando, Ida: The Dynamics of the Nurse Patient Relationship. G. P. Putman's Sons, New York, 1961.

Paynich, Mary Louise: Cultural barriers to nurse communication. Amer. J. Nurs., *64:*87, February, 1964.

Peters, Ann de Huff, and Chase, Charles L.: Patterns of health care in infancy in a rural southern county. Amer. J. Public Health, *57:*409, March, 1967.

Pratt, Lois, Seligman, Arthur, and Reader, George: Physician's views on the level of medical information among patients. Amer. J. Public Health, *47:*1277, October, 1967.

Roberts, Doris, and Hudson, Helen H.: How to Study Patient Progress. Public Health Service Publication No. 1169, U.S. Government Printing Office, Washington, D.C., 1964.

Robischon, Paulette: The challenge of crisis theory for nursing. Nurs. Outlook, *15:*28, July, 1967.

Rothberg, J. S.: Why nursing diagnosis? Amer. J. Nurs., *67:*1040, May, 1967.

Ruesch, S., and Kies, W.: Non-verbal Communication. University of California Press, Berkeley, 1956.

Schwartz, Doris: Some thoughts on quality in nursing service. Int. Nurs. Rev., *14:*24, March-April, 1967.

Steward, R. F., and Graham, Josephine L.: Evaluation tools in public health nursing. Nurs., Outlook, *16:*50, March, 1968.

Suhrie, Eleanor B.: The importance of listening. *In* Stewart, Dorothy, and Vincent, Pauline (eds.): Public Health Nursing. William C. Brown Company, Publishers, Dubuque, 1968, Chapter 14.

Sundberg, Alice: Influencing prenatal behavior. Amer. J. Public Health, *56:*1218, August, 1966.

Ujhely, Gertrude: What is realistic emotional support? Amer. J. Nurs., *68:*758, April, 1968.

Wiedenbach, Ernestine: Family Centered Maternity Nursing. 2nd ed., G. P. Putman's Sons, New York, 1967.

Wilson, Robert N.: Patient-practitioner relationships. *In* Freeman, Howard, *et al.* (eds.): Handbook of Medical Sociology. Prentice-Hall, Inc., 1963.

Community Health Nursing in the Agency Structure

ESSENTIAL ELEMENTS OF AGENCY ORGANIZATION

Community health nurses function in many different types of institution, each of which sets both opportunities and constraints that govern the way nursing operates within its structure. The rapid rate of change in the responsibilities and activities of health institutions, along with the impact of an expanding theoretical base in administrative practice, has resulted in a situation in which specific patterns of organization in any given agency have a very short life indeed. Not without some foundation in fact is the quip, "If the boss calls be sure to get his name." For these reasons, the organization of nursing in the agency structure will be discussed in terms of the essential elements with which the community health nurse should familiarize herself, rather than in terms of specific extant patterns. In particular, the discussion will be concerned with the ways that the agency structure:

1. Determines the scope and nature of nursing responsibility.
2. Defines channels of accountability for nursing efforts.
3. Provides for professional direction.
4. Allows for communication and coordination of effort.

Conditions that Define the Nature and Scope of Nursing Responsibilities

AGENCY COMMITMENTS

Agency commitments will vary in accordance with the sponsorship of, and the basis of the authority for, the agency. For example, the health

74

department, by virtue of its legislative authorization, must concern itself with the health of the population as a whole. The school health unit, on the other hand, is specifically concerned with the health of school children, sometimes with the health of school personnel, and with certain specified services for preschool-age children. The Visiting Nurse Association (or other voluntary agency involved in nursing services) may limit its concerns in many ways, acting as it does within the purposes stated in their articles of incorporation.

These commitments may be stated or implied in legislation that authorizes the agency's action, as in the case of government or quasi-government bodies or, as with the Visiting Nurse Association, in the statement of purpose included in the agency's articles of incorporation.

In government agencies, these commitments are explicitly or implicitly stated either in the legislation which authorized the agency or in regulations which supplement this legislation. The commitment of the health department, welfare department, or school health service is to be found in state or federal health, education, and welfare legislation. In addition, there is likely to be a set of regulations that further defines the nature of the agency commitment. For example, the authority under which the federal health services in the United States operate emanates from the basic mandate of the Preamble to the Constitution: the federal government is obligated to "promote the general welfare." This authority is further defined by other powers specifically reserved by the Constitution for the federal government, such as the authority to regulate commerce with foreign countries and among the states and the power to levy taxes.[1] The implied commitments in these legislative statements are realized through many specific legislative enactments such as the Social Security Act or the Economic Security Act.

Other health and health-related legislation or regulations may still further define the commitment of the agencies and their various subunits. For instance, in the Economic Opportunity Act, which provides for the development of community action programs that may involve health and that are sponsored by the Office of Economic Opportunity, there is specific reference to the groups to be served and to the involvement of the recipients in the decisions relating to action taken. State education laws may specifically require medical examinations, hearing tests, or vision tests at prescribed intervals; or they may define the relationship that must obtain between the health and education authorities with respect to the school health program.

The commitments of a particular agency are further clarified in policies, regulations, and agreements that specify conditions that must be met. For example, a school health manual, prepared jointly by the schools and the health department, may spell out the responsibilities of each agency.

Sometimes there are commitments that have grown up informally; they have never been put in writing or explicated in conference, but they are nevertheless binding as a result of custom. A Visiting Nurse Association, for instance, may have an informal understanding with a local hospital to provide certain supportive services to clinic patients who are required to carry out prescribed therapeutic measures at home.

The community health nurse should, as far as possible, familiarize herself with the conditions under which the agency is authorized to function and with the nature of the commitment that the agency has undertaken as shown in reports of the governing board, in the agency's legislative or board authorization, in the agency's bylaws and annual reports, and in policy statements or informal agreements. The community health nurse will then better understand her own place in the agency structure. She will consequently have a basis from which to project her own particular style into those activities that are subject to more selective and flexible development.

AGENCY OPERATING POLICIES

Within the general framework of the agency's commitments, each agency further develops certain operating policies and patterns that will affect the nature of the community health nurse's responsibilities.

There may be an operating principle which dictates that nursing services will be generalized—that is, that the assignment of each nurse or nursing group is in terms of *families* to be cared for rather than in terms of *specified patient groups*. For example, if 20 nurses are functioning in the agency, each of the 20 is expected to care for the families assigned to her whether the primary problem concerns maternal and child health, longterm or acute illness, psychiatric or behavioral disturbance, or a communicable disease. Each nurse or nursing group would function as a generalist in the health field.

In other instances, or at given points in time, the community health nurse may be assigned to specialized functions. The nurse on a special tuberculosis project may serve only those requiring diagnostic, preventive, or curative care. A pediatric nurse specialist may have a defined case load made up of those whose pediatric problems require unusual depth in nursing care. School nursing may be provided on a specialized basis, with only some nurses assigned to this service; or it may be provided as part of a generalized program, with all nurses participating.

At present, generalized assignment is much more common than is specialized assignment in all but the school nursing services. The generalized pattern was developed because it was felt that families found it easier to deal with a single worker, that travel time and administrative costs were reduced, and that the family-centered approach, rather than a disease-centered approach, was more effective in working with the kinds of problems most often encountered in the community health setting.

Recently there has been some interest in the development of nurse specialists in various fields. This attention is based on the premise that the increasing complexity of care justifies the use of one whose expertise is deeper, but narrower in range. This is undoubtably true in certain settings, especially in the hospital or in the special intensive care clinics. For example, in an "all out" type of clinic, dealing with high-risk mothers and infants, the nurse-midwife may be able to accomplish more with some families than could the generalized nurse. Furthermore, the introduction into the case load of the community agency of large numbers of older patients needing relatively simple care over a long period of time suggests the need for a specialized staff who are temperamentally and technically adapted to this kind of work.

In the community health setting, it is important not to lose the family-oriented approach, even though the service is rendered by a specialist. Through group planning or shared visiting, the generalist may "back-stop" the specialist (and vice versa) to allow the care to be truly family centered and as comprehensive as possible.

Other agency policies may also define the kinds of groups admitted to care and the types and extent of care rendered. For example, agency policy may dictate that no family may be admitted unless they are under some kind of medical supervision, or certain treatments may be deemed by a medical review or advisory committee as unsuitable for administration by nurses in the home setting. These policies are usually clarified during the nurse's orientation to the agency.

SUPERVISORY JUDGMENT

Sometimes the nature of the responsibility undertaken will rest on the supervisor's estimate of the readiness of a particular nurse to carry a given responsibility. For example, the supervisor may decide when a community health nurse may head a nursing group or assume certain community organization or group teaching responsibilities. Such judgments are usually made jointly by the nurse and the supervisor and are based on the training and experience of the nurse and on the complexity of the immediate situation.

Channels of Accountability Defined by Agency's Organization

In any professional activity, there are two kinds of action for which the nurse must be accountable: one is the action taken to accomplish a *function* and the other is the action taken in carrying out professional *practice*. Thus, the nurse must account for the way in which she contributes to the management of the prenatal patient and her family during the maternity cycle in terms of the degree to which the agency's program objectives are realized. At the same time, she must account for the way in which she exercised her professional practice in the accomplishment of this responsibility—that is, she must be aware of the relevance, effectiveness, and the safety of the nursing process itself. It is important to understand the dyadic nature of this accountability, since it is reflected in the ways that the community health nurse reports on what she has done; it also determines the person to whom she looks for the direction and evaluation of her work.

ALL-NURSE HIERARCHY

Nursing may be organized within an agency in what is essentially a professional hierarchy. The members of the nursing-care group may report to and be guided by a nursing supervisor in all aspects of work, and the supervisor may, in turn, report to a nurse director. The nurse may plan and work with a multidiscipline group in carrying out her work, but for the effectiveness and quality of her work, she is accountable only to a nursing line of authority. This is the usual pattern in voluntary agencies whose function is restricted to nursing and some additional personal care services such as physical or occupational therapy.

With such organizations, it is usual for each supervisor to have a designated number of staff nurses under her supervision; in general services in the United States, this number is most often somewhere between six and eight. This ratio of supervisor to staff nurse tends to differ in specialized service, such as school nursing, where it may be lower, and also in highly specialized projects, where it may be higher. The average ratio in the United States is considerably above the level found in some other countries; in Great Britain, for example, the ratio usually approximates one supervisor to 20 staff nurses.

Multidiscipline Hierarchy

In other instances, nursing may be organized primarily around a multidiscipline functional area under the direction of someone other than a nurse. Many health department activities and special projects follow this pattern. This functional pattern may also pertain in agencies where the nursing service provided is more advisory than direct. Such is the case in a state health department where the nurse advisers may work most directly with the chief of the service in which the nurse is advising. Thus the nursing consultant in mental health may be assigned to the bureau of mental hygiene, and the nurse in maternal and child health is assigned to the bureau of family health; the nurse reports directly to the director of the service unit, and her work is directed and judged by him with respect to its program effectiveness.

When this pattern of organization pertains, it is important that there also be a channel through which the nurse can secure guidance and evaluation of the nursing *practice* facets of the work. She needs a method of accounting for the pertinence, safety, and currency of nursing itself. Professional guidance of this nature can be provided only by a member of the particular profession involved, be it nursing or engineering or medicine or administration. The agencies generally provide a nurse adviser or a director of nursing services who works directly with the nursing staff and also with the non-nurse service leader to ensure the quality of nursing performance.

Professional Direction Must Come from Professional Sources

In addition to accounting for the work she is doing with respect to a given program or agency, the community health nurse must constantly evaluate and expand her general professional competence. As previously noted, in this she needs to have available the support of a member of her own profession who is more qualified by training or experience, or both, and who can help in this evaluation and growth process.

This presents no particular problem when the channels of accountability go through an all-nurse hierarchy, for the program accounting and staff developmental measures tend to merge. When there is an established nurse consultant or nurse advisory system that provides for consistent and continuing professional review and counseling, there is likewise little difficulty. When the nurse finds herself in a situation when neither of these situations pertains — for example, if she is a school nurse working alone — it may be necessary for her to identify some source for such help on her own initiative. The school nurse may request to be included in the staff education activities of the local health department, she may request advisement from the supervisory staff in that agency, or she may find a state consultant nurse in the field of school health who can provide some help. When such help is requested, the administrator should be informed and should understand that securing assistance with professional practice problems does not in any way interfere with the usual administrative channels of responsibility.

Patterns of Communication Are Usually Based on Custom

Although an organization chart shows channels of reporting and responsibility, the patterns of communication within an agency rarely follow the same channels. It is important to know how people communicate in a particular agency. For instance, do nurses tend to go directly to specialized consultants in an agency, or do they go first to their own supervisor? Does the staff nurse freely consult with a physician responsible for service, or does information generally go through the supervisor? Are there multidiscipline meetings or case conferences to which the nurse may go? Are there regular nursing staff meetings?

The general trend is definitely toward the greatest possible freedom in communication, with the problem, rather than the organization chart, deciding the best way to obtain needed opinion and guidance.

As noted, it is not possible to describe even briefly all the extant and desirable agency organizational patterns within which nursing functions. However, it should be remembered that there are three general conditions that the agency organizational structure should always assure. These are:

1. An opportunity for the community health nurse to identify herself with the functional or service group and also with those in her own profession.

2. Freedom to communicate with the many agency and community groups that have some concern with the work of the nurse.

3. Professional guidance for the professional aspects of the work.

THE HEALTH-CARE GROUP

At the direct care service level, the health system is organized for the purpose of providing to individuals or groups personal and environmental services, including curative, preventive, ameliorative, rehabilitative, and health promotional measures. This is the level at which the nurse is visiting families at home, holding conferences with school personnel, attending safety committee meetings, providing therapeutic and educational nursing to a clinic population, or interpreting the usefulness of family health nursing services to a local physicians' group.

Multidiscipline and Multiagency in Composition

There are three general types of members of the direct care group in which the nurse is working:

1. Personnel employed by the agency and responsible for a certain aspect of the general functional area that is the focus of the service. For example, in the school health program the sanitarian deals in matters relating to hygiene of the school environment, safety, and accident prevention; in the health department the nutritionist and the social worker have certain responsibilities in the care of the geriatric patient and his family.

2. Recipients of service and other members or representatives of consumer groups who may have prescribed or elective responsibilities for certain aspects of the program. For the community health nurse, the family is of course the most frequent example of this type of membership. In addition there may be volunteer workers or citizens' committees that are officially appointed or that serve on an informal basis as advisers or helpers.

3. Professional or citizen representatives not within the agency but integrally related to the purpose of the service. Some examples of this type of member are the family physician who is responsible for the medical supervision of the family receiving nursing care at home; the physician, hospital nurse, or medical social worker involved in the posthospital care of patients also under the care of the community health nurse; and the representative of a parent-teacher association who is helping to plan for an accident prevention educational program in the school.

Changing and Regrouping Membership

Because health care deals with many types of problems, each of which is seldom duplicated, the group providing care must constantly be adapted to the requirements of the specific setting or condition. For this reason, what is often referred to as *the public health team* may not be a formal and static structure but rather a group (or team, if you will) organized around a particular problem or function; and the members of the group will change as the problem changes. For example, if well-child supervision is provided through clinics administered by the health department that also provides nursing supervision to others in the family, the health-care team may be composed essentially of the agency workers and the recipients of service. If, however, a comprehensive children and youth project sponsored by, say, a university begins to assume responsibility for aspects of the well-child program for some segments of the population, the team for this subpopulation will be expanded to include appropriate university and project representatives.

Frequently there are groups within groups: the nursing staff may be organized into groups that include two or more levels of training, with the less-prepared personnel usually (but not always) falling under the direct supervision of the better-prepared nurse. Also, physicians may have physician assistants, social workers may function with social work aides, and engineers and sanitarians may share responsibility for environmental control measures.

Changing Leadership

As group membership changes, the leadership may also change. For example, in problems involving medical care—that is, involving illness or the diagnosis of illness—the physician will undoubtedly be the acknowledged leader. When the problem is one of changing health behavior, such as the reduction of smoking in a school group, the leadership may rest with a health educator; when the problem is family health-care management—that is, increasing the family's ability to foresee and handle health problems—the nurse may be the leader.

Health Professionals Who Are Frequent Coworkers

Certain types of community health personnel appear with sufficient frequency to warrant discussion.

The family physician is in many instances responsible for the medical management of patients receiving nursing care from a community agency. When this is the case, the community health nurse will plan with him for the care of his patients, working within the framework of both his orders for therapy and agency policy regarding the kinds of responsibilities that may be taken by the community health nurse.

For instance, a particular patient may need injections of a drug which is not suitable for administration by the patient or by a family member but which the physician feels could be administered safely by the community nurse from the Visiting Nurse Association. The nurse would provide such treatment only within specific written orders of the physician. The Visiting Nurse Association may have a policy regarding administration of drugs by their staff, or they may require that a special medical committee of the agency review and advise them regarding the safety of administering this particular drug in the home situation. Thus, both the doctor's prescription and the agency's policy determine exactly what will be done.

The nurse based in another agency is frequently involved in decisions regarding family care in the community setting. For some families, the interludes of hospital care are sufficiently frequent to make the hospital-based nurse a frequent member of the care group. The nurse in the school, in the industrial setting, and in the physician's office may be similarly involved. Frequent nurse-to-nurse contact helps synthesize the care provided from these various nursing sources.

The public health physician may fill many roles. He may serve as an administrator, directing the total or some part of the health program of the agency; as a provider of preventive or curative services in schools, industry, or clinics; or as an epidemiologist investigating the conditions related to the occurrence of disease or accident. He may also serve as a consultant to other professional workers in the agency or in the community: for example, a psychiatrist may advise with general practitioners, nurses, or comprehensive clinic personnel on matters relating to public health. The public health physician usually has special training in both public health and preventive medicine.*

Sanitarians or *sanitary inspectors* in public health work form a group that is second in size only to that of nurses. The sanitarian works closely with individuals and communities to promote and protect public health by controlling environmental hazards. He investigates domestic waste and sewerage systems and sanitary conditions in hotels, restaurants, motels, nursing homes, and sometimes, in schools. He interprets and enforces sanitary regulations, serves as a public health educator in matters relating to his field of work, and supports and promotes many programs in public health.

The public health sanitarian's emergence as a professional worker is in response to the broad responsibilities required in his field. Although many sanitarians do not have extensive formal training, the trend is toward strong preparation in biologic and sanitary sciences and in public health. The American Public Health Association statement recommends training to the baccalaureate level, including courses in social and physical sciences, and in addition, two years of work related to a specific field of sanitation such as bacteriology, entomology, parasitology, public health administration and law, epidemiology, principles and practices of water supply and sewage disposal, and biometry.[2] The number of sanitarians meeting these requirements has risen sharply in recent years.

The social worker has long been recognized as an important contributor to health action, and in recent years the number of social workers employed in community health agencies has increased markedly. The National Association of Social Workers has developed a working definition of social work, a definition that is under constant review. Social work has been described as the "disciplined use of self in relationship with an individual or group" that has as its purpose effecting change both in the individual and in his environment and in the interaction between them in order to achieve self-realization and effective social contribution.[3]

The boundaries between social work and nursing in the community setting are not always easily defined. However, in case discussion it is usually possible for both social worker and nurse to delineate those situations which are more readily handled by the one or the other.[4] In addition to sharing in direct care, the social worker may serve as a consultant to the community health nurse in those areas in which the

---

*American Public Health Association, through its Committee on Professional Education, develops descriptions of the work and desirable educational qualifications for various types of personnel which are revised periodically. The community health nurse would do well to familiarize herself with these statements as they appear in the *American Journal of Public Health.*

social worker is particularly expert, or she may help determine the need for social work services for specific families.

The health educator is an increasingly important member of the health-care team as the care of the conditions from which people suffer requires more and more knowing participation on the part of the family and the community. The health educator's professional preparation usually includes a strong orientation in the behavioral sciences and education as well as in public health. The health educator is in a position to help with community organization for health action (the motivation of families and groups and the organization of instruction).

In some countries, short-trained health educators who have had six or nine months of preparation may be used to deal with limited areas of health education.

As with the social worker, the boundaries between the work of the health educator and the nurse in direct service to families and groups are seldom clearly drawn. Again, the distinction lies in the degree of expertise required in a given situation rather than on the delineation of different areas of action or responsibility.

The public health nutritionist contributes to the appraisal of the nutritional problems of the family or community and to dietary management of nutritional problems. She may provide direct services to individuals or groups, or she may serve primarily as an adviser to other staff members. The community health nurse will have frequent need for such assistance.

The physical therapist and occupational therapist are also apt to serve in a dual capacity, providing service to families and groups and advising others on the staff. In the care of the longterm patient and his family, the physical therapist assumes an especially important place. In some instances the physical therapist may be the one who "carries" a case, with the nurse providing only supportive service.

Other frequently encountered members of the health team include the lay administrator; the sanitary or public health engineer; the public health dentist, who is usually a specialist in preventive dentistry; the speech therapist; and the psychologist or behaviorial scientist.

Multilevel Community Health Nurse Group

In addition to the many special health disciplines that are part of the health-care system, increasingly within nursing itself there exists a diversified nursing group. This group may exist within the single agency when one or more community health nurses join in the provision of care with registered nurses, licensed practical nurses, and short-trained nursing personnel such as home health aides, school nursing aides, or clinic nursing aides.

The organization of such a nursing group differs from one agency to another. The nursing-care group may be organized into functional units, each unit being responsible for a designated population or patient load; or the nursing-care team may be organized on what might be called a "requisition basis."

In the first instance, the operational group might consist of a public health nurse, one or more registered nurses without public health preparation, and varying numbers of practical nurses or home health aides. The group would function under the leadership of a designated team leader who would probably be the nurse with the highest level of preparation.[5] She would take responsibility for seeing that appropriate family-care plans were developed, and that nursing needs of the population served by this unit were being met within the limits of the responsible agency. In most cases, the supervision of workers with respect to immediate patient and family care is carried out by the team leader, but "developmental" supervision—that is, the overall evaluation of the performance of the worker that provides the basis for advancement, salary change, and professional advancement—is apt to be retained by the supervisor.

In the second instance (i.e., organization on a "requisition basis") the auxiliary workers are organized as a separate cadre under the direction of a supervisor who is responsible for their training and supervision. Each nurse takes responsibility for a designated district; this involves the development of a case load, which she manages. When it appears that auxiliary care is indicated, the nurse and the supervisor arrange for the assignment, and the nurse undertakes some of the on-the-spot supervision and special training of the of the auxiliary worker.

Whether the nursing-care group is organized as a continuing team or on an *ad hoc* basis, it is important that the members involved plan together for nursing care, communicate frequently, seek help from one another, and share in evaluating the progress of the patient and the results of the nursing care.

Multiprofessional group care has characterized community health services from the beginning. Although group functioning may have been approached intuitively rather than systematically, the community health nurse has traditionally worked closely with the family physician, the social worker, the nutritionist, and the hospital personnel, involving them in the decisions regarding care. Case conferences have been described in the literature of public health nursing for many years.

The use of a multilevel nursing group in providing direct care has been a little slower to develop in the community setting than it has in the hospital setting, perhaps because of the constraints imposed by the nature and locale of the care. For example, the type of care required by a particular family may involve several different levels of skill or the special skills of different health disciplines. Yet, because the care is provided in the home or in a nonhealth environment such as a school or an industrial plant, the problems of travel to the patient may make it impracticable to have more than one worker present. Even though only about 10 percent of the care given to a particular family requires professional level skill, it may nevertheless be necessary for the professional nurse to provide 100 percent of the care, since it cannot be delegated without undue costs in travel time. Furthermore, since much of the work of the community health nurse involves longterm relationships with families or groups and since many of the services are of an interpersonal, rather than of a technical, character, the effectiveness of the service may be reduced if too many people are directly involved. Thus it may be that the community health nurse will undertake types of service that in the hospital setting would be the responsibility of the social worker or the physical therapist or the nurse's aide.

However, the transfer of much care of the sick from hospital to home, the expanded opportunities for service afforded by Medicare and Medicaid, and the improvement of planning for patient care that places the hospital and the community health agencies into closer partnership have sharply increased the opportunities for and feasibility of using multilevel nursing personnel in the community setting.

Operative Care-Group Characteristics

Simply increasing the number and variety of health-care personnel available for the care of people may expand the types and extent of service available to the population. It will not, however, automatically produce the most comprehensive care that is possible. The way in which those involved in care are organized and the relationships and patterns of work that are developed by them make the difference between multiple, fragmented services and the planned, reinforcing activity that *should* characterize a care group.

Ideally the care group functioning in the community health setting should possess four characteristics:
1. Shared goals.
2. Comfortable and complete communication.
3. Merged resources.
4. Adaptive interchange of roles.

SHARED GOALS

If a group is to make an organized effort to effect some change in a person or in his environment, there must be agreement as to what changes are desired. For example, if the nurse designing a prenatal nursing program in a suburban area has the objective of improving parental skills and supporting an already adequate medical surveillance system, whereas the health director's objective is that of reducing maternal and infant deaths, it is doubtful that their efforts with respect to implementing the nursing program will be mutually reinforcing. There would be sharp differences in the way in which families were selected for care, the amount and type of nursing support provided, and the selection of the method of approach (*i.e.,* the choice of a group or an individual approach).

The sharing of goals is not likely to be achieved by chance. Sometimes goal setting in the care groups is undertaken in rather formal terms. In an agency which has accepted a "goal-oriented management" pattern or in community groups that have a similar goal-oriented approach, there is apt to be great stress laid on goal setting at all levels of care. On the other hand, in dealing with a busy family physician, the achievement of goal sharing may be very informally approached by agreement on a joint course of action that implies, rather than defines, a particular goal.

COMFORTABLE AND COMPLETE COMMUNICATION

Comfortable and complete communication permits the kind of sharing of ideas and opinions that makes for productive joint effort. Communication is a skill integral to all of the helping professions, but these skills are all too often applied in a much more consistent and thoughtful way in relationships with clients than in relationships with coworkers. It is important to recognize and overcome the barriers to communication as they operate in the care-group situation.

Perhaps no barrier is more important and pervasive than limitations of time. It takes time not only to find out what another worker has already done with a family but also to keep others informed in turn. One must be convinced that this time is well spent.

Interprofessional barriers may also interfere; for instance, the nurse, or the physician, may see the physician as the one who takes final authority in all health matters, which may be interpreted to mean that he makes all of the care decisions. This perception might lead to the nurse's withholding of contributions in favor of ascertaining the physician's wishes, or it may result in the physician's feeling that it is not important for others to understand why he wants a particular course of action followed. As important as this "single source of decision" fallacy is the attitude that no member of a professional group should "interfere" with the work of other professions. Thus a social worker might feel it is not her prerogative to suggest that a family, whose care is primarily the responsibility of the community health nurse, might benefit from being pushed toward more self-help in the nursing phases of care. Such interprofessional barriers must be diminished.

Barriers may be created by the mechanisms that have been developed for interchange of information. The impersonal form; the required, but unnecessary, approval for referral; the use of formal abstracts as a substitute for the telephone call or a personal visit; or the substitution of written procedures for face-to-face joint decisions about care may seriously impede intra-group communication.

Some community health nurses develop their own means of informal communication. For instance, she may make it a habit occasionally to drop in at physicians' offices to say "hello" and to ask whether there is any patient-care problem with which she could help. In the course of this friendly visit, the nurse gets to know the physician's feelings about prenatal care or the handling of adolescent behavior problems. The nurse would probably not obtain this information if her contact with the physician were limited to reporting nursing action taken on behalf of his patients. Informal communication devices may be equally effective in relationships with nurses in doctors' offices or in other agencies, with the social case worker, or with the counseling staff in the school.

MERGED RESOURCES

In the community health setting there are great economies to be achieved in the *merging of resources* of the several groups involved in health care. Thus, for instance, the school nurse might undertake a special program on the effects of cigarette smoking at the same time that the local health department is waging a special antismoking campaign. *Merging* of resources should not be confused with *simple addition*. Merging implies planning for the entire effort; using the person, the timing, and the approach that is considered most effective in a particular instance; and having the knowing support of one another's efforts on behalf of the recipients of care.

ADAPTIVE INTERCHANGE OF ROLES

Perhaps the most striking characteristic of organization within the modern health-care group is the high degree of interchangeability in functions and the blurring of the roles of various members.

Thus the social worker, rather than the nutritionist or the public health nurse, might advise an expectant mother on the fundamentals of appropriate family diet in the course of discussing the problems of money management; or the nurse, rather than the psychiatric social worker, might help the family understand and deal with the special stresses incident to the return of a hospitalized psychiatric patient.

The decision as to who does what may be based on convenience or expediency—that is, which worker happens to be present at a given point in time—or it may be made on the basis of the kind of relationship one worker has already developed with the family or group and on the positive or deterrent effect this relationship is likely to have with respect to the immediate situation.

In any case, when roles are interchanged, it is essential that there be good "backstopping." For instance, the social worker would brief the nurse carrying what is theoretically a social work responsibility.

The harmony and efficiency with which the health-care group functions will largely determine the degree to which it is possible to provide truly comprehensive and continuing health care. As a key participant in the health-care group, the community health nurse has a special obligation to contribute to and to work within the goals of the group as a whole; to understand and appreciate the contributions of other members; to make and use opportunities for interpersonal and technical interchange; and to lead or to follow as the situation requires. Most of all, the community health nurse must realize that the development of an effective health-care group requires and deserves her time and thoughtful concern.

REFERENCES

1. For a fuller description of this topic, see Chapter 2. *In* Mustard, S., and Stebbins, E. L. (eds.): Introduction to Public Health. 4th ed., The Macmillan Company, New York, 1968.
2. Educational and other qualifications of Public Health Sanitarians. American Public Health Association, Committee on Professional Education, New York, 1956.
3. Bartlett, Harriet M.: Social Work Practice in the Health Field. National Association of Social Workers, New York, 1961, p. 22.
4. Murdagh, Jessica: There is a difference. Nurs. Outlook, *16:*45, October, 1968.
5. Brink, Carol: Supervising group practice in public health. Amer. J. Nurs., *68:*344, February, 1968.

SUGGESTED READINGS

Anderson, Margaret M., Glasser, Betty Ann, and Manning, Mary Jane: Nursing and social work roles in cooperative home care and treatment of the mentally ill. Nurs. Outlook, *11:*112, February, 1963.

Arnold, Mary F.: Perception of professional role activities in the local health department. Public Health Rep., *77:*80, January, 1962.

Bates, Barbara, and Kern, M. S.: Doctor–nurse teamwork: what helps? what hinders? Amer. J. Nurs., *67:*2066, October, 1967.

Beloff, J. S., and Willett, M.: Yale studies in family health care. III. The Health Care Team. J.A.M.A., *205:*663, September, 1968.

Bergman, Rebecca Lyons: Team nursing in public health. International Journal of Nursing Studies, *1:*179, December, 1964.

Brink, Carol: Supervising group practice in public health. Amer. J. Nurs., *68:*344, February, 1968.

Clack, F. B., and Wishik, Caroline: New staff for public health. Public Health Rep., *83:*150, February, 1968.

Health occupations supportive to nursing. Amer. J. Nurs., *66:*559, March, 1966.

Heath, Alice M.: Health aides in health departments. Public Health Rep., *82:*608, July, 1967.

Home Health Aide Service in Relation to Public Health Nursing. National League for Nursing, New York, 1965.

Jamison, Eileen F.: Non public health nurses in public health. Nurs. Outlook, *14:*56, August, 1966.

Murdagh, Jessica: There is a difference. Nurs. Outlook, *16:*45, October, 1968.

Parramore, Beatrice, and Yeager, Wayne: Team nursing in public health. Nurs. Outlook, *16:*54, 1968.

Phillips, Elizabeth: Group approach to nursing service. Nurs. Outlook, *13:*45, August, 1965.

Potts, Dorothy, and Miller, Carl: The community health aide. Nurs. Outlook, *12:*33, December, 1964.

Robinson, Sally: Is there a difference? Nurs. Outlook, *15:*34, November, 1967.

Stein, Leonard I.: The doctor-nurse game. Amer. J. Nurs., *68:*101, January, 1968.

CHAPTER
6

Community Health Nursing in the Community Structure

In order to guide her own work effectively, the community health nurse, whether a beginner or a seasoned administrator, must understand how community health nursing fits into the various parts of the community health-care system.

The health-care system may be defined, for the purposes of this discussion, as the complex of people, structures, facilities, and relationships that has been developed within a community to provide health care to individuals, groups, special populations, or to the community as a whole. Thus the system would include health professionals of all types; other individuals and groups, including consumers of health care, who are taking health action for themselves or on the behalf of others; the health and health-related institutions, including hospitals, health and welfare departments, school health services, and voluntary agencies; and the mechanisms through which all of them relate to one another.

GENERAL CONSIDERATIONS

Community health nursing operates under a variety of sponsorships: government authorities, ranging from local to international in coverage; voluntary agencies; and private industry or health groups. Each of these types of sponsor has particular commitments and particular ways of organizing to meet these commitments. Within this total system, community health nursing is involved at three levels: the direct-care (operational or practicing) level, the institutional or agency level, and the community level. Each level has its own particular conditions, opportunities, and constraints.

Provision for Health Care Through the Government Structure

Government concern with health is a worldwide phenomenon; virtually every country has some provision for health care under government sponsorship. Community health nursing within a government agency may be placed in departments of health, welfare, or education or, in smaller numbers, in many other government units. Although government agencies do not provide all, or even most of, the health care of the people of the United States, they do have a broad mandate. It is generally accepted that with respect to health, the government is obligated to assure as far as possible that adequate and safe care reaches all segments of the population in amounts and quality calculated to preserve and promote health. Sharing the same broad obligation, community nursing in the government setting is also geared to the public as a whole.

Community health nursing is represented in the health efforts of all three tiers of government: local, state or provincial, and national. In each of these three levels, nursing is adapted to the degree of responsibility characteristic of that particular government level.

THE LOCAL AGENCY

The local government agency – the city or county health department, welfare department, or school system – represents the delivery point for the majority of governmentally sponsored community health nursing services. The local health department is usually considered to have major responsibility for identifying the health needs of the community and for mobilizing and coordinating the many resources that are used to meet these needs.[1] Each local government will design its own health program, distributing responsibility among the various departments of government in a manner that is suited to the particular situation. In many communities there is a board of health, an officially authorized body usually made up of both lay members and members of the health professions. The responsibilities of the board of health are variously defined, ranging from advisory to decisional.

THE STATE AGENCY

The state may and usually does delegate considerable power to local units of government, but it still retains the ultimate responsibility and authority for the public's health. A policy statement of the American Public Health Association defines four major functions of the state health department:

1. Providing leadership for the advancement of public health through analyzing the health condition and health needs of the population, and planning a program designed to meet these needs.
2. Providing financial assistance to localities, including the distribution of state aid and the administration and distribution of federal grants-in-aid.

3. Setting standards by such activities as the administration of public health laws, sanitary codes, and licensing programs.

4. Providing health services to areas not otherwise served, in cases of emergency, or when the service requires a degree of specialization not available locally.[2]

The state department of health is expected to take the lead in coordinating the health efforts of all government agencies functioning within the state. This category includes such agencies as departments of welfare, mental health, and licensing.

The state's authority in health matters derives from the sovereign powers reserved to the states under the Constitution. In most states several agencies carry health programs, but the state health department is generally recognized as the agency primarily responsible for public health within the state.

THE FEDERAL AGENCY

Health agencies in the federal tier of government have two types of responsibility: the first is concerned with acting on problems that cannot be logically or feasibly dealt with by the states, and the second is concerned with supporting and improving the health care provided through state and local health authorities. This responsibility is met through the following activities:

1. Maintaining a health intelligence system for the nation as a whole in coordination with the states and with international health sources. This includes the collection of data by the National Center for Health Statistics and the maintenance of interstate and national data required for the control of communicable diseases, air pollution, and similar problems that transcend state boundaries.

2. Setting national health policy and providing the legislative arm of government with information and technical assistance required as a basis for developing adequate and appropriate legislation. Most health professionals feel that the national health policy is as yet not very clearly defined.

3. Providing financial aid to state and local health groups through grants-in-aid, contracts, project grants, and other funding mechanisms.

4. Supporting state and local health efforts through a system of continuing technical consultation to the states; allocation of highly specialized personnel to deal with exceptional state or local problems that require a degree of expertness not available in the states; and developing standards and supportive guides, criteria, and other materials for use by the state and local agencies.

5. Providing direct services to groups—for example, Indians, Eskimos, members of the armed forces, and veterans—to which the federal government has a specific commitment.

6. Conducting or supporting research in health care.

The Voluntary Agency Is Less Restricted

Unlike the government agencies, voluntary agencies are not bound by the responsibility for the total population. The voluntary agency, which can be local, state, or national in scope, is an expression of public concern with problems not being fully met by personal or government action. As such it may elect to deal with only a particular disease, a demonstration service, or a small segment of the population.

The voluntary agency derives its authority from its board of directors. It functions within the legal restrictions regarding incorporation and fund raising and within the general welfare and public health laws of the particular state. The board of directors sets policy, provides broad directional leadership, and takes final responsibility for the conduct of the agency's business. These boards of voluntary health or nursing agencies are usually made up mostly of representative citizens who serve as volunteers; members of the health professions constitute a minority in the total membership. There is currently some concern that these boards have failed to secure adequate representation from certain segments of the population; in particular, representation from the low-income or minority groups.

The voluntary agency is expected to work within the framework of the total health effort: to relate its work to the work of others, to avoid unnecessary duplication, and to recognize all needs that fall within the purview of its commitment. This relation to the total health effort is essential if the voluntary agency is to meet its obligation to spend prudently and for the purpose intended the money it receives from contributions or contracts.

As previously noted, voluntary organizations in the United States may be local, regional, or national in coverage. The major voluntary nursing services are organized on a local level. (In contrast, in Canada and in Great Britain the major voluntary nursing services are organized on a national level.)

There is little consistency in the nature of the programs undertaken by voluntary agencies: the quality or comprehensiveness of the services afforded and the nature of their relationship to other community efforts vary. The tendency has been for voluntary agencies to undertake new or untried programs and, in some instances, services that have a low priority in government programs but that are still felt to meet a human need; such programs may later become part of a government program. Many of those engaged in the voluntary health movement feel that a major contribution is the opportunity it offers individuals to express their concern for others and to engage in social action through their voluntary contributions.

The recently established program undertaken by the National League for Nursing in coordination with the American Public Health Association for the accreditation of home health agencies may have a significant effect on the quality of voluntary nursing services. This accreditation may serve as the basis for the certification of voluntary agencies as providers of services to individuals under the Medicare program. The National League for Nursing also includes a Council of Public Health Nursing Agencies, which serves as a stimulus to improvement and as a forum for the exchange of ideas. National health agencies that include nursing concerns are likely to be members of the National Health Council; this also provides an opportunity for unified efforts toward improvement. However, the number of nurses in such national health agencies (other than those nurses in the member nursing organizations) is very small.

The professional association has special responsibilities for increasing the societal contribution of the profession, for improving the quality of professional practice, and for protecting and speaking for the practitioner as a negotiator or interpreter. This responsibility is reflected in the aims of the American Nurses' Association as stated in its articles of incorporation:

The purposes of this corporation are and shall be to promote the professional and educational advancement of nurses in every proper way; to elevate the standard of nursing education; to establish and maintain a code of ethics among nurses; to distribute relief among such nurses as may become ill, disabled or destitute; to disseminate information on the subject of nursing by publications in official periodicals or otherwise; to bring into communication with each other various nurses and associations and federations of nurses throughout the United States of America. . . .[3]

To meet these responsibilities, professional associations develop educational programs, materials, or other means of improving the quality of professional practice; and represent the profession in the total group of health professions and in their relationships with government and voluntary health and legislative groups.

Private Sources of Health Care Serve the Majority of Americans

For many, the phrase "medical care" means care by the family physician and, if he recommends it, further care by a medical specialist in private practice. The majority of physicians work as private entrepreneurs; that is, in solo practice. Hospitals coordinate their efforts with the physician's efforts in a variety of ways, such as housing physicians' offices in the hospital or allotting hospital privileges, which permits the physician to care for his patient while the patient is in the hospital.

The rapid development of group practice has produced a different kind of family health care in which a group of specialists engage in joint practice and share in the care of patients and families. An extension of this is the large, prepaid-insurance supported medical-care center. (The Kaiser Foundation Health Plan or the Health Insurance Plan of New York City are examples of this kind of program.) Such groups operate with a large and varied supportive staff to supplement the physicians' work, and the physician complex operates somewhat like an agency. These groups may operate on a nonprofit basis, in which case they come under state regulations governing nonprofit agencies; accordingly, if funds are provided by insurance, the group functions under the insurance regulations of the state.

Health care is an important fringe benefit in industry. Many industrial concerns and privately sponsored health or welfare services provide nursing services to their employees or their members. Such services may be included because of job considerations: that is, they may reduce compensation insurance costs, or increase productivity by caring for minor health problems or by reducing absenteeism. These services are often considered to be a fringe benefit that is important to the workers involved and a point for negotiation between industry and labor unions.

Authority for such health service is provided by the board of directors of the organization, either directly or through delegation to the executive or management officers of the corporation. This authority may be written into the directives of the company, or it may be incorporated into the bylaws or regulations of an organization.

Programs vary widely from industry to industry, and occupational health nursing reflects this. The health service may be primarily a first-aid station effort, or it may be a comprehensive and carefully planned health-care program with intensive counseling and preventive services for workers and their families.

The Roles of Health-Care Sources Are Blurred

The traditional roles of these many partners in organized health care are becoming more and more blurred. Private or voluntary sources, such as universities or groups of physicians, undertake responsibilities formerly considered the province of government. Federal agencies, at one time restrained from by-passing the state health structure, now deal directly with local governments or voluntary groups. Projects under voluntary agency management may have what appears to be responsibility that has traditionally rested with the public authorities.

Realignment of responsibilities and programs is a continuous process. Interposed among these structures is a relative newcomer to the organization family: the community-based citizen advisory or controlling group. Nursing agencies, especially voluntary agencies, have traditionally leaned on citizen advisory groups. However, in the past these groups have been represented by boards, committees, or advisory bodies who related to a particular agency or phase of the health effort. Recently, though, citizen groups have become much more powerful and involved in larger spheres of responsibility. Many laws providing for funding of health programs require that the planning and evaluation of the work be undertaken by a representative group that must be made up of general representatives of the public as well as of professional personnel. The Nurse Training Act and the Community Action Program of the Economic Opportunity Act are examples of legislation requiring such general citizen involvement.

At present, problems of health care appear to be dealt with largely on an expedient *ad hoc* basis, any accredited or responsible agency or care source feeling free to move into any program for which they have a fancy and for which they can mobilize the necessary money and personnel.

This convenient "no system" approach is understandable. The public, impatient with any delay, is demanding that its institutions apply quickly what is known about health. Thus there is often a failure to consider at what level of organization or through what type of structure the most effective and economical total result could be achieved.

Furthermore, health problems refuse to stay put within given geographic boundaries or service units: often a safe and plentiful water supply cannot be assured by a single state authority; nor can a single agency, such as a hospital or a health department, deal with the multiple problems of the geriatric patient and his family. Thus new and unconventional methods that will work effectively under these new conditions must be devised. Perhaps some clearer and more timely definition of roles will come as the efforts sponsored by the Community Health Planning Act progress further.

Community Health Nursing at the Local Level

Nursing in the local community may be fragmented, especially in urban areas. In 1946, what was then the National Organization of Public Nursing (since incorporated into the National League for Nursing) issued a statement (reaffirmed at a 1952 conference on the home care of the sick) suggesting three types of community organization for public health nursing:

1. All public health nursing services, including care of the sick at home, administered and supported by the health department. This is the usual pattern for rural communities.

2. Preventive services carried by the health department with one voluntary agency working in close coordination with the health department carrying responsibility for nursing care of the sick and for some special fields. This type of organization is the most usual one found in large areas.

3. A combination nursing service jointly administered by official and voluntary agencies with all field service given by a single group of public health nurses. Such a combination of services is especially desirable in small cities.[4]

These recommendations were designed to reduce the proliferation of community nursing services and were based on the concept of provision of service solely by public health nurses, each of whom carried a generalized program and served a designated population group. However, subsequent developments make it unlikely that these recommendations will continue to be relevant. School nursing services have continued as separate entities in many communities, and both school nurses and school authorities appear reluctant to change this situation. Moreover, the introduction of Medicare has catapulted health departments, as well as visiting nurse associations, into extended care of illness in the home. Among the new clients are a good number who require nursing care at a less-than-professional level. In longterm illness care, some of the tasks and responsibilities may be frustrating or limiting to the public health nurse and more suited to the carefully selected short-trained home health aide. As a result, the number of practical nurses and short-trained nursing personnel in community health is increasing rapidly.

At the same time, high-impact programs—large-scale projects for disadvantaged families, tuberculosis control, and comprehensive-care centers and the consequent realignment of medical and nursing functions and activities—have created the need for a community nurse with a higher degree of expertise in a particular clinical area than can be expected of the generalized nurse. Directors of special purpose projects may recruit and appoint their own specialized nursing staff. Even when the nursing staff of the project is appointed by an existing health agency, the project may be organized as a virtually autonomous service.

Thus in the local health system, community health nursing may be expected to function in many different organizations and structures. While community health nurses tend to be concentrated in the health department, in the school, and in the visiting nurse associations, there may be a considerable number of community health nurses working alone or in small groups in the urban area. It is important to devise some method of relating these many nursing efforts to avoid unnecessary duplication and to protect the family from the constant incursion of different nurses, all trying to help but all needing to establish a relationship, to fill in a record, and to meet the special concerns of their own agency; all, in short, expecting some response from the family. On the other hand, in the rural area this situation may be reversed. Rather than having a plethora of reiterative or multiple nursing services, the nursing staff may be isolated from the stimulation of other nurse practitioners; and the need may be to relate to and plan with nurses outside the immediate community as well as within the narrower local range.

It seems, then, that the "generalized nursing" organization in the local community health agency is not always the definitive answer. It is true that in the past, a generalized public health nurse was thought to be able to provide all of the necessary curative, preventive, and health promotional nursing family care needed in the home; specialists might be used in clinics or for single-service aspects of care, but family nursing care would remain with the generalist. Furthermore, the generalist would be employed either by the health department or by a combined (two components) agency. When populations were large or when there was a strong and simple dual voluntary and government nursing system, the two-agency system could prevail. Now the answer isn't quite that simple.

The Combination Agency

One possible effective local public health structure is the combination agency; that is, two or more agencies under official and voluntary auspices that have joined forces in order to provide more economical and more effective public health nursing.[5] In 1966 there were 85 combination agencies, employing 2305 nurses.[6]

In such situations, the combination agency absorbs the general responsibilities of all its constituents. Funds come from some combination of taxes, fees, voluntary contributions, endowments, or joint fund raising group such as the community chest. Authority for the various functions in the combined agency is drawn from the same sources as pertain to the constituent agencies. The boards of directors of the voluntary agencies and the appropriate government authorities draw up agreements to define the respective responsibilities and to coordinate planning and action.[7]

A combined public health nursing service is usually one that is jointly administered by both government and voluntary agencies with all field service rendered by a single staff of public health nurses. However, many transitional programs exist, and the patterns of combining efforts range all the way from two independently organized units consolidated only by the employment of a single director of nurses and the joint use of a supervisory and consultant staff to a complete amalgamation of the two units. The following patterns are typical:

1. Administration by a single agency with other agencies buying the service that it sponsors. For example, a social welfare division may buy home nursing service for recipients of old age pensions from a visiting nurse association, or the community chest may provide funds for the local health department to pay for visiting nurse service or practical nursing care to the chronically ill; this care would be supervised by the public health nursing staff.

2. Independent funds and control but coordinated service. A visiting nurse association might raise its own funds, determine its own scope of service, and set personnel policies for the staff employed by that association, while the health department also maintains a separate budget and policy-making procedure. However, within this framework both parts of the nursing service function under a single director; and the individual nurse, whether employed by the visiting nurse association or by the health department, carries out the functions of both agencies so that the service rendered to a single family is given by a single worker. Coordination is maintained at the policy-making level by planning committees, councils, or other policy-making bodies.

3. Completely integrated programs with pooled funds and staff and with a joint directing board. In this instance, responsibility for certain aspects of the work may have to be allocated to one or the other of the component groups; for example, the health department or board of health cannot legally delegate its specific responsibilities to a voluntary group, nor can an incorporated voluntary group relinquish its responsibility to account for the expenditure of its funds and to maintain adequate financial records.

In the development of combined agencies that afford services from both government and voluntary sources, certain principles might be considered:

1. The policy of voluntary effort on behalf of health should be maintained.

2. Relative responsibilities and commitments of each constituent should be clearly defined and agreements should be confirmed in writing.

3. The organization should provide for adequate medical direction and for a qualified nursing director responsible for the total nursing effort.

4. Provision should be made for full utilization of representative consumer and professional groups to assure sound community-based planning.

5. The program should be based on the objective of meeting the nursing needs of the total population regardless of place of residence or ability to pay for care.

Other Consolidations of Nursing Effort

MERGERS OF VOLUNTARY AGENCIES

As home-care responsibilities increase, visiting nurse services are also faced with tremendous expansion and modification of their usual services. What may have been a placid well-established small visiting nurse association is suddenly confronted with a burgeoning (and paying!) home-care load with mountains of forms, regulations, billing procedures, and unmet requirements for certification for federal funds for Medicare patients. Even though the requirements established by the Public Health Service as a guide to the states in certifying agencies and the National League for Nursing criteria for accreditation as a home agency are certainly minimal, they are still beyond the facilities of some small visiting nurse associations.[8, 9] Therefore, there has been considerable pressure for small voluntary agencies to combine to effect economy and permit more adequate supervisory and consultant staffing. Thus the number of voluntary agencies may be reduced while the available services increase.

URBAN DECENTRALIZED HEALTH CENTERS

In many urban areas, especially in cities where there are defined poverty areas, decentralized health centers are being established in an effort to bring health care closer to the people served. In this setting it is felt that nursing service may be more quickly responsive to the needs of people and close enough to get the kind of feedback from the population that is essential for planning the health program. Sometimes nurses and auxiliaries from various agencies are jointly assigned to these centers, and, helped by the members of the community, they work as a group on the total community health nursing needs. When this happens, the agencies involved set up formal or informal agreements, but usually the nurses in the center have considerable latitude in working out their mutual responsibilities.

HOSPITAL-BASED HOME-CARE PROGRAMS

Increasingly in the United States, hospital-based services are finding a need for a community health nurse. The hospital-based home-care program may purchase nursing service from the local health department or visiting nurse association, use the existing agencies as a source for referral, or establish an independent home visiting service.

The rapid expansion of out-patient services (there were more than 148 million—749 per 1000 of the population—out-patient visits in 1967) has made health planners increasingly aware of the need to improve and modify the care provided and to relate out-patient services more closely to the home and the community.[10]

In this setting, the community health nurse may deal directly with families in the home or in the hospital or clinic setting, or she may serve as a liaison with other community nursing and health services.

A further factor is the trend toward more patient-oriented care in the hospital. Those responsible for in-patient hospital services are also increasingly concerned with the home and community facets of care. This places additional responsibility on the hospital nursing staff for relating to the home and to other community agencies. As a result, the incorporation of community health nursing into hospital-based programs is moving ahead rapidly.

Special Problems

CARE FOR PRIVATE PHYSICIANS' PATIENTS

Although it is true that families in lower income levels are most likely to have serious health problems and are least likely to be under the care of the private physician, once outside the big city complex, the proportion of people in all economic classes under private medical care shifts upward.

At present in the United States, community nursing support to private physicians is minimal. It is true that voluntary nursing organizations offer their services to the families served by the private physician and keep the physician informed about the services available to him. In a few instances there have been efforts to provide more consistent support.[11] However, there has been no movement in the United States to parallel that in Great Britain where the health visitor or district nurse may be "attached" or "partially attached" to a group of physicians. Under this scheme, developed by the health authorities in conjunction with private medical practitioners, a health visitor is assigned to work directly with a group of general practitioners. The physicians' case load becomes her population; there are usually about four general practitioners and a population of from 6000 to 10,000. Her function is not to be "extra hands" for the doctor but to carry her own nursing responsibilities in support of the overall medical patient-care plan.[12-14] Her work is described in one statement as comprising largely work with children and mothers and with the elderly. Although not without administrative problems, this type of arrangement appears to be quite satisfying to nurses and to the physicians with whom they work.

The extension of group practice (an estimated 15 percent of the physicians in practice in 1967 were in group practice) would appear to offer an excellent opportunity for more intensive nursing support for private physicians, thereby extending community health nursing service in an efficient and potentially useful way.[15]

In the absence of any formal arrangement, the community health nurse may visit the physician's office periodically, confer with him and his office nurse, and keep a two-way information flow going.

THE ISOLATED "MINI" NURSING GROUP

The urban community health nurse working alone or without immediate nursing supervision or in a very small group (in a school, in industry, or in a project, for example) may find it difficult to relate to the whole scene in community nursing. Hopefully when there are larger community health nursing groups, they will offer assistance; they may include these smaller groups or solo workers in staff educational activities or, if indicated, offer to provide consultant or supervisory help.

The nurse in the rural health department is more likely to be tied into an advisory network provided by the state health departments and thereby gain some continuing support. Sometimes the small rural visiting nurse association can also make arrangements to benefit from this advisory assistance. Even if this rather formal commitment is not possible, definite liaison plans should be set up for the exchange of information.

Sometimes community health nurses or groups of community health nurses may resist too close an affiliation with other services. The nurse in a combined service and research project may feel her interests do not extend to the community as a whole and that others will not understand or appreciate her research concerns. The nurses in schools or industry may find it inconvenient to meet with other groups, or indeed, the health department and visiting nurse association may have been feuding for years!

Even if the good of the community were not sufficiently compelling to urge the stronger organization to woo the reluctant group into dialogue and decision, self-interest would make it sufficiently worthwhile. To plan any community health nursing program apart from others in the community is decidedly foolhardy.

COMMUNITY HEALTH NURSING AT THE STATE LEVEL IS MORE SPECIALIZED

Although the state is a strong unit in the three tier system of government agencies, it is seldom a very strong facet of the voluntary health system, since the latter tends to concentrate on national and local units. (A few community health nurses are employed in voluntary agencies such as the state units of the National Tuberculosis Association or the American Heart Association.) For this reason, at the state level, governmentally sponsored nursing tends to be the more developed.

In most state government agencies, the primary nursing responsibility is one of leadership and planning rather than of direct service. A few states provide direct nursing services to communities that do not have organized government community nursing programs or where the population is so scattered as to make local nursing units too small to be efficient. In this case, even though employed and directed through the state health department or other government agency, the community health nurses work in the same manner as in a local agency. They have the same responsibility for reconciling community health nursing with other nursing efforts and of looking at the health needs and health-care provisions as a whole, just as would the nurse employed and supervised locally.

Nursing concerns in a state or provincial health department are not limited to community health nursing. For example, the supply of nurses in all fields and the supervision of nursing homes are major health problems in the state health departments.

Nurses in special fields who serve as consultants and advisers are included in many units of state government. Units that have substantial concerns with nursing, such as welfare, education, or grants management, may not have a nursing staff specifically assigned to that unit but may instead have an arrangement with a nursing unit that provides them with whatever nursing advisement and support may be required.

Nurses are also important members of state planning bodies and state action groups such as regional medical programs for heart, cancer, and stroke. They may be either employees of the group or nursing leaders who serve on an intermittent basis as members of commissions or committees.

The state health department is the principal health agency of the state, and the nursing staff of the state health department shares its general responsibility for leadership. Typical responsibilities of community health nursing in state health departments are:

1. To study and recommend, in conjunction with other groups concerned, action relating to the overall nurse manpower supply. This involves such activities as arranging for nurse manpower surveys; evaluating the adequacy of training facilities and making recommendations for change; helping communities to adapt to change in the nurse manpower supply; and working with professional associations, hospitals, and others to develop required data.

2. To relate nursing to the larger health effort of the state by advising with other health or health-related bureaus, departments, agencies, or organizations on nursing phases of their work so as to ensure coordination and effective utilization of the available nurse supply. This includes participation in the development of the overall plan and administration of the total health programs, including administration of grants to local communities.

3. To assist and supplement the efforts of local government and voluntary and private groups engaged in nursing. This involves such activities as providing supplementary general or specialized staff to advise on professional or administrative problems in nursing, establishing uniform record systems, and providing computer services for reporting.

4. To improve the quality of nursing efforts within the state. This will include such activities as developing criteria or guidelines; establishing recommended or required personnel requirements for employment or for certification or licensing; and engaging in, or arranging for, ongoing educational programs for employed or to-be-employed nursing staff.

5. To promote coordination of all state-wide efforts for nursing, whether sponsored by government, voluntary, professional, quasi-professional, or private agencies.

Because of the nature of these tasks and responsibilities when local health services are well established, the nursing staff at the state tier is apt to consist primarily of specialists or consultant personnel. In a few states where local services have not been developed, the state employed staff may include a larger number of direct service personnel.

COMMUNITY HEALTH NURSING AT THE NATIONAL LEVEL SUPPORTS AND SUPPLEMENTS STATE AND LOCAL EFFORTS

Within the national health network, nursing takes its place in assuring the vitality and relevance of policies and plans for the national nursing effort, in strengthening and improving the quality of state and local nursing efforts, and in conducting nursing programs that require a nationwide approach.

In the national government structure, nursing is integrally related to virtually every unit and program having substantive health content. There is a chief nurse officer, formerly located in the Surgeon General's office but currently in the Bureau of Health Services and Mental Health Administration, who is concerned with broad policy and program development. The Division of Nursing in the Bureau of Health Professions, Education, and Manpower Training plays a major role. Nursing leadership formerly supplied through the nursing staff of the Children's Bureau is now effected through the nursing section of the Maternal and Child Health Service, the Bureau of Health Services, and the Mental Health Administration. The Veterans Administration Hospital system provides for both direct nursing care and certain contract community services for its beneficiaries. Each of the regional offices of the Department of Health, Education, and Welfare has a nursing complement to plan and implement the nursing phases of programs in support of regional, state, and local health action. Employee health services are well-developed in the various agencies of the federal government. Many other agencies of the federal government have nursing concerns and nursing staff.

In the direct care services — such as services to special population groups or to employees — afforded under federal sponsorship, community health aspects of health care correspond to those at a local level. For instance, although federally supported, the army health nurse assigned to an army post is expected to relate not only to the army preventive medical service but also to the community in which the post is located.

Typical responsibilities of the combined nursing effort in the national government structure include:

1. To build nursing into national health policy, plans, and action. This involves anticipating nursing implications of national developments: for example, anticipating the nursing impact of the Medicare and Medicaid legislation or of new approaches such as the recent decision to maximize independence by encouraging mothers of dependent children to work rather than to rely on welfare aid. This might be expected to increase nursing responsibilities with respect to counseling working mothers, assisting in day care centers, and working with mother substitutes. New plans and policies regarding manpower development, support of research, foreign aid, or civil defense are other examples of action that has distinct nursing implications. This requires that nursing provisions be built into legislation or policy statements. It may also require the mobilization of national resources to brief, train, or advise state and local nursing groups, and also the development of criteria, manuals, or supportive educational materials that might be required.

2. To provide consultation, advisement, and training. Federal agencies working through the regional offices of the Department of Health, Education and Welfare and through special institute-like structures, such as the Communicable Disease Center, offer continuing or *ad hoc* consultation and training services to the states and to local health, education, and welfare groups. The nursing advisers of the regional

health, education, and welfare offices maintain a continuing relationship with the states in their region.

3. To administer nursing aspects of national programs authorized by legislation. Notable are the programs developed under provision of the National Nurse Training Act and the programs developed under the National Manpower Act.

4. To coordinate and support research pertinent to nursing. This includes provision for "internal" research essential to the agency's work, administering various research grants programs, and providing for scientific review panels for grants falling within the nursing purview and for a continuing surveillance of projects supported.

5. To provide health services to groups to which the federal government has a special commitment. This includes nursing services to the military forces, to veteran and special groups such as Indian or Alaskan populations, and to employees of the government. It also provides for nursing support in surveillance and action in health problems that are of interstate or international scope. Migrant health problems have long been a matter of national concern, and nursing has a strong part to play, in both technical and administrative consultation, in meeting the national obligation to this group.

The organization of nursing effort in national voluntary agencies is not cohesive. Many national voluntary agencies employ nurses, and most have some regular channel for securing nursing advisement as needed. For example, the American Public Health Association and the National League for Nursing maintain a close and continuing interchange, as do the American Medical Association and the American Nurses' Association. Some foundations and national voluntary agencies that have continuing programs involving nursing employ one or more nursing advisers to develop the nursing phases of the program. The National Health Council has provided opportunities for conferences of nurses employed in national health agencies, thereby allowing for the interchange of ideas and information.

NURSING AT THE INTERNATIONAL LEVEL

Programs of intercountry nursing aid have greatly increased throughout the world during the past 30 years, and most have a strong nursing complement. This interest appears to stem in part from the conviction that medical skills cannot be fully implemented unless they are extended by skilled nursing service and, also, in part from the high acceptability and the tangible nature of nursing itself. These efforts may be bilateral (independent arrangements between two countries) or international (developed by an international body such as the World Health Organization or the International Council of Nurses).

The World Health Organization has had a designated nursing unit, as well as nursing advisers, in each of their six regions of the world since the creation of the organization in 1948. During the period from 1958 to 1968 the World Health Organization sponsored more than 160 specific nursing projects and participated in an additional 230 general projects that included nursing. They have provided international workshops, country surveys of nursing needs and resources, and continuing nursing guidance to countries.[16] Efforts are directed toward long-range planning, the establishment of sound country plans for nursing, and supportive legislation. The nature of the nursing aid supplied has ranged from direct nursing services at the staff level in projects to consultation with a country's government. As countries develop their programs, the trend is toward more advisory support and less direct service.

The principal bilateral aid agency in the United States is the Agency for International Development. Although this agency has changed names and organization many times, it has existed in some form since 1942 when bilateral aid started within the Institute for Inter American Affairs. In the 24 years between 1942 and 1966, nursing assistance was provided in 47 countries on 5 continents. Typical programs are strikingly similar to those of the World Health Organization: developing basic nursing education; educating special groups, especially those likely to become leaders; and assisting in the development of nursing legislation and national standards.[17]

The Peace Corps is a government agency designed to afford professional and other citizens of the United States an opportunity to serve as volunteers in a people-to-people assistance program. Nurses serving in the Peace Corps are paid only travel expenses and a living allowance. They serve primarily in direct service capacities in countries whose health services are poorly developed or very much understaffed.

The International Council of Nurses, the League of Red Cross Societies, and various foundations, such as the Rockefeller and the Kellogg foundations, have sponsored international nursing activities. These activities vary as the agency's or foundation's program goals change to adjust to new developments and new problems.

Missionary societies throughout the world contribute much to the development both of community health nursing and of nursing in general. The trend toward consolidation of efforts of missionary operations has allowed for more substantive approaches in many countries.

Whatever the sponsorship, certain threads appear consistently throughout reports of international nursing actions. These may be summarized as follows:

1. The recipient country must have the final decision regarding the action to be taken.

2. Emphasis is upon longterm development of the country's own resources. Thus the stress is on developing leaders and teachers rather than on meeting only immediate needs.

3. Nursing must be related not only to the overall health plans and needs but also to the general development of the country. Nursing efforts must therefore reinforce and support efforts to upgrade the food supply or to promote local (village) development or rural health centers.

4. The nurse from the "provider" country must be prepared to make the adjustment to the cultural change and not expect the recipient country to adapt to her culture patterns. The nurse in international work must be prepared to work with a different language, different methods of

medical treatment, different interprofessional relationships, and different social customs.

5. Programs must be flexible to adapt to rapid change in the situation, since many countries are telescoping 50 years of advancement into 10.

6. Not frequently mentioned, but of primary importance, is the fact that the efforts of all "provider" countries for a particular country should be coordinated to unify and maximize their contribution. Relatively brief observation would suggest that this is currently one of the weakest links in the provision of intercountry assistance.

CRITERIA FOR THE ORGANIZATION OF NURSING IN THE HEALTH-CARE STRUCTURE

Nursing is woven into the whole fabric of the community health structure. The organizational accommodations that are made to facilitate and enhance the community health nurse's contribution will not in themselves guarantee good working relationships or efficient operation. However, understanding how nursing fits into the total structure will enable the nurse to make judgments that are based on consideration of the total health effort. Furthermore, good organization of nursing within the care group, the agency, and the community provides the basis for coordinated planning, economical use of available staff, and mutual reinforcement of efforts of the many units contributing to the total health effort.

Some criteria might be suggested as a basis for evaluating the way in which nursing fits into the larger health-care structure. Desirable organization for community nursing in the care group, the agency, and the community should:

1. Provide, within the limits of available resources, comprehensive and continuing nursing care to all who need it through the integration of nursing with all appropriate health and medical-care services.

2. Recognize the fundamental obligation of the government health authority to concern itself with the total health care of the population regardless of the auspices or financing under which the various segments of care are provided.

3. Provide for a planned combined approach of all involved in care to assure the provision of basic health services, to avoid unnecessary duplication or confusion in the services provided, to hold ineffective time to a minimum, to encourage experimentation, and to make full use of voluntary, private, and government resources.

4. Provide a "closeness" in services to people, allowing for ready access, easy communication, and prompt responsiveness to the needs of the consumer.

5. Recognize not only the responsibility and the right of the public, including users of community services, to share decisions regarding health planning and action but also the importance of having representation from all segments of the population in decisional bodies.

6. Ensure economical and appropriate utilization of the varying skills of each level and unit of nursing in order to conserve nurse resources.

7. Permit the nurse to work as a close member of functional health teams while at the same time maintaining identification with nursing as a whole in the agency or community.

8. Provide for medical direction in all work involving medical care.

9. Provide for nurse leadership of nursing phases of the work, including nursing direction of nursing practice.

10. Allow sufficient flexibility and adaptability to meet changing conditions or special needs.

Although the community health nurse may not be able to change the organizational structure within which she works, fully understanding this structure may enable her to work to the best advantage with the opportunities and limits it imposes. It may also be possible to develop compensating mechanisms: for example, if the agency does not provide professional nursing direction, a nurse advisory committee or a state nursing consultant or a supervisory nurse from another agency may serve as a substitute.

In addition to adapting to the existing structure, the alert community nurse may find opportunities to influence the structure by trying out new ideas in her own area and by participating in committees of the agency, the professional associations, and other community groups that are in a position to make recommendations or to effect change.

REFERENCES

1. Policy statement: The local health department services and responsibilities. Amer. J. Public Health, 54:131, January, 1964.
2. APHA Policy Statement—The State Public Health Agency. Amer. J. Public Health, 55:2011, December, 1965.
3. American Nurses' Association. Certification of Incorporation, 1917.
4. Desirable Organization for Public Health Nursing for Family Service. Public Health Nursing, 38:387, August, 1946.
5. Nurses in Public Health. U.S. Department of Health, Education and Welfare, PHS Publication No. 785, U.S. Government Printing Office, Washington, D.C., 1967, p. 10.
6. Progress Report on Combination Services in Public Health Nursing. National League for Nursing, New York, 1955, p. 1.
7. Ibid., p. 33.
8. Conditions for Participation for Home Health Agencies. U.S. Department of Health, Education and Welfare, Social Security Administration, U.S. Government Printing Office, Washington, D.C., 1966.
9. Community Nursing Services: Guide for Preparing Accreditation Reports. National League for Nursing, New York, 1968.
10. Public Health Reports. 83:944, November, 1968.
11. See, for example, Lindberg, Helen G., and Carlson, Betty: A public health nurse in the private physician's office. Nurs. Outlook, 16:43, April, 1968.
12. Fry, John, Dillane, J. B., and Connolly, M. M.: The evolution of a health team: a successful general practitioner-health visitor association. Brit. Med. J., 5428:118, January, 1965.
13. Butterworth, J., and McDonagh, V. P.: General practitioner and health visitor. Lancet, 1:549, March, 1964.
14. Marsh, G. N.: Group practice nurse. Brit. Med. J., 1:489, February, 1967.
15. Philp, J. R.: Dimensions of health care in the changing scene. In Comprehensive Health Care for Children and Families: Report of a Conference. University of Michigan School of Public Health, Ann Arbor, 1967, p. 13.

16. The Second Ten Years of World Health Organization. WHO Chronicle, *22:*267, July, 1968.
17. Taking a Look at Cooperation—An Assessment of 24 Years of AID Technical Assistance in Nursing. U.S. Department of State, Agency for International Development, Department of State, Washington, D.C., 1966.

SUGGESTED READINGS

Anderson, Gaylord: Men, methods and materials in public health. Amer. J. Public Health. *56:*19, January, 1966.

Arafeh, M. K., Fumiatti, E. H., Gregory, M. E., Reilly, M., and Wolff, I. S.: Linking hospital and community care for psychiatric patients. Amer. J. Nurs., *68:*1050, May, 1968.

As They See It—The Role of Health and Welfare Councils in Comprehensive Community Neighborhood Planning. U.S. Department of Health, Education and Welfare, Division of Community Health Services, P.H.S. Publication No. 1488, U.S. Government Printing Office, Washington, D.C., 1966.

Blum, H. K., and Leonard, A. R.: Public Health Administration—A Public Health Viewpoint. The Macmillan Company, New York, 1963, Chapter 4.

Cohen, Hedwig: Accreditation of community nursing services. Amer. J. Public Health, *57:*2138, December, 1967.

Community Nursing Services: Guide for Preparing Accreditation Reports. National League for Nursing, New York, 1968.

Conditions for Participation for Home Health Agencies. U.S. Department of Health, Education and Welfare, Social Security Administration, U.S. Government Printing Office, Washington, D.C., 1966.

Creelman, Lyle: Quality care in the right quantity. Int. Nurs. Rev., *15:*102, April, 1968.

Govan, Elizabeth S. L.: Voluntary Health Organization in America. Royal Commission of Health Services, Queen's Printer, Ottawa, Canada, 1966.

Griffith, E. I.: What is the future role of the V.N.A.? Nurs. Outlook, *16:*29, November, 1968.

Hanlon, John J.: Principles of Public Health Administration. 5th ed., St. Louis, The C. V. Mosby Company, St. Louis, 1969, Chapters 11 and 12.

Hastings, J. E. F., and Mosley, W.: Organized Community Health Services. Royal Commission on Health Services, Queen's Printer, Ottawa, Canada, 1966.

Health in America. The Role of the Federal Government in Bringing High Quality Health Care to All the American People. A Report to the President by the Secretary of Health, Education and Welfare, Washington, D.C., 1968.

Health is a Community Affair. National Commission on Community Health Services, Harvard University Press, Cambridge, Mass., 1967, Chapters 8 and 9.

Kelly, Eunice: A combination nursing service in DuPage County. Nurs. Outlook, *8:*206, April, 1960.

Kennedy, Joanna: Community nursing revived. Nurs. Outlook, *13:*52, July, 1965.

Levine, Sol, White, Paul E., Paul, Benjamin: Community interorganizational problems in providing medical care and social services. Amer. J. Public Health, *53:*1183, August, 1963.

Lindberg, Helen G., and Carlson, Betty: A public health nurse in the private physician's office. Nurs. Outlook, *16:*43, April, 1968.

Miner, E. L.: Public health nursing and a provincial medical insurance plan. Canad. J. Public Health, *57:*527, November, 1966.

Mitch, A. D., and Kaczala, Sophie: The public health nurse coordinator in a general hospital. Nurs. Outlook, *16:*34, February, 1968.

Muller, John N., and Bierman, P.: Cooperation between departments of health and welfare. Public Health Rep., *71:*833, September, 1956.

Mustard, S., and Stebbins, E. L. (eds.): Introduction to Public Health. 4th ed., The Macmillan Company, New York, 1968, Chapter 2.

National Voluntary Health Agencies: Profiles of 19 Member Agencies of the National Health Council. National Health Council, New York, 1969.

Nursing concerns in home health services in health insurance for the aged. Amer. J. Nurs., *65:*72, November, 1965.

Policy Statement: The Local Health Department—Services and Responsibilities. Amer. J. Public Health, *54:*131, January, 1964.

Policy Statement: The State Public Health Agency. Amer. J. Public Health, *55:*2011, December, 1965.

Porterfield, John (ed.): Community Health Services. Basic Books, Inc., Publishers, New York, 1966, Chapter 1.

Ryan, Philip: Role of voluntary agencies in planning to meet the health needs of older persons. Amer. J. Public Health, *51:*878, June, 1961.

Sanders, Irwin T.: Public health in the community. *In* Freeman, Howard, Levine, Sol, and Reeder, Leo G.: Handbook of Medical Sociology. Prentice-Hall, Inc., Englewood Cliffs, 1963, p. 369.

The second ten years of world health organization. W.H.O. Chronicle, *22:*276, July, 1968.

Standards for Organized Nursing Services. Amer. J. Nurs., *65:*76, March, 1965.

Strickler, M., Bassin, E. G., Malbin, V., and Jacobson, G. F.: The community based walk-in center: a new resource for groups underrepresented in outpatient treatment centers. Amer. J. Public Health, *55:*377, March, 1955.

Suchman, Edward A.: Sociology and the Field of Public Health. New York, Russell Sage Foundation, New York, 1963, Chapter 3.

Taking a Look at Cooperation—An Assessment of 24 Years of AID Technical Assistance in Nursing. U.S. Department of State, Agency for International Development, Washington, D.C., 1966.

CHAPTER

7

The Family as the Unit of Service

As early as 1932, an official publication of the then National Organization for Public Health Nursing stated: "*The cardinal principle* of public health nursing which must permeate all considerations of visit content is that *family* health work is the basis upon which all factors rest."[1] The concept of the family as the unit of service was accepted well before the publication of that document and has been reiterated frequently since that time. Yet despite such widespread acceptance, there are many indications that this approach is not always used; practice does not always follow precept. Indeed, the recent proliferation of special program projects that serve only individuals in specific age groups or with particular health problems might make implementation of this approach even more difficult. Thus one must examine whether the concept of the family as a unit of service is as valid today as it has been in the past.

THE FAMILY IS STILL A NATURAL UNIT OF SERVICE

There are several arguments for considering the family as the unit of service in community health nursing:

1. *The family is considered the "natural and fundamental" unit of society.*[2] Farber describes the family as ". . . a collective enterprise based on relationships defined by birth and marriage . . . a kinship organization mobilized to endure."[3] The long duration of the family experience, which exists in some form throughout the world and includes virtually every individual, the intimacy of the contacts, and the social and legal obligations imposed by family membership make the family an institution that involves the majority of the population. For this reason the preservation and improvement of family functioning is frequently a major concern in public policy.

The level of general family functioning—the degree to which the family can move as a unit to deal with its problems and can maximize the fruition of the potential of each of its members—will profoundly influence capability in health matters. The quality of family functioning is therefore a central concern of the community health nurse.

2. *The family as a group generates, prevents, tolerates, or corrects health problems within its membership.* Health problems may be caused by family behavior or by family relationships. For example, disease or defect may be transmitted from parent to child, or emotional imbalance in a family may be conducive to emotional illness in one or more of its members. On the other hand, the skill and confidence of a family operating in unison may not only facilitate the long tedious treatment associated with a crippling condition but also lend emotional strength to the afflicted member and contribute to the social and emotional development of others in the group. It is usually the family, rather than the individual alone, that exerts the energy necessary to achieve health goals.

3. *The health problems of families are interlocking.* The health of any one member of the family is highly likely to affect the health of others. The mentally retarded child may affect the health of his siblings because he requires an inordinate amount of parental time and energy, or the terminal illness of a parent cared for at home may impair the health of the daughter who is home nurse as well as wife and mother. Emotional problems in particular appear to be reinforced by family interaction. Such a situation is illustrated by the familiar picture of the critical parent, a self-critical spouse, and a resistive impulsive child.[4] Whatever happens to one member of the family has some effect upon the family system as a whole and occasions a whole series of accommodations on the part of the other family members.

4. *The family provides a crucial environmental force.* Each individual member constantly interacts with the physical, social, and interpersonal milieu created by his family. The individual responds in his own way to slovenly housekeeping or to compulsive conformity to rigid norms, to positive family attitudes of social responsibility or to a sense of social alienation. Each individual in turn affects the family environment by his own presence. That is, each person serves either to reinforce or to contest the values or attitudes held by the others, to preserve or to modify the existing physical environment, and to strengthen or to weaken the cohesiveness of the family as an operating unit. This continual interaction, which for the most part is within a closed system, influences and molds the individual in myriad ways.

5. *The family is the most frequent locus of health decision and action in personal care.* In the long run it is most often the family unit, not the individual or the health professional, that decides whether or not to seek or to use health care. Children, of course, must rely on parental action for their health needs. Additionally, however, the husband's influence may have much to do with his wife's decision to seek care early in pregnancy or to see that the children receive proper immunization. The grandmother may influence child rearing practices and may either encourage specific home remedies as a substitute for medical attention or,

alternatively, encourage prompt use of medical services. It is often necessary for the nurse to mobilize the family to provide financial assistance in critical situations or to help evaluate the need for going to a doctor or a clinic.

The family is by far the most frequent provider of health care. Care for minor ills, longterm illnesses, or disability, and prehospital and posthospital care for acute illness are generally provided at home by family members. In many instances no care other than family care is required or sought. Alpert, for example, requested that 78 low-income families (selected at random from a case pool of 500 families) record on a calendar the day-by-day health of their members; they were to include notes of *any* indisposition and how it was remedied. They discovered that the low-income families in their study sought professional medical help in only 4.7 percent of the episodes of illness; the remaining 95.3 percent of illnesses — most often described as respiratory or gastro-intestinal ailments, fever, headache, or accidental injury — were presumably treated by the families themselves. Hence the ability of the family to provide nursing care for its members is an important factor in health care.[5]

6. *The family is an effective and available channel for much of the community health nursing effort.* The community health nurse has the opportunity to develop sustained and close relationships with the families she serves. This relationship in turn enables her to "get through" quickly when service is being provided, to establish communication conducive to appropriate self-reporting on the part of the family, and to support and encourage family, as well as individual, development and growth. Furthermore, the number of individuals who are reached by care is greater when the family is the unit of service. The family itself becomes the means of extending a nurse's influence to those members she cannot personally see. Through use of the family approach, she is able to fulfill her obligation to reach the total community.

Of course, there are instances when the individual, rather than the family, can and perhaps should be the unit of service. The increasing complexity of care may require the use of clinical specialists in nursing. When care is of a highly specialized and technical nature, it may not be possible to use a general nursing staff. The specialist's training, on the other hand, is not geared to the broad spectrum of problems found in most families. The specialist can and should work within the context of the family; that is, she can take into account family concerns that affect the care of her patient and try to modify them when they are inimical to the patient's care. Whereas the community health nurse may consider the *family* as her patient, the clinical specialist may consider the *individual* as her patient with the family constituting only an influence on her patient's care.

Also the expanding use of the crash program directed at limited phases of health care creates an increasing number of administrative structures and agency purposes that are focused on the individual, not the family. To be consistent, the community health nurse in this setting must likewise focus primarily on the individual. There is no doubt that this method of delivering health care sets some constraints on the relationship between nurse and family; but on the other hand, the selectivity of concerns may possibly lead to a greater depth in the nurse-patient relationship.

The potential present advantage of using the family as the unit of service for community health nursing seems clear. However, there will be some situations in which the family approach is not possible. Hopefully, when the family is not in fact the unit of service, the nursing care will nevertheless be guided by a general concern for the family as a whole.

THE FAMILY AS THE PATIENT

The Family Is a Product of Time and Place

Although some sort of family is virtually a universal phenomenon, the ways in which the family is organized and the societal tasks which are assigned to it will vary with time and place. Thus the family in a highly industrialized country, in a middle class neighborhood, and in this highly technical era is likely to be structured in a rather loose way. The roles of children, mother, and father are not likely to be clearly defined or rigidly fixed. Increasing technology and urbanization may encourage both father and mother to be wage earners, and consequent adjustments in familial roles will have to be made. Out-of-home concerns and activities may assume greater importance for all members of the family, and the strength of family influence on the individual may be diluted. The economic function of the family may be subordinated to its social function. Conversely, in the agricultural village of a developing country, the family may be organized as an extended group with clearly defined roles for each member and with strong emphasis on the family as a producing economic unit.

Family size is apt to reflect social conditions; the size of the average family rises in good times and falls in poor times. An exception to that simple rule is the increasingly common case of the family which responds to rising aspirations in good times by curtailing its size. For example, in the United States in 1910, a period of rapid expansion, the birth rate was high. It dropped abruptly in the 1930's during a period of economic depression and rose sharply after World War II in a "catching up" period, as shown in Table 2. Since 1960 the rate has been falling again. Some attribute this latter trend to rising expectations accompanied by family planning; others ascribe it to the greater availability of birth control measures; still others believe it is sheer fashion. The fact that the number of women of childbearing age (15 to 44) was slightly smaller (21 percent of the population in 1957 and about 20 percent in 1967) apparently does not account for the decrease, since the fertility rate (the number of live births per 1000 women aged 15 to 44) has also dropped from 118 in 1960 to 96.7 in 1965. The trend lends credence to the idea that the causes are, after all, socially determined.[6]

Subcultures, too, influence the nature of the family. Bronfenbrenner points out that parental role differentiation tends to decrease as one goes

Table 2.   Live Births and Birth Rates per 1000: 1910 to 1966

Year	Total live births	Births per 1000 population	White	Nonwhite
1910	2,777,000	30.1	–	–
1920	2,950,000	27.7	26.9	35.0
1930	2,618,000	21.3	20.6	27.5
1935	2,377,000	18.7	17.9	25.8
1940	2,559,000	19.4	18.6	26.7
1942	2,989,000	22.2	21.5	27.7
1945	2,858,000	20.4	19.7	26.5
1947	3,817,000	26.6	26.1	31.2
1950	3,632,000	24.1	23.0	33.3
1955	4,104,000	25.0	23.8	34.7
1960	4,258,000	23.7	22.7	32.1
1961	4,268,000	23.3	22.2	31.6
1962	4,167,000	22.4	21.4	30.5
1963	4,098,000	21.7	20.7	29.7
1964	4,027,000	21.0	20.0	29.2
1965[1]	3,767,000	19.4	–	–
1966[2]	–	18.5	–	–
1967(est.)[3]	3,600,000	17.9	–	–

[1]*Health, Education and Welfare Trends.* U.S. Department of Health, Education and Welfare, U.S. Government Printing Office, Washington, D.C., 1965, p. S–6.

[2]*200 Million Americans.* U.S. Department of Commerce, Bureau of the Census, U.S. Government Printing Office, Washington, D.C., November, 1967.

[3]*The Facts of Life and Death.* U.S. Department of Health, Education and Welfare, P.H.S. Publication No. 600, U.S. Government Printing Office, Washington, D.C., 1967, p. 6.

up the socioeconomic scale.[7] He also notes that the greater permissiveness, the freer expression of affection, and the indirect discipline that characterize the wider culture are bringing the child rearing practice of the various socioeconomic groups closer together.

The Family Develops Its Own Life Style

Within the constraints of its societal roles, each family develops its own set of values, its own patterns of behavior, and its own style of life. In some families there is little or no communication between husband and wife and between parents and children. Each lives locked in a private world of thought and feeling, even though the physical aspects of group life go on. In other families there may be much communication and interchange, perhaps at an acting out level where shouts, tears, and recriminations are balanced by tenderness, laughter, and sharing. In still other families, undemonstrative outward behavior may conceal a depth of understanding and affection not quickly apparent to the observer.

Families also develop their own power systems, which may either be balanced, in that father, mother, and children have their own areas of decision and control, or be strongly biased so that one of the members gains dominance over the others.

In some instances, power distribution is related to role: the mother may make all decisions relative to management of the home and care of the children, while the father makes decisions regarding the economic aspects of family life. Power struggles within the family are not uncommon, and the effect of such a contest may reach every family member.

Time orientation may also vary. For some the focus is on the present, and problems that may arise in the future have little meaning. If the family has been living precariously, the future may have little significance in comparison to the immediacy of securing food or paying the rent.

THE FAMILY OPERATES AS A GROUP

In the business of daily living, the family develops its own ways of operating. In dealing with common problems, one family may have developed a pattern of facing the problem as a group, deciding together what they will do. For example, if Father has a job opportunity in another town, the whole family may talk about the pros and cons of the move, each helping to arrive at a decision. Or the pattern may be that one person decides: Father, if the problem involves work or discipline; Mother, if the matter is in the realm of health care or home management; or the children, if the problem falls within the stated limits of their own activities. Also, it is possible that one person in the family may make all decisions.

Families must find ways to manage children, money, time, housework, and all the myriad things that are required in today's world. Some may have a habit of coping, dealing as a matter of course with problems as they arise. The poor mountain family may manage to survive despite a year of poor crops and little outside work, to find a way to get to the health center when no ready transportation is available, or to improvise a bed for a sick child who ordinarily shares a bed with other children. Other families give up when trouble strikes and wait helplessly for something to happen or for someone to come and help.

THE FAMILY ACCOMMODATES TO THE NEEDS OF THE INDIVIDUAL

Within the family, each individual is functioning not only as a member of the group but also as a unique human being with his own destiny to fulfill. By some means each member must assert himself in a way that allows him to grow and to develop. Sometimes individual needs and group needs seem to find a natural balance; and self-expression is balanced by consideration for others, power is equitably distributed, and independence is permitted to flourish.

At other times individual and family needs may not be easily reconciled, and conflict or withdrawal may result. The adolescent's need for self-determination may run counter to his parent's need for social acceptance, and the result may be a continuing battle.

THE FAMILY RELATES TO THE COMMUNITY

The family develops a characteristic stance with respect to the community. For some this relationship is wholesome and reciprocal: the family utilizes the community institutions and contributes whatever it can to community betterment. Sometimes there is a firmly rooted sense of family responsibility to the community, which often stems from a family tradition of "charitable" endeavor.

Other families feel a sense of isolation from the community. They maintain a proud "we keep to ourselves" attitude. Too, the reaction may be an entirely passive one of adapting to the community and taking the benefits that are offered without either contributing to, or demanding change from, the community.

The Family Growth Cycle

Families, like individuals, have their own growth cycles. Young marrieds build a home and (hopefully) an enduring relationship that is capable of withstanding the daily demands for tolerance, maturity, understanding, and love. As the family grows and children are born, new parental tasks arise. Among them are the acceptance of the sovereignty of their offspring and the provision of guidance that will enable their children to live independently. Next, a couple readjusts to the empty nest—the difficult period after the children have grown and moved away. They face retirement and possible resettling and try to cope with the special problems and increasing dependence of age. When the family does not mature—when the mother stays the spoiled young fiancée or when the parents cling too long or too tightly to the growing children—the developmental lag may have profound influences on health.

In sum, the family is the unit to which community health nursing is most often addressed. It is a functioning group that is composed of individuals held together by bonds of kinship; a unit in which the action of any member may set off a whole series of reactions within the group; an entity whose strength may be the greatest single supportive factor when one of its members is stricken with illness or death.

HEALTH TASKS OF THE FAMILY

The health tasks of the family are the nurse's primary concern. These health tasks include:

1. Recognizing interruptions of health development such as illness or a child's failure to thrive. The family monitors the concepts of illness and health. For example, backache may constitute an illness in one family but be an expected normal occurrence in another. To the degree that this monitoring is based on reliable information and on optimistic, but reasonable, expectations regarding health, it will serve to facilitate healthful development.

2. Making decisions about seeking health care. The family must decide whether to see a physician, to ask a druggist's advice, to institute home remedies, or to "just wait and see" each time a family member is indisposed. Usually the family is the first to recognize any deviation from normal health, and when necessary, it must take the first step toward getting into the health-care system.

3. Dealing effectively with health and nonhealth crises. Crises are inevitable in any family. Severe or incapacitating illness, death, childbearing, and hospitalization affect all families at some time. Nonhealth crises, such as unexpected unemployment, military service, or moving into an unfamiliar community, also have an effect on health, since if poorly met, these occurrences place great emotional strain on the family as a group as well as on the individual family members.

4. Providing nursing care to sick, disabled, or dependent members of the family. Only a small fraction of illnesses are cared for in hospitals or other institutions. Care of minor ills, personal care of the very young or the very old, care of the sick before and after hospitalization, or care of ambulatory patients who require special treatments that can be provided at home all represent health-care demands commonly placed upon the family. Home care may range in complexity from providing dialysis to caring for a child with a head cold.

5. Maintaining a home environment conducive to health maintenance and personal development. The home should represent a safe place in the physical sense: an environment in which elderly members are protected from the likelihood of falls by stair railings and in which young children are not exposed to rat bites or tempted by accessible switches on the gas stove. It should also provide an emotional and social environment conducive to development: an atmosphere of confidence and mutual concern, a modicum of beauty, a place to play, and toys to play with.

6. Maintaining a reciprocal relationship with the community and its health institutions. Health care of the family requires the intervention of a variety of community-based individuals and groups ranging in kind from the neighbor who baby-sits to the sophisticated teaching hospital.

In relating to the community and its institutions, the family (and the institutions as well!) must arrive at some realistic base of expectations. They must learn to appreciate their rights as individuals and at the same time to appreciate the limits inherent in the community or institutional situation. The family has a right, for example, to expect that those who provide care be qualified and that health services be run efficiently. On the other hand, the family should expect to take the responsibility for getting children to school on time, for putting their garbage in a covered can, for getting children immunized at the proper time, for keeping clinic appointments as scheduled (or letting the clinic know they can't come), and for understanding the limits of resources that may be understaffed and overloaded.

Increasing reference is made to the importance of community involvement as one step toward social health. Opportunities for everyone to help make decisions about community programs—to give to, as well as take from—are not always made available to all segments of the population.

These family health tasks are obviously of great importance, and the community health nurse must be deeply concerned with increasing the capability of each family to deal with them. It is not enough to improve the family's ability to care for an elderly incapacitated patient at home while ignoring the need for changing a home environment that is not conducive to the physical or emotional health of its other members. Nor does it seem consistent to work for the community goal of increasing family capability in dealing with its health tasks by dealing only with that often chance-selected proportion of families that receives nursing care. This problem is of sufficient importance to justify special multi-agency planning and action that is calculated to reach a substantial portion of the families in the community.

THE COMMUNITY HEALTH NURSE'S ROLE

Promote Family Development

The community health nurse's responsibility is not limited to using the family as a resource for health care; it also includes the provision of general support for family development. As she builds nursing care on the family's own abilities and supplements their action when the problem is too much for them to manage alone, the nurse is constantly aware of the opportunity for strengthening the family, better equipping it to deal with future problems of health care and family management.

Thus, when teaching the expectant mother to select foods that offer adequate protective elements for herself and the coming baby, there is an opportunity to examine the dietary regimen of the whole family, to discuss family mealtime as a vehicle for social as well as physical nourishment, and to consider the managerial elements of shopping, food storage, and preparation.

By building special information into the structure of family functioning, it is possible to contribute to general family development via the provision of immediate health care. Also, careful teaching may contribute substantially to the family's "can do" orientation in health matters; and the nurse's "reaching out" and supplying prompt and responsive tangible help or careful referral procedures can strengthen the family's confidence in, and its ability to use, community institutions.

In planning her service to families, the community nurse must work within the framework of the whole structure of family health tasks. She must also understand that the resolution of many health problems will depend upon a family's skills in areas other than health. The family that utilizes health-care services too late and too infrequently may be reflecting a general failure to relate to the community. Through her efforts to solve a particular health problem, the community health nurse can help ameliorate other negative factors.

Maintain Objective Judgment

A family approach doesn't just come naturally. The shift from the concept of care for the individual in the context of the family to the concept of family as patient is not an easy one. Much of the clinical education of health professionals is carried out in large medical centers that are primarily concerned with serious and acute illness or disability and in which the individual is the natural service unit. Thus the habit of the individual approach is apt to be well established.

Furthermore, the community health nurse is more likely to have come from a middle class background and have family values and ways of dealing with family problems which inevitably differ from those of the families for whom she cares. She may ascribe to others those values which she herself holds. For example, in a prosperous population, she may not realize the social pressures placed upon the wife of the executive and may feel that too much of the mother's child rearing responsibility is being assigned to employees.

At times the nurse may not be able to separate herself from her own family experiences. If she herself has been caring for a disabled mother while also working full time, she may project her own resentments or frustrations into the observations she makes in the course of her work. She may have stereotyped ideas of what makes a "good" mother or a "cooperative" family.

Also, in many cases the nurse is younger and less experienced in many family tasks than is the group she serves. If the nurse has just transferred from student to worker status, she may feel inadequate to the demands made upon her for understanding or for decision making.[8] A sense of inadequacy may also arise from the feeling that she herself could not muster as much strength and wisdom as the family has done. She may feel overwhelmed by their problem, lack confidence in her capacity to help, or have a sense of hopelessness that interferes with her judgment.

Furthermore, she may seldom see tangible results of her labors. In the hospital, the patient looks more comfortable, his treatment is producing the desired result, and there is a feeling that all that has been prescribed has been dispatched with efficiency. Helping a family in the home, however, is often a much less tangible task. How can one help reduce the anxiety of a mother whose husband is out of work and who has never before experienced the "indignity" of making a welfare application? How can one help the overworked young mother who also has the responsibility for caring for a senile parent that wanders away and needs constant surveillance? When "help" of any tangible kind is not possible, the nurse's role may prove frustrating; she may feel "I can't do anything for this family!"

With greater experience and knowing supervision, these problems usually become manageable. But there may be times when the nurse's doubts about her ability to help make it difficult for her to work productively with the family as a unit.

REFERENCES

1. Principles and Practice in Public Health Nursing. National Organization of Public Health Nursing, the Macmillan Company, New York, 1932, p. 57.
2. United Nations. Universal Declaration on Human Rights.
3. Farber, B. et al.: Kinship and Family Organization. Wylie and Sons, New York, 1966, p. 8.

4. Interlocking problems of child and parents. Feelings, Ross Laboratories, Columbus, Ohio, vol. 10, no. 2, March-April, 1968.
5. Alpert, Joel J., Kosa, John, and Haggerty, Robert: A month of illness and health care among low income families. Public Health Rep., *82:*705, 705, 3, August, 1967.
6. Trends. U.S. Department of Health, Education and Welfare, U.S. Government Printing Office, Washington, D.C., 1965, pp. 5-6.
7. Bronfenbrenner, Urie: The changing American child — a speculative analysis. Journal of Social Issues, *17:*6, 1961.
8. Corwin, R.G.: The professional employee: a study of conflict in nursing roles. *In* Skipper, J. K. and Leonard, R. C. (eds.): Interaction and Patient Care. J. B. Lippincott Co., Philadelphia, 1965, p. 341.

SUGGESTED READINGS

Collins, Rosella D.: Problem solving: a tool for patients too. Amer. J. Nurs. *68:*1483. July, 1968.
Cotten, Dorothy W.: The Case for the Working Mother. Stein and Day Publishers, New York, 1965.
Duvall, Evelyn W.: Family Development. J. B. Lippincott Co., Philadelphia, 1966.
Geissmar, Ludwig and LaSorte, Michael: The Multiproblem Family. Association Press, New York, 1964.
Gunn, Alexander: The life of preschool children when mother works. Nurs. Times, *64:*631, May, 1968.
Hill, Reuben: The American family today. *In* Katz, Alfred and Felton, Jean S. (eds.): Health and the Community. The Free Press, New York, 1965, Part II: Chapter 1.
Jackson, Joan K.: The role of the patient's family in illness. Nurs. Forum, *1:*118, Summer, 1962.
Komorosky, Mirra: Blue Collar Marriage. Vintage Books, New York, 1962.
McKinley, Donald G.: Social Class and Family Life. The Free Press, New York, 1964.
Missildine, W. H.: Feelings. Ross Laboratories, Columbus, Ohio, vol. 8, no. 9, October 1966.
Parsons, Talbott: The stability of the American family system. *In* Bell, Norman and Vogel, Ezra (eds.): Modern Introduction to the Family. The Free Press, New York, 1960, Chapter 7.
Pittman, Rosemary: The man in the family. Nurs. Outlook, *16:*62, April, 1968.
Russman, Leonard: Levels of aspiration and social class. Amer. Sociol. Rev. *18:*233, 1953.
Shostak, Arthur and Gomberg, W.: Blue Collar World: Studies of the American Worker. Prentice-Hall, Inc., New Jersey, 1964.
Spence, Sir James *et al.*: A Thousand Families in New Castle on Tyne. Oxford University Press, Inc., New York, 1954.
Willie, Charles V.: The structure and composition of "problem" and "stable" families in a low income population. Marriage and Family Living, *25:*440, November, 1963.

The Longterm
Patient at Home

Chronic Illness

Longterm illness is a major public health problem in virtually every industrialized country of the world. Chronic diseases are a major cause of death. Deaths from cardiovascular disease in the United States rose from a rate of 494.4 deaths for each 100,000 of the population in 1950 to 509.8 deaths in 1964; and during that same 14-year period, deaths due to malignant neoplasms rose from 139.8 deaths per 100,000 people to 151.6.[1]

Perhaps even more important, though, is the fact that longterm illness is a primary cause of disability. In the period from July 1964 to June 1965, it was estimated that 87.3 million people—about 46 percent of the population—had one or more chronic diseases; in one of every four instances, these diseases limited activities to some degree.[2] Although longterm illness is more prevalent in older age groups, there is a substantial problem with younger groups as well. In a recent study of chronically ill patients who were receiving public health nursing care in 18 counties of New York State, almost a fourth were under 15 years of age.[3]

Even though heart disease, malignant neoplasms, stroke, and diabetes represent the most frequent chronic conditions, the prevalence figures for many other chronic disease entities are equally impressive. It is estimated that at least two million Americans suffer from chronic obstructive respiratory conditions such as emphysema, chronic bronchitis, asthma, bronchiectasis, and certain forms of chronic pneumonia; that 2 percent of those 40 years old or older have chronic glaucoma, and that 3 percent of the population is mentally retarded.[4] Despite dramatic reductions in incidence, tuberculosis continues to be a problem. There were 47,767 new cases reported in the United States in 1966[5]—a rate of 24.4 per 100,000 of the population.

Chronic Disease Includes Developmental, Functional, and Disease Entities

The problems of chronic disease range from mental retardation to the disabling traumatic effects of accident; from heart disease, cancer, and stroke to loss of hearing or sight; and from tuberculosis to psychiatric illness. These disorders are bound together by chronicity and by similarities in the social and medical problems they present. Kurlander offers a useful operational definition. He defines chronic disease as meeting one or more of the following criteria:

1. It is permanent.
2. It leaves a residual disability.
3. It is caused by nonreversible pathologic conditions.
4. It requires special rehabilitative training of the patient.
5. It requires long supervision of care.[6]

Public Concern for the Chronically Ill

In addition to the 1965 amendments to the Social Security Act, which produced Medicare and Medicaid, there has been much other federal legislation that bears directly on the care of the chronically ill.

The Mental Health Act of 1946 (since amended several times) has provided grants-in-aid programs for the development of services in the various states. The 1956 amendment provided for grants for investigations, experimental studies, and research projects.

The Community Mental Health Act of 1963 allotted 150 million dollars to states for the construction of community mental health centers.

The 1965 amendments to the Public Health Service Act contained provisions for greatly extending the facilities for the care and study of heart disease, cancer, and stroke.[7] This action was the outgrowth of the President's Commission on Heart Disease, Cancer and Stroke, which was composed of physicians, agency representatives, laymen, and scientists. This commission, convened in 1964, recommended a nationwide network of diagnostic, treatment, demonstration, and research centers.[8] The purposes of this legislation are:

1. Through grants, to encourage and assist the establishment of regional cooperative arrangements among medical schools, research institutions, and hospitals for research and training; this includes demonstrations of patient care in heart disease, cancer, stroke, and related diseases.

2. Through such cooperative arrangements, to afford the medical profession and the medical institutions of the nation the opportunity of making available to their patients the latest advances in the diagnosis and treatment of chronic diseases.

3. By these means to improve generally the health, manpower, and facilities available to the nation.

The law specified that the program was to be developed in the context of existing services, making full use not only of government agencies and hospitals but also of private medical facilities and voluntary agencies. Significant is the fact that the commission felt that it would take some time to plan such a program. Thus the first three years were designated as planning years at the end of which grants were to be awarded to implement those study proposals expected to provide the bases for action. The acquisition of new knowledge (through research) was thereby tied to the need for designing methods for utilizing what the researchers learned. Also implicit in the law is the assumption that regional boundaries, rather than political boundaries, will be used in setting up the resulting health programs. For the first three planning years, 348 million dollars were allocated to be disbursed on the basis of plans submitted by appropriate authorities.

The 1965 amendments to the Social Security Act also provided for increased appropriations for crippled children's programs (a large share of these funds were earmarked especially for mentally retarded and multiple-handicapped children), for the training of professional personnel in the care of crippled children (training of the mentally retarded was given priority), and for grants to states to plan assaults on mental retardation.

The Community Health Nurse's Role in Control of Chronic Illness

PRIMARY PREVENTION IS THE DESIDERATUM

Obviously the best way to combat any adverse condition is to prevent it. However, opportunities for primary prevention of chronic conditions are often limited because either the etiology of the disease is obscure or preventive measures have not yet been developed.

The association between smoking and chronic respiratory disease and lung cancer offers an opportunity for primary preventive action by means of educating the public about the hazards of cigarette smoking. Efforts to prevent exposing the expectant mother to infectious disease, radiation, or inadequate obstetric care may help prevent injury to the fetus. Genetic counseling that leads to voluntary restriction of conception may help reduce the transmission of certain genetic faults. However, primary prevention of many diseases such as epilepsy, muscular dystrophy, multiple sclerosis, and some mental retardation must wait for further research.

No matter how inadequate and incomplete the information may be, the community health nurse should be familiar with the associative health factors accepted by the medical profession, even though these factors cannot be considered as causative or solely responsible for the occurrence of a particular condition. In some instances possible causes may be many. For example, epilepsy may be associated with a congenital malformation; with the development of scar tissue following brain injury; or with measles, mumps, or whooping cough. Many preventive measures rely on a sort of shotgun approach: in trying to get at whatever seems to have some association with the development of the disease condition, one encourages general health measures that are, in the meantime, likely to reduce the stress on the functioning organism. The following are examples of measures considered useful:

1. Discouragement of smoking, particularly of cigarette smoking, and of unnecessary exposure to polluted air.

2. Adequate prenatal and delivery care.

3. Avoidance, through immunization, of infectious disease.

4. Genetic counseling for those families in which there is a history of diabetes, mental retardation, or other heritable conditions.

5. Prompt care of predisposing conditions such as obesity, elevated blood pressure, anemia, and stress.

6. Accident control in the home, school, industry, and in the city streets.

SECONDARY PREVENTION OFFERS
MORE OPPORTUNITIES AT PRESENT

Secondary prevention is concerned with the early recognition and treatment of conditions in order to make them less destructive. In this area, medicine can move more surely and effectively. Among nursing measures recommended for secondary prevention are:

1. Encouraging regular comprehensive medical surveillance including emotional and developmental assessment, as well as physical assessment, throughout life and with increased frequency at points of greater vulnerability such as early childhood, adolescence, pregnancy, late middle age, and the period of senility.

2. Employing formal and informal screening measures in the home by the family, in school, in industry, and in the community. Although screening measures do not diagnose illness, they do serve to identify those who need more definitive study. Self-examination of the breast or the evaluation of changes incident to arthritis are screening measures adapted to the family level. General screening, multiphasic screening, or screening for special conditions, such as tuberculosis, cancer, heart disease, or behavioral disorders, may be conducted on a community-wide basis. (The nurse's role in family and community screening is discussed more fully elsewhere.)

3. Participating in specific testing programs to identify asymptomatic disease. School and industry-wide tuberculosis testing frequently involves the community health nurse, as do recent programs to detect cervical cancer in women.

4. Using ongoing services as a means of uncovering conditions requiring further investigation. For instance, in the course of prenatal visits to an expectant mother, the nurse may find a family member who has symptoms suggestive of cancer; or she may discover a child who is developing unusually slowly or who is exhibiting bizarre or unexpected behavior. Sometimes such observations offer a dramatic contribution to health care. Hanchett and Johnson have indicated some of the observational responsibilities implicit in the care of the cardiac patient, and the

descriptions of "little strokes" suggest again the importance of knowing both what to look for and how to report it.[9, 10] Such "case finding" is admittedly opportunistic, but a sensitive eye can uncover many conditions needing further study.

5. Alerting vulnerable groups to the need for early recognition of symptoms of particular chronic conditions. For example, low-income groups and certain older age groups might be considered especially vulnerable to tuberculosis, and educational health channels could be geared to inform them of the need for utilizing available diagnostic facilities and of the importance of observing symptoms of the disease. Reaching such populations may require a variety of channels such as the incidental contacts made during visits, the spread-the-word method of teaching in which individuals are encouraged to be health emissaries, and the utilization of ready-made groups such as parent-teacher groups, farm cooperatives and Four-H clubs. Although every member of the health team will be engaged in these efforts in some way, the nurse's share will be considerable, especially in the less populous areas where such efforts tend to be rather informal.

6. Strengthening ongoing preventive services. Efforts directed toward prenatal care, school examinations, and the prompt use of the family medical adviser for preventive as well as curative care are examples of programs that could be strengthened in order to encourage community participation.

NURSING THE CHRONICALLY ILL IS FAMILY-FOCUSED

The nature and the direction of nursing provided to the family with a chronically ill member will be determined by the impact of the condition on individual function and also by the degree to which the family is able to cope with the problem, given its present resource.

Not All Chronic Illness Is Disabling

Many chronically ill persons are able to carry on their usual activities despite the existence of a chronic condition. They may be able to manage quite well without assistance from community service; or if under community care, they may not require the services of the community nurse. Eighty to eighty-five percent of those afflicted by epilepsy, to take one example, may be expected to lead an essentially normal life; about half of those under care become entirely free from seizures.[11] Most diabetics are also able to carry on their usual activities with little or no assistance.

The great majority of those with chronic illness will be at least ambulatory. Lavendowski, in selected communities, found that of those on the nurse's case load, 62.9 percent were ambulatory, 23 percent were partly ambulatory, and only 14.5 percent were bedridden or confined to a wheel chair.[12] Furthermore, even when care is required, the patient or family may be fully capable of assuming the responsibility.

The Burden Is More Than Physical

In many families the impact of chronic illness may be felt not primarily in physical impairment but rather in the associated familial, psychologic, social, or economic concomitants. Five phases of the chronic illness situation may be identified.

The prediagnosis phase of chronic illness may be fraught with uncertainty and stress. The threat of disablement or disfigurement, a concern about the costs of care, and worry about interruption of work or school may conspire to create tension. If the family has not built strong supportive relationships, the patient (or the parent or other responsible person) may try to "protect" others in the family from knowing the facts, even though he may feel alone and unsupported.

The phase of acceptance of the condition may be stressful. The patient's first reaction may be shock, rage, or despair. "Why me?" is the inevitable and unanswerable question of each. However, sometimes the reaction is one of simple relief at having a hidden worry transformed into a reality that can be confronted. As the illness progresses, acceptance is usually achieved, although with varying degrees and types of accommodation ranging from extended dependency to patient martyrdom.

The phase of action, when treatment and care are initiated, may also create some anxiety in the patient or in the individual administering care. Until the skills of observation and of personal and therapeutic measures are well established, the anxiety may be tempered by action itself; "doing something" lends a sense of some control over the situation.

The phase of the long hard pull is often characterized by periodic discouragement or, in the case of a family nurse, just plain fatigue. The home nurse or the patient may become irritable, impatient, and careless in carrying out care. At this point, support becomes very important.

The phase of separation may be reached either when care becomes too complex for the family to manage and nursing-home or hospital care is required, or when death is imminent. For the family, separation will mean grief and, frequently, some feelings of guilt. For the patient, hospitalization can imply rejection, and as it often is proof of a downhill course, it can precipitate despair. By means of action in the following areas of nursing intervention, the community nurse can support the patient and family throughout the course of chronic disease:

1. Maintenance of function in patient and family.
2. Support of the patient's care regimen.
3. Maximization of the comfort and safety of the patient.
4. Coordination of community and family-care efforts.
5. Reduction of patient and family stress occasioned by illness and by eventual separation.

MAINTENANCE OF FUNCTION IN BOTH PATIENT AND FAMILY

For the care of longterm illness, a well-known slogan applies: "It's not how long you make it; it's how you make it long." The quality of life of the longterm illness patient is very much affected by the degree to which he can do those things he considers important and maintain his independent and contributing role in the family.

Physical Function.   The maintenance of physical function means independence to the patient. Nurses are familiar with the need to maintain adequate range of motion in postsurgical care of the mastectomy patient. The struggle for any patient to control those activities necessary for daily living—to come as close as possible to feeding himself, to wash his face, and to comb his hair—is an important one.

In the out-of-hospital situation, the direct nursing care must be predominantly a family responsibility, and the resultant demand on the family is great. Success may be limited, and the cost in energy and time can be high. It may take long plodding care to enable the stroke patient to talk or to feed himself. Such nursing intervention in the hospital or nursing home is the primary job of the personnel, and the scheduling of the institution is geared to providing this needed care. In the home, family members have other pressing responsibilities, and intensive care of the chronically ill member can be disproportionately demanding of energy and time.

Moreover, professional personnel are available only on an intermittent basis, and they too are occupied with competing demands for nursing time. There may not be special personnel, such as a physical therapist, available to help a family either directly or in a consultant capacity. Thus, the community health nurse must:

1. Determine, through conference with others involved in care, reasonable goals that can be set for the restoration of function for the patient.

2. Increase her own skill by working with agency personnel, such as physical therapists, or by self-initiated training wherein she arranges to participate in rehabilitative care in the hospital or to undertake formal class work.

3. Evaluate and increase the competence of the family or the auxiliary worker to carry out the required care.

4. Supervise and encourage the family and the auxiliary worker as they carry out the required procedures.

Social Function.   Social functioning is as important to the quality of life as is physical functioning. To the patient with limited vision who is accustomed to reading a great deal, it may be very important to find substitutes, such as Braille or listening to recordings, with which he need not rely on someone else.

The ability to contribute—to help with preparation of a meal or to do handwork for others—may also play an important role in the maintenance of social functioning. Too, providing social stimulation can help make the days of the chronically ill more pleasant. The nurse's visit, during which she talks to the patient about events and plans, may assume great importance.

It is imperative to avoid patient immobilization that may contribute to a decline in functioning capacity. In encouraging activity, the nurse must enlist the family. Valuable support may be provided by volunteers; teenagers are especially good at reading to patients, for example. Voluntary agencies may be able to provide direct services to patients through their own volunteers; these agencies may also be a source of consultation, teaching materials, and educational opportunities for the nurse.

Family Function.   In some cases, good patient care may lead to poor family health care. The care of the disabled person must be fitted into the overall family commitment so that the health or development of other family members is not jeopardized.

The community health nurse should be alert and responsive to signs of interference with family functioning. The mother who can't find time to spend with a teenage daughter because of the responsibility of caring for the grandmother, and the woman who neglects to get care for a persistent headache or for unexplained uterine bleeding because she "hasn't time" to think of herself are both courting family disaster. The daughter caring for an aged parent may feel she has become a drudge rather than a person, and her sense of life's passing her by may lead to a more serious human loss than would a little less personal or less detailed care of the older person.

Through better planning and the enlistment of others in care and by supporting the family when they feel guilty about "selfish" actions that are really essential to the maintenance of family functioning, the community health nurse can do much to help families balance their dual responsibility.

SUPPORT OF THE PATIENT'S CARE REGIMEN

An important aspect of nursing the chronically ill is to assess and maintain adherence to the prescribed treatment regimen. Maintaining the prescribed treatment regimen may be a difficult task. In a recent study of 213 patients with diabetes, 76 percent were judged to be in poor control. Estimates reported in recent studies of adherence to a medication regimen for tuberculosis range from 29 percent to 86 percent. Even allowing for differences in the criteria for adherence used by the various investigators, it is likely that there are wide variations in performance.[13, 14]

In longterm care, the need for adherence may make heavy demands on the patient and the family. The drugs prescribed may be numerous and hard to distinguish from one another. In many instances several drugs may have to be tried before finding an effective one. In the interim, the patient may become discouraged at the lack of progress.

Recently there have been attempts to establish or to predict the likelihood of whether or not a particular person will follow prescribed treatment regimens. However, at present there does not appear to be any clear trend in the findings of these reports.[15] The patient's knowledge of the disease and of the treatment does not seem to be consistently related to performance. In fact, Watkins and others reported that in a study of 60 diabetic clinic patients at home, those in poorer control knew more about the disease than the rest of the group.[16.] It seems likely from these and similar studies that conformity to a prescribed regimen will show considerable variation and that a family-by-family assessment of the forces for and against compliance is necessary.

Despite the apparent inability to pin down just which patients are likely to be delinquent or exactly what it takes to prevent delinquency in care, the following approaches seem justified, pending further research:

1. Be sure that the patient and family understand the importance of the treatment. Even if they do not know much about the disease or the

reason for the treatment, the patient should understand that in tuberculosis, for example, taking the pills is the crucial factor in his treatment and that irregularity may render the drug ineffective.

2. Be sure they *know how to do* what is required. Explicit instructor demonstration and "play back" by the patient and family are crucial. Krysan points out that the nurse may find it difficult to understand how complex the treatment may seem to her trainee. The diabetic, for instance, needs to know the principles of asepsis in order to give his own insulin safely and to care for his equipment. To recognize symptoms of hypoglycemia and to carry out the procedure of urine examination, he must understand the difference between the cure and the control of disease and the need for lifetime follow-up. Then too, he must master the measuring of dosage, be able to estimate "fair exchange" in allowable foods, and appreciate the relationship between insulin and low metabolism. All of this information is rather a lot for a nonscientific trainee group!

3. When treatment extends over a long time, provide *frequent reinforcement* and encouragement. Especially in the "long hard pull" phase of the illness there may be a tendency to be less careful in carrying out the regimen, or there may be a temptation to experiment with self-selected tactics, unorthodox methods, or well-advertised over-the-counter drugs. Inasmuch as drugs are administered by the nurse or family in the absence of an on-the-spot medical or nursing supervisor, considerable responsibility is placed upon the community health nurse to familiarize herself with the possible complications and contraindications for any drug prescribed. A conference with the responsible physician or the hospital nurse may provide the necessary information. In some instances a medical committee of the agency or a special nursing consultant may be a good source. However it is accomplished, the nurse must be sufficiently informed to carry out the procedure required and must take whatever time necessary to become fully informed.

MAXIMIZATION OF THE COMFORT AND
SAFETY OF THE PATIENT

Keeping the patient comfortable has a high priority. In many instances, comfort-giving care is the most imperative need of both patient and family. The skill with which the patient is bathed, fed, and gotten into and out of bed has much to do with his ability to tolerate discomforts that cannot be removed. Skin care, positioning, and carefully controlled exercise to avoid fatigue all help prevent more serious discomfort. "Keeping mother comfortable" is reassuring to the family as well as to the patient. To achieve this end, the community health nurse can help by:

1. Providing personal care for a short part of the day or at intervals when the need is great.

2. Teaching and supervising the family, the home health aide, or any other care provider.

3. Referring the family to other care sources such as the Visiting Nurse Association, or Red Cross or adult education classes in home nursing.

4. Assisting the family in finding sources for needed equipment or supplies. A community loan chest may supply a hospital bed; the local chapter of the American Cancer Society may provide dressings.

5. Teaching the family to notice and report immediately any change in the patient's condition. It may be wise to leave a list of things especially important to observe and the number to be called should the necessity to report any change arise.

It is important, also, to protect the chronically ill patient from the possibility of infection. Contact with family or friends who "just have a cold" or with children who have been exposed to an infectious disease should be discouraged. Even a common cold may be serious for the victim of emphysema.

Other safety measures may also be required, such as placing potent drugs out of the patient's reach or keeping a small light burning so the patient will not stumble if he must get up at night. Taking extra care with heating pads, lamps, or other electric equipment may be necessary; special care is required if the patient is disoriented or confused.

COORDINATION OF COMMUNITY AND FAMILY-CARE EFFORTS

Coordination saves time and enhances service. The chronically ill person is probably using multiple sources of care in a constantly changing configuration. He may be now in, now out of the hospital; now under the care of a diagnostic and treatment center; and now under the supervision of the family physician. The physical therapist, occupational therapist, speech therapist, neurologist, cardiologist, and psychiatrist may be constant or intermittent providers of care. Any change in the treatment pattern, then, may involve several people.

Often, but by no means always, the responsibility for coordinating these many facets of care rests with the community health nurse. When this is the case, she must try to achieve the following:

1. A plan for care that is known and accepted by all the practitioners and family members involved. The nurse herself will probably want a written plan for care, but it may not be feasible to formalize the multiprofessional plan in this way, especially when care is given by a family physician rather than through an organized (institutional) care source. However, through conference, exchange of progress notes, or by some other means, the nurse must be sure there is indeed a clear and unified plan of action.

2. The prompt exchange of essential information. Telephone communication, as well as written exchange, may be important.

3. Periodic group review of progress and group decision regarding the continuing or revised care plan.

REDUCTION OF PATIENT AND FAMILY STRESS

Reduction of stress adds to the family's ability to cope with the illness and the eventual separation. There is inevitably some stress associated with chronic disease, especially in those instances in which the condition is catastrophic or highly disabling. Families will vary in the strength they can muster to deal with this stress and in the amount of "outside" support they require. The degree and type of support will also depend upon different points in the disease.

A question frequently raised is "Should the patient be told the truth?" As Brauer points out, this is far from a simple question.[18] The answer must be carefully considered by the physician and the family as well as by the nurse. Indeed, the question must be "Which patient, what truth?"

The apparent stoic who demands "the truth" may actually be hoping for reassurance rather than facts. The family, too, may react to the truth in different ways. If the diagnosis is catastrophic and the outlook dim, they may in some instances act as though the patient were already dead; or they may become so frightened that they are unable to provide the support needed by the patient. Furthermore, so much of chronic disease remains a mystery that "the truth" may turn out to be wrong—for instance, when the patient survives far beyond the time expected.

The *how* as well as the *why* of helping the family at this point assumes critical importance. In general, it seems useful to encourage open expression of feelings about these critical periods in one's life: the patient should know that his rage or depression is acceptable behavior in the nurse's eyes; and the family must know that they can discuss their own disappointments and frustrations freely, without fear of being judged, as they struggle to adapt their life to the new demands and limits imposed by the chronic illness.

The community health nurse may help reduce stress by reassuring the family members that they are able to deal with the situation and that help is available. Her stance of confident matter-of-fact expectation may provide great strength to them, since one of the important approaches to reassurance is the provision of an "anchor": someone to whom the family can turn when they need help. This may be the nurse; or in the case of the diabetic patient whose major problem is dietary, it may be the nutritionist. When a home health aide provides the major part of the care, the professional nurse may take a "backstopping" stance, so that the family will turn first to the home health aide. Properly briefed by the professional nurse, the aide may prove a close and welcome support.

Action may also be suggested as an antidote to stress. Finding out about a prosthesis if breast mastectomy is likely, restructuring the home situation so the disabled stroke patient can do more for herself and for others, and helping with tasks that are within the patient's physical limits are therapeutic actions.

Providing occasional respite from responsibility may reduce stress. Care of the chronically ill person, especially when he is greatly incapacitated, can be a grueling task. It is not surprising that families become tense and upset during the "long hard pull" phase, when the illness seems likely to drag on forever. The Victorian picture of the overworked unappreciated dutiful daughter who gives up all hopes of marriage and career has somewhat faded as community resources have improved, provision for care has increased, and cultural values have changed. However, there are still instances in which the unmarried daughter or the geographically nearest relative assumes a disproportionate burden. Plans for travel, for further education, for home improvements, or for social activities may have to be postponed or relinquished. No matter how willingly the task is undertaken, some resentment or despair is likely to exist.

Less serious, but still troublesome, is the problem of never being able to get away for a vacation or even for a shopping spree. If care is demanding and prolonged, some relief should be found for the responsible care provider and family. Sometimes another relative can take over for a few weeks, a home health aide can be assigned for one or two half days a week, or short-term nursing-home placement can be arranged. The nurse can support the family by assuming a listening role, by encouraging the family to see their problems in realistic terms, by helping them to accept assistance, and by referring them to case work or to other counseling service when necessary.

Not surprisingly, nonmedical problems may be a source of stress. One great concern of families is the fear that they cannot meet the financial obligations imposed by prolonged illness. They may be justifiably worried about medical and hospital bills, about the inability of the patient to continue to contribute to the family income, or about future expenses such as that incurred by the need for nursing-home care. The nurse can help by referring the family to sources of information about insurance benefits or about community facilities for care, including the special provisions under the Social Security Act for illness and for total or partial disability. The nurse should familiarize herself with the general provisions of legislation affecting the chronically ill so that she can judge whether or not the family should investigate these possibilities of further help. Provisions for the care of veterans and for industrial compensation coverage are other examples of possible sources of financial aid. When the nurse's information is inadequate or the financial problems complex, the help of the social welfare staff should be sought.

The Nurse's Role During the Stressful Separation Phase. Frequently families must face the ordeal of separation because of death or because the patient needs hospital or nursing-home care either permanently or for an extended period.

When the separation is due to the need for special care not possible in the home, there may be a strong feeling of guilt on the part of the family, a feeling that somehow they should have managed. The patient may feel rejected and hurt at being "sent away," and he may be fearful of the new experience. He may openly and bitterly blame the family for taking this step and plead for a change in plans. Perhaps even harder for the family is the situation in which the patient—a very retarded child or a disturbed adult—may not understand what is happening.

The nurse can help the family and the patient to verbalize their concerns; she can reassure the family that they have indeed considered all possible alternatives; and she can interpret the contributions and conditions of the facility to which the patient will go.

Henderson has pointed out the responsibility of nurses to help patients achieve a peaceful death, and Quint has looked at the problems the nurse faces in dealing with this terminal phase of care.[19, 20] Because the community health nurse is often not present at the time of death (when the patient is likely to be in the hospital), her opportunity lies in mobilizing the efforts of the family in support of the dying patient and in supporting the family in their "grief work."

The community health nurse can help the family to *appreciate and support the efforts of the hospital or nursing home personnel* to make this an "affirmative" time for the dying patient—as Saunders puts it, "to help the patient *live* until he dies."[21] To the family, the staff may seem callous and unaware of the gravity of the situation. Too, the family may fear the effects of the liberal use of narcotics; they may not understand the basic rationale that dictates maximum control of pain for the patient at this time. They may feel that the staff is "cruel" in answering the dying patient's queries honestly, that this takes away any hope the patient may have for recovery. An opportunity to talk to the personnel responsible for the institutional care can reassure the family and help them to support and feel comfortable about the steps that are taken.

If, as may be the case, the family really does experience insensitive or evasive handling by the staff in a nursing home or hospital, they may be helped by knowing how difficult it is for the staff, as well as for the patient and for the family, to face the fact of death. An interview with the hospital personnel may ameliorate the problem.

The patient's style in facing crises, including this one, may be to put on a good face and appear cheerful and self-contained, reserving for himself the process of confrontation with this problem of dying. Other patients get much relief from talking about death, discussing their feelings and concerns. These latter may especially need reassurance that steps will be taken to control the pain and that they will not be allowed to die unattended.

Often the family is at a loss as to how to behave in the face of death. They may adopt a false cheerfulness, or they may fail to acknowledge the situation and talk constantly about "when you are well," or "after you are home again." This behavior may, in fact, be the worst thing for the patient, who would like to clear up the untidy ends of his life before he dies. The family may let their consternation and fear of death show, thereby deepening the patient's anxiety and heightening his guilt at making the family suffer. The family may also try to circumvent their grief by looking upon the dying patient as though he were already dead—not including him in any of the family deliberations or decisions and assuming that the patient has no interest in the world outside. Conversely, the family and the patient may show unexpected understanding and courage, needing only the reassurance of knowing that the nurse is standing by to help in any way she can.

It is important for the family to realize that when most people find death close, it becomes the more welcome; and the interval just before death may be free from the usual constraints, worries, and complexities of life.

For everyone faced with losing a loved relative, there is a sense of bereavement and loss, however expected and even welcome the death may be. In this process, the individual accepts the idea of loss in advance, grieves for a reasonable period, and then returns to his usual pursuits. The manner and the time of grieving will be a highly individualized thing depending on the closeness of the severed relationship; the usual crisis management patterns of the individual; his degree of self-reliance; and the external demands and forces—such as work or care of children—that may exert a countereffect to the grief.

The community nurse's task is to help the family members understand the validity of their sorrow and to help them with the anticipation of difficult small things that attend this period: for example, deciding in advance who might help in sorting and disposing of the personal effects of the patient, what funeral arrangements will be made, and what relatives should be called.

The rites of passage that attend death may in themselves be beneficial. The business of the funeral, the demands on the bereaved, and the rituals may mitigate the internalization of their grief, thereby making it easier to bear. If, as is sometimes true, these rites seem to be excessive (as when the low-income family arranges for an expensive funeral), they must be understood as an ameliorating gesture that, for the family, has great significance.

The family can be helped to support one another and to use this experience constructively. Parents may share a firm religious conviction in life after death, which makes the loss bearable. An understanding of death is important to children's development, and they should be helped to see it as a natural event. Some children, and in particular adolescents, may find this experience a devastating one without parental help. They may need help in understanding that their own aggressive hold on life is not necessarily shared by those whose life is behind them and who may be ready for death, that there is a time for dying as well as a time for birth and for marrying and for growing up. The adults must try to understand and deal with their children's fears and anxieties, as well as with their own. Sometimes children show their fear and withdrawal by adopting what appears to be a callous attitude toward the event. They may say things that the family feels are cruel or unfeeling. The very young, in their unfamiliarity with the finality of death, may manifest what seems to the parents to be a casual acceptance of their loss. In all of this, the community nurse can be a steady supporter, readily helping the family with practical and simple suggestions and conveying her own understanding of, and sympathy with, their grief.

REFERENCES

1. Health Education and Welfare Trends. U.S. Department of Health, Education and Welfare, U.S. Government Printing Office, Washington, D.C., 1965, p. 9.
2. *Ibid.,* p. 11.
3. Lavendowski, M. C.: Survey of Public Health Nursing Visits to Chronically Ill Patients. Part 2. New York State Department of Health, Albany, 1964, p. 5.
4. Emphysema—the Battle to Breathe. U.S. Department of Health, Education and Welfare, PHS Publication No. 1715, U.S. Government Printing Office, Washington, D.C., 1967.
   Cataract and Glaucoma, U.S. Department of Health, Education and Welfare, PHS Publication No. 793, U.S. Government Printing Office, Washington, D.C., 1963.
   Mental Retardation, U.S. Department of Health, Education and Welfa e, PHS Publication No. 1152, U.S. Government Printing Office, Washington, D.C., 1966.
5. Reported Tuberculosis Data 1966. U.S. Department of Health, Education and Welfare, PHS Publication No. 638, U.S. Government Printing Office, Washington, D.C., 1968, p. 1.
6. Kurlander, Arnold R.: Chronic and degenerative disease: *In* Porterfield, J. H. (ed.): Community Health Services. Basic Books Inc., Publishers, New York, 1966, p. 67.

7. Social Security Amendments of 1965, Public Law 89-97.
   Title IX of the Public Health Service Act, Public Law 89-239.
8. President's Commission on Heart Disease, Cancer, and Stroke. U.S. Department of Health, Education and Welfare, Public Health Service, U.S. Government Printing Office, Washington, D.C., 1965.
9. Hanchett, Effie, and Johnson, Ruth: Early signs of congestive heart failure. Amer. J. Nurs., *68:*1456, July, 1968.
10. Little Strokes: Hope Through Research. U.S. Department of Health, Education and Welfare, PHS Publication No. 689, U.S. Government Printing Office, Washington, D.C., 1962 (rev.).
11. Epilepsy. U.S. Department of Health, Education and Welfare, PHS Publication No. 938, U.S. Government Printing Office, Washington, D.C., 1965.
12. Lavendowski, *op. cit.,* p. 11.
13. Williams, T. F., *et al.* The clinical practice of diabetes control in four settings. Amer. J. Public Health, *59:*441, March, 1967.
14. Kuemmerer, J.: Adherence to Medical Recommendations for Oral Anti-Tuberculosis Drugs. Doctoral thesis, Johns Hopkins School of Hygiene and Public Health, 1968, p. 10.
15. McDonald, M. E., *et al.:* Social factors in relation to participation in followup care of rheumatic fever. Pediat., *62:*503, 1963.
    Curtis, E. E.: Medication errors made by patients. Nurs. Outlook, *9:*290, May, 1961.
    Schwartz, Doris.: Medication errors made by elderly chronically ill patients. Amer. J. Public Health, *57:*452, 1962.
16. Watkins, Julia, *et al.:* Study of diabetic patients at home. Amer. J. Public Health, *57:*452, March, 1967.
17. Krysan, G. S.: How do we teach four million diabetics? Amer. J. Nurs., *65:*105, November, 1965.
18. Brauer, Paul H.: Should the patient be told the truth? *In* Skipper, J. K., and Leonard, Robert C. (eds.): Social Interaction and Patient Care. J. B. Lippincott Co., Philadelphia, 1965, p. 167.
19. Henderson, Virginia: Principles of Nursing. World Health Organization, Geneva, 1960, p. 3.
20. Quint, J. C.: Obstacles in helping the dying. Amer. J. Nurs., *66:*1568, July, 1966.
21. Saunders, Cecily: The last stages of life. Amer. J. Nurs., *65:*70, March, 1965.

SUGGESTED READINGS

Adams, Mary, Downs, Thomas, and Denke, Hazel: Nursing referral outcomes for post hospitalized chronically ill patients. Amer. J. Public Health, *58:*101, January, 1968.
After a Coronary. American Heart Association, New York, 1964.
Arthritis and rheumatic disorders: manual for nurses, physical therapists and medical social workers. Arthritis Foundation, Medical and Scientific Committee, New York, 1966.
Barsch, R. H.: The handicapped rating scale among parents of handicapped children. Amer. J. Public Health, *54:*1560, September, 1964.
Birth Defects: The Tragedy and the Hope. The National Foundation, New York, n.d.
Blum, H. L., and Keranan, G. M.: Control of Chronic Diseases in Man. American Public Health Association, New York, 1966.
Bulkeley, Katherine: Home care for chronically sick patients. *In* Stewart, Dorothy, and Vincent, Pauline (eds.): Public Health Nursing. William C. Brown Company, Publishers, Dubuque, 1967, Chapter 38.
Conley, Veronica, and Olson, Stanley: Regional medical programs. Amer. J. Nurs., *68:*1916, September, 1968.
David, Wilfred: Chronic respiratory diseases: the new look in the public health service. Amer. J. Public Health, *57:*1357, August, 1967.
Davis, Milton, and Eichorn, R. L.: Compliance with medical regimens: a panel study. J. Health Hum. Behav., *4:*240, Winter, 1963.
The Early Detection of Cancer. World Health Organization Chronicle, *20:*323, September, 1966.

Epilepsy: Hope Through Research. U.S. Department of Health, Education and Welfare, U.S. Government Printing Office, Washington, D.C., 1965.

Flexible fashions—clothing tips and ideas for women with arthritis. U.S. Department of Health, Education and Welfare, PHS Publication No. 1814, U.S. Government Printing Office, Washington, D.C., 1968.

Hanchett, Effie, and Torrens, Paul: A public health nursing project for adult patients with heart disease. Public Health Rep., *82:*683, August, 1967.

The Health Consequences of Smoking. U.S. Department of Health, Education and Welfare, Public Health Service, U.S. Government Printing Office, Washington, D.C., 1967.

Hulka, B.: Detection of cervical cancer among the medically indigent. Public Health Rep., *81:*143, February, 1966.

Kegeles, S. S., and others: Survey of beliefs about cancer detection and taking Papanicolaou tests. Public Health Rep., *80:*815, September, 1965.

Kurlander, Arnold R.: Chronic and degenerative disease. *In* Porterfield, J. H. (ed.): Community Health Services. Basic Books Inc., Publishers, New York, 1966.

Lester, E. *et al.:* Information and referral services for the chronically ill and aged. Public Health Rep., *83:*295, April, 1968.

Lilienfeld, A. M., and Gifford, A. J.: Chronic Diseases and Public Health. The Johns Hopkins Press, Baltimore, 1966.

May, E. E., Wagonner, N. R., and Boettke, E. M.: Homemaking for the Handicapped. Dodd, Mead and Co., New York, 1966.

President's Commission on Heart Disease, Cancer and Stroke. A National Program to Conquer Heart Disease, Cancer and Stroke: Report of the President's Commission on Heart Disease, Cancer and Stroke Vol. 1, U.S. Government Printing Office, Washington, D.C., 1964.

Reynolds, Frank W., and Barsom, Paul: Adult health: services for the chronically ill. The Macmillan Company, New York, 1967.

Runswick, Harriet: Teaching self examination of the breast. Nurs. Times, *64:*737, May, 1968.

Schwartz, Doris: Nursing needs of chronically ill ambulatory patients. Nurs. Res., 7:185, 1960.

Schwartz, Doris, Henley B., and Zeitz, L. Care of the Elderly Ambulatory Patient. The Macmillan Company, New York, 1964.

Strokes: A Guide for the Family. The American Heart Association, New York, 1969.

Sultz, Harry A., *et al.:* The Erie County survey of long-term childhood illness. Amer. J. Public Health, *58:*491, March, 1968.

Watkins, Julia, *et al.:* Study of diabetic patients at home. Amer. J. Public Health, *57:*452, March, 1967.

Delegation of Nursing Care

DELEGATION OF CARE IS MODIFIED BY THE COMMUNITY SETTING

Team leadership has become a common element in nursing practice in hospitals, and the general approach to team leadership has become a part of the basic nursing curriculum.[1] However, there are some differences when the concept of a nursing group or the delegation of care to another single individual is transferred to the nonhospital setting.

Surveillance Cannot be Constant and Immediate

The person to whom nursing care is delegated in the home, clinic, or nursing home must be able to function much of the time in the absence of any professional supervisor. Although intermittent observation and case discussion are possible, the professional nurse is rarely within call at the time the care is actually given; and she is not able to observe on a continuing basis the condition of the patient, the relationship within the family, or the apparent results of nursing care. This condition sets certain demands on the level and nature of the training and supervision required by those to whom care is delegated.

A Broad Range of Responsibilities

The auxiliary worker in the hospital is likely to be assigned to a particular service or ward and to deal with one category of patient. Even though the patients themselves differ just as much as in the community, the technical skills required and the nursing needs that arise from the nature of the disease encompass a narrower range. Thus, training in the hospital can be specifically related to the demands of a particular diagnostic or age group.

However, in the community setting, more reliance must be placed on constantly repeated on-the-spot specific training of the auxiliary worker; her generalized training provides the necessary background and makes it easier to adjust to the frequent change in the nature of the case load.

The Care Group Is Diverse

Families represent the major member of the care group in the community setting, and even when the direct nursing care is delegated to a nonfamily care agent, the family shares the responsibility. In addition to the families and other informal resources, the care-group members may include licensed practical nurses, home health aides, homemakers, clinic or school aides, job trainees, students in nursing and in related professional fields, and volunteers at all levels and with all kinds of preparation. Those in this group are likely to come under the immediate supervision of a designated nurse. On a "swap" (*i.e.,* interprofessional reinforcement) basis, peers not responsible to the nurse may include health educators, sanitarians, public health representatives, physician's assistants, physical therapists, occupation therapists, recreation therapists, and dental hygienists, who may provide some nursing care as an incidental part of their own work.

The alert community health nurse may thus extend her own usefulness through collaboration. In the theater, when ticket sales are slow, there is a practice referred to as "twofers" — that is, the patron gets two tickets for the price of one. The well-organized community nurse can apply the same principle through the use of coworkers; her one visit to the prenatal patient counts as two if the reinforcement she would usually provide during a second visit is given as an incidental part of the scheduled visit of a nutritionist or social worker.

CARE-GROUP CONFIGURATION VARIES

Often in the community setting it is not feasible to have a regularly organized "permanent" team with a professional nurse serving as the leader. The budget for auxiliary personnel may be low, and the allocation of auxiliaries may have to cut across populations served by several nurses. Moreover, auxiliaries may vary so widely in background, responsibility potential, and training that they must be placed very selectively. The composition of the team may change frequently because of the source of the assistant group. When the labor pool is very limited or when the provision of nursing care is linked with job training, new categories of worker may be added to or subtracted from the team as social programs develop. The addition of general health representatives or physician's assistants may require new adjustments, since their preparation may closely parallel that of the professional nurse.

Lateral, as well as Hierarchic, Delegation Is Frequent

Although the members on the health team are at least as numerous in the hospital as in the community setting, there is less need in the hospital for lateral delegation—that is, the delegation of nursing responsibilities to other professional workers—because of the constant availability of nursing staff. In nonhospital care, especially in rural or small town settings but increasingly in urban areas as well, there may be great economy in the exchange of duties among professional peers. The sanitarian may be in the school at a point between nursing visits, or the social worker in an urban setting may be visiting a family also carried by the nurse; and when this is the case, there may be considerable economy to both family and agency if, for example, the sanitarian checks to see whether or not the children referred for further study as a result of a vision-testing program actually did receive further care.

GENERAL PRINCIPLES OF GROUP CARE REMAIN CONSTANT

Despite the differences in the conditions of the delegation of nursing care in the community setting as compared to the hospital, certain general principles remain constant.

The Decision to Delegate Depends on Need and Feasibility

Whether the nurse will undertake nursing care herself or delegate it to another will depend in part on the patient: the demands of the treatment, the need for personal or supportive care, and in part, the feasibility of using other resources. Criteria for delegation include:

1. Given the training and supervision that is practicable, the treatment, observations, and judgment required must be within the competence of the individual to whom the delegation is made. The Code for Professional Nurses includes this statement: "The nurse has an obligation to protect the public by not delegating to a person less qualified any service which requires the professional competence of a nurse."[2]

2. Others must be available to provide care. *Available* in this instance should be interpreted in the functional rather than the absolute sense: private practice nurses, visiting nurses, home health aides, or homemakers who can be secured at a cost the family can afford to pay; relatives that are willing as well as able to provide the needed care; immediate family members that can provide the required care without damage to their own health.

3. The patient needs care that cannot be given by himself, or the family is unable to provide the total care. "Unable" families may include those who cannot provide care without occasional or periodic relief or whose attitudes are so negative that the care would be detrimental to the patient.

4. The physician, family, and community must accept the use of auxiliary personnel.

Training Must be Adequate

The individual giving nursing care must be adequately trained for the tasks to be performed. Such training cannot be assumed to have indefinite staying power and will need frequent reiteration, especially if the span of task variety is great or if a particular task may be undertaken intermittently after long intervals. Thus the aide who has once been taught to give insulin to a diabetic patient but who has not provided that type of care for several months may need retraining before it is safe to entrust her with this care under the relatively uncontrolled conditions of the home.

When the delegation is lateral, the same responsibility for training exists, although of course it must be more subtle! The social worker must understand the basis on which the nurse is working with a particular family with respect to developing the independence of the patient; the sanitarian checking on the school lunch program must know what to check in order to supplement the nurse's information and relate his findings to the overall nursing plan.

Collaboration Must be Based on an Explicit Care Plan

The plan for care should be developed by all of those involved and should be clearly spelled out. Even when more than one person is directly involved in the provision of care (for example, when a home health aide is providing care to the disabled member of the family while the community health nurse is providing health counseling services to the family as a whole), it is particularly important that both of these members of the care group clearly understand the total plan. It is important, too, that the family and the responsible physician be aware of the general care plan and of the functions of the various members of the care group.

The Family Should Identify a Primary Care Agent

To avoid confusion for the family and the possible mismanagement of the nursing plan, it is highly desirable that the family identify one primary source of nursing care and that, as far as possible, services to the family be routed through this source. As has already been pointed out, the primary care provider need not be the community health nurse; professional personnel may be in a backstopping and supervisory position, supporting but not supplanting the principal care agent.

Supervision Must be Adequate

Even though the supervision provided to the practical nurse, aide, or family member in the home, nursing home, or clinic is not a constant on-the-spot procedure, it must be both planned and sustained to ensure that the nursing tasks are carried out with safety and effectiveness. This should take more forms than the simple inspection and correction of inadequate practice. Such measures as case conferences, counseling sessions, record audit, and practice training sessions may supplement the observation and advisement of the helper at work.

Periodic Reappraisal of Nursing Needs

Reappraisal of nursing needs at intervals—usually not exceeding three months, in the absence of any changes that suggest an earlier reconsideration—is essential both to safeguard the patient and family and to use available nursing-care resources to the best advantage. Sometimes the best therapy for the family is the reduction or withdrawal of "outside" nursing care when it appears to be hampering the move toward independence. Sometimes the family reaches a point when the burden is not bearable, or some change in the health (or related circumstance) of a family member can affect the ability to provide needed care. Reappraisal, like all nursing appraisals, should involve the several members of the care group—the patient, the family, the physician, the nurse, and all other participants.

DIFFERENT HELPERS NEED DIFFERENT KINDS OF HELP

Interprofessional Reinforcement Demands Communication

Interprofessional reinforcement must be based on consistent and persistent communication and planning. If the entire staff responsible for a population group meets periodically to discuss and evaluate their progress in contributing to the health of the population serviced, the natural interchange may produce a sense of goal and also a high level of understanding of one another's functions and problems; and the exchange of ideas may consequently facilitate a greater coordination of action.

When such formal interchange is not a part of usual agency practice, the community health nurse may be able to establish her own means of achieving a similar result. Case conferences with the social worker may become discussions of the problems of the community as a whole; reporting a sanitation problem may become the occasion for discussing with the sanitarian the general tack the nurse is taking to improve school health; and dropping in to visit the nurse in the physician's office in order to check on a specific family may produce broader mutual efforts on the patient's behalf.

The Family Nurse

When the family is providing nursing care, they need training that is just as thorough and systematically organized as that provided to the paid auxiliary. Often by the time the nurse arrives, the family has already been involved with care and has developed its own methods of dealing with some of the nursing-care problems. Because of their familiarity with the patient and with the home equipment, they may appear to be much more knowledgeable than they actually are with respect to the details of care. The nurse's "class" in the home is often a class of one student, and as a consequence the situation will require an appropriately informal approach. However, care must be taken lest the informality result in a failure to achieve the systematic coverage provided under the more formal training afforded the paid auxiliary.

In training family members for nursing responsibility, it is important to take nothing for granted and to check out their knowledge, skills, and attitudes as carefully as possible in order to be sure they have the *know-how* needed to provide safe and adequate care. The family must also develop what might be called *"know-when."* They need to know when to call for help should the situation change and they become unable to provide the needed care; for the aged patient with chronic bronchitis, the family nurse who has a cold should know that this is the time to get someone else to provide the personal care required, since the patient's vulnerability to infection is exceedingly high.

The nurse role is also different from the family role, and sometimes the family member must know when to be a nurse rather than a spouse or a daughter. As a daughter, the family nurse may feel she wants to do everything possible to keep her elderly parent comfortable and assured that her children would "do anything for her." As a member of the nursing group, she must realize the importance of balancing the demands of the patient against the demands of other family members; it may be more important that the teenage daughter have the living room for socializing with her own group than that grandmother have the reassurance of being wanted in every family function. Also, as a nurse the daughter must balance her desire to cause her mother no pain with the nursing goal of greater independence which may involve painful exercises that the patient undertakes very unwillingly.

The family nurse must also realistically assess her own and the family's capability in the situation and face the fact that demanding care required over a long period may wear the best of tempers thin. She must be helped to recognize and accept the need for occasional relief; and she should be helped to find such relief within the family, the neighborhood group, or through community resources. The nurse herself may occasionally take over the care. It is the nurse's responsibility to assure the "relief help" that they are also adequately prepared for the required tasks. The community health nurse must be as concerned with the health and well-being of the home nurse as she is with that of the patient.

In some communities, voluntary agencies or groups may maintain a loan closet so that families may borrow needed sickroom equipment. The development of such a loan closet is not a simple matter; and it should not be undertaken unless there are adequate provisions for securing equipment that is safe, for keeping the equipment in good repair, for transportation, and for keeping records. However, when such a loan closet can be developed and staffed by volunteers, it may be a great help to the family. The nurse might well encourage such an activity, but in general it is too time-consuming an activity for the nurse to undertake herself.

Paid Auxiliaries

There is an almost limitless amount of experimentation in the use of short-trained workers today. Constant and imaginative efforts are being made to tap hitherto untapped manpower resources for use by the health agencies. In particular, efforts are being directed toward recruiting men, persons in disadvantaged groups, and married women with grown children. This has produced a nursing-care group of great diversity.

LICENSED PRACTICAL NURSES

The number of licensed practical nurses has undergone a greater increase than that of all other types of registered or licensed nursing personnel; they were formally recognized in 1940. However, their use in public health agencies has been less than in the hospital. In 1966 there were 870 full-time and 37 part-time licensed practical nurses employed in public health agencies.[3] The practical nurse may work under the direction of a professional nurse or a physician.

Most practical nurses now entering the field have completed a formal course of study and have been licensed to practice by the appropriate government licensing agency. Thus it is possible to have some general idea of what might be expected of them and on what basis continuing or reinforcing training efforts should be planned. Although there are still many practical nurses who were licensed under waiver—who were certified as capable on the basis of experience and recommendation in the early years of licensing in each state—there are relatively few such "waivered" nurses in public health practice. However, even though practical nurses have had training and are licensed to practice, it must be recognized that schools differ greatly and that individuals differ in the degree to which their school experiences are reflected in on-the-job practice. Thus it is important for the nurse, when she is the supervising agent, to evaluate the capabilities of the practical nurse with respect to the assignment she has been given. When the physician is the supervising agent, the nurse may offer to assist the practical nurse if the physician feels that this is necessary. Many practical nurses working as solo practitioners under the supervision of physicians appreciate the opportunity to discuss their problems with the community health nurse and may benefit considerably from such an interchange.

The community health nurse will have considerable discretionary power in the use of practical nurses. For this reason it is important that she be familiar with the state laws governing their practice and with the agency's policies relative to the use of practical nurses.

UNLICENSED SHORT-TRAINED WORKERS

The number of unlicensed short-trained workers employed in community health work is increasing very rapidly. In 1968 there were almost 800 agencies sponsoring homemaker or home health aide programs in 41 states, and there were approximately 8000 full-time or part-time homemakers or home health aides.[4]

The emphasis on the use of the home health aide in conjunction with Medicare and Medicaid programs that provide for extended home care catapulted agencies into new patterns of staffing, with a resultant greater reliance on short-trained workers. Concomitantly, increased experimentation in the utilization of nursing personnel and improvements in administrative practice produced a marked increase in the use of nurse aides in clinics and in schools.

These workers may be trained on the job; or they may have had prior training in programs of community agencies, in vocational schools, or in American Red Cross classes in home nursing. When trained on the job, most workers are paid for the training period. Almost always they work under the direction of a registered nurse.

The community health nurse will in many instances be responsible for the continued training and supervision of this group; she may even be responsible for planning or implementing the initial training program. Although the educational background of such workers will vary greatly—all the way from primary education to some college preparation—the majority will be recruited from among those with fairly low educational achievement.

Whether during a pre-employment period or on the job, the training provided should be systematically organized and clearly defined as to content. Some states have guides for such training.[5] In most cases it is not wise to depend upon the method of generalized teaching and allowing the student to make the applications of theory in actual practice, since the ability to apply generalizations and to make judgments is usually related to educational level. Teaching should be explicit and there should be plentiful opportunities for practice. Sometimes this means that the agency must set up a teaching area or arrange to use the classroom facilities of other agencies. When initial training is provided elsewhere, it may be possible at the outset to arrange for supplementary content to meet the needs of a particular agency; for example, students trained in the Red Cross home nursing course may be given an additional unit on assisting with screening procedures carried out in the school.

In the selection of such short-trained workers, it is important to find those who are capable of warmth and respect in their relationships with others and who have shown an ability to take responsibility in the management of their own lives. These characteristics appear to be more closely related to successful performance than does educational attainment, although it is essential that the aide be able to read. Good grooming is also important.

In the assignment of short-trained workers, actual skill may be no more important than the personality or the "style" of the worker. Some aides, for example, may be very good with elderly patients but have little patience or skill in dealing with children; others may be very effective with low-income groups but not yet possess the social skills to be comfortable in the middle- or upper-income family.

Usually there are fewer short-trained workers than could be used with benefit to families under care, and it may be necessary to decide whether to limit the number of families admitted for such service or to limit the amount of care that can be provided to each of the families being served. This requires good judgment on the part of the responsible nurse as well as a continuing search for family or other informal resources for care.

Since many short-trained workers provide services other than nursing care in the home, it is important that both worker and family understand the extent to which such services as cleaning, cooking, and shopping are a legitimate part of the aide's job. This will vary with the preparation of the aide, the availability of aides, and the goals of the service. The worker may be primarily trained and assigned as a homemaker, and nursing care may be a minor part of the job. Such housekeeping care may be essential in making home care possible, thereby reducing the demand on scarce and expensive hospital beds. In other instances the service may be offered primarily for nursing care, and other resources must be found for the housekeeping chores. Early clarification may prevent later misunderstandings that could be traumatic to the family and to the worker.

For job trainees, nursing may offer a means to social change. There is an increasing recognition that work is an important element in social adjustment. For those who have never gained work skills or who have lost them through long unemployment, work may be a valuable means of social therapy. For many, the health field, which appears to have an insatiable appetite for human services, offers an opportunity to learn or to relearn the skills of work. For young people on "learn and earn" programs, work offers an opportunity to stay in school and, at the same time, to learn how to live in the land of work. For others, it offers the hope of economic independence.

Many short-trained workers are recruited from very low-income groups. When this is combined with a lack of work adjustment, it creates special problems in training and assignment. However, the short-trained worker's very lack of social advantage may offer an unusual service opportunity: in working with other low-income families, the worker's feeling that he "has been there" may lead to a level of communication that is difficult for the middle class professional to achieve.

The responsible supervisor must accept the commitment to make this situation work. It is essential that the supervisor realize, for example, that members of the group may not be accustomed to meeting time deadlines; getting up and getting to work in the morning may be a new and very difficult habit for them to master. Their idea of suitable dress may not have been geared to the demands of a work situation. They may never have had a telephone at home; moreover, they may have seldom used one, and simple directions like "call the nurse should you need help" may be quite anxiety-producing. They may have had little occasion to question or to change their way of doing things. The ways of nurses, health professionals, and agencies may not make very much sense to them, and their anxiety may lead them to avoid a confrontation by just not reporting for work or by going home instead of going on to make a home visit because they "chickened out" at the last moment. The nurse must anticipate and understand the reasons for these possible responses and be willing to go 90 percent of the way, rather than only half way, in sharing the responsibility until new habits are established.During the training and indoctrination period, the supervisor must be willing to accept a standard of efficiency very different from that of more advantaged groups. When other aides are employed, it is important to enlist their help in this important task and to forestall a sense of injustice based on the observation that "that bunch can get away with anything, but just let ME try it!" They should understand that while the training and readjustment period may be long and demand what seems like limitless patience and effort on the part of the rest of the staff, eventually every worker will be expected to accept his full share of responsibility and to perform at a level that is a source of pride to all.

Careful interpretation of the reason for the rules and understanding, acceptance, and support combined with a firm insistence upon reasonable performance standards will set the stage for learning. Simplified, explicit, and amply reiterated instruction; the liberal use of visual aids and manipulative materials; and plentiful opportunities for practice will get the learning task done. Readily available explicit written or verbal statements of the exact nature of the tasks expected in a particular job will help forestall failure.

Some of this group will not make it to regular full-time employment. Some will be absent. Some will be hostile. But some will develop a new confidence and self-respect and a degree of work competence that makes the whole program worth every frustrated, discouraged moment.

Volunteers

Volunteers have taken many important roles in the development of health services in America; they have been members of boards, fund raisers, and also providers of nursing care. Voluntaryism is a rewarding and enriching experience for most people. The use of volunteers as extenders of patient-care services affords citizens a channel for public service and simultaneously helps to get the needed work done.

Volunteer workers should not be used to fill positions that would normally be filled with paid staff. To do so might impede the proper development of the basic services that the community should have. Volunteers can, however, provide many enrichment services such as visiting with the home-bound patient, helping with screening procedures in order to relieve overburdened teachers and nurses, and staying with children or elderly people while the homemaker shops.

The selection of volunteers should not be limited to any particular group. There has been a tendency in the past to recruit volunteer assistants that were largely from the middle or upper socioeconomic groups, preponderantly women, and most often, older women. This kind of selection does not take full advantage of the potential for human service that lies in "ordinary" individuals who would like to help. One recommendation of the 1963 President's Commission on the Status of Women reads as follows:

Volunteer's services should be made more effective through coordinated and imaginative planning among agencies for the necessary training, placement, and supervision, and their numbers augmented through tapping the large reservoir of additional potential members among youth, retired people, members of minority groups and women not now in volunteer activities.[6]

The special skills of the high school youth who can find his cause in tutoring a home-bound child under the guidance of the visiting teacher; the man whose children are older and who can now find time and can gain the skills to be a part-time substitute father for a fatherless and alienated child; and the low-income family that can share their know-how in purchasing and preparing foods on a minimum outlay are all valuable community resources that should be coordinated in the provision of nursing care.

Volunteers may be located one by one as people are encountered who have the desire to help, or they may be recruited from other organized groups such as church groups, Boy Scouts, Girl Scouts, or Rotarians.

The training of volunteers should be undertaken as conscientiously as the training of any other helping group. When training is provided by other than agency sources—for example, by the Red Cross or a central volunteer bureau—the nurse should familiarize herself with the training afforded and be prepared to supplement it.

Utilization of volunteer workers should be geared to the special capabilities of the individual, but in no case should it be based on an expectation that volunteer service is a "sometime thing" without the same degree of responsibility expected from paid staff. Such an assumption is an injustice to the serious volunteer and a danger to the service. Job descriptions should be developed for volunteer assignments in order to make expectations clear and to provide a ready guide for the worker. Supervision of volunteer activities involving any direct care of patients should be under the professional supervision of the nurse. Non-nursing supportive jobs, as well as certain administrative chores, may be under the direction of a volunteer supervisor.

Everybody Needs to Belong

Whether professional nurse, practical nurse, aide, or volunteer, everyone involved in the nursing effort should have a sense of identity with the agency and its purposes and with others in the care group. Some identifying insignia may be useful. A strong orientation to the purposes of the agency and to the people it serves, the participation in meetings with others in the care group, and being kept "in the know" about new developments and problems of the agency are all important measures for reinforcing agency identification. In this, the community health nurse, as the professional worker most often responsible for coordinating these multiple efforts, will have to take a major role. If her planning for and with these sources of service is systematic and sensitive, the dividends can be very high indeed.

REFERENCES

1. Kron, Thora: Nursing Team Leadership. 2nd ed., W. B. Saunders Company, Philadelphia, 1966, p. 6.
2. Code for Professional Nurses. American Nurses' Association, New York, 1962.
3. Facts About Nursing, 1967. American Nurses' Association, New York, 1967, p. 174.
4. Nurs. Outlook. *17*:31, February, 1968.
5. One example is the publication entitled Guide for Home Health Aide Services in New York State. New York State Health Department, Albany, 1968.
6. American Women. President's Commission on the Status of Women, U.S. Government Printing Office, Washington, D.C., 1963, p. 26.

SUGGESTED READINGS

Bellin, L. E., Killen, Mary, and Mazuka, J. J.: Preparing public health subprofessionals recruited from the poverty group—lessons learned from an OEO work study program. Amer. J. Public Health, *57*:242, February, 1967.

Disosway, L. M.: Reappraising the role of the practical nurse. Nurs. Outlook, *12*:40, February, 1964.

Grant, Murray: Health aides add new dimensions to home care programs, Hospitals, *40*:63, December, 1966.

Groeppinger, Jean: Why a home health aide? Amer. J. Nurs., *68*:1513, July, 1968.

A Guide for Utilization of Personnel Supportive of Public Health Nursing. American Nurses' Association, New York, 1967.

Hammond, Edith: Home care and improvisations. In Stewart, Dorothy, and Vincent, Pauline (eds.): Public Health Nursing. William C. Brown, Dubuque, 1968.

Hicks, Florence: Training neighborhood health aides. Amer. J. Nurs., *65*:79, April, 1965.

Homemaker Services. Nurs. Outlook, *17*:31, February, 1968.

Homemaker Services—How It Helps Children. U.S. Department of Health, Education and Welfare, Children's Bureau Publication No. 443, U.S. Government Printing Office, Washington, D.C., 1967.

Home Nursing Textbook, 7th ed. American National Red Cross. Doubleday and Co., Inc., New York, 1963.

Huntington, W., Miller A., and Gordon, J.: Use of teenage student volunteers in a local health department. Public Health Rep., *76*:665, 1961.

Licensed practical nurses in nursing services. National League for Nursing, New York, 1965.

Martens, Ethel G.: Culture and communication: training Indians and Eskimos as community health workers. Canad. J. Public Health, *57*:495, November, 1966.

Neumann, Alfred, and Young, Marjorie: Evaluation of homemaker service programs in Massachusetts. Amer. J. Public Health, *57*:128, January, 1967.

The Patient Returns to the Community: A Guide for a Voluntary Service in the Community. U.S. Department of Health, Education and Welfare, Veterans Administration Pamphlet 10–83, U.S. Government Printing Office, Washington, D.C., 1966.

Pearl, Arthur, and Reissman, Frank: New Careers for the Poor—The Nonprofessional in Human Services. The Macmillan Company, New York, 1965.

Reissmann, Frank: The Helper Therapy Principle. Social Work, Vol. 10, No. 2, April, 1965.

Training the Homemaker—Home Health Aide in Personal Care. U.S. Department of Health, Education and Welfare, Public Health Service Publication No. 1656, U.S. Government Printing Office, Washington, D.C., 1967.

Trautman, Mary Jane: We volunteered as visitors. Amer. J. Nurs., *68*:341, February, 1968. Vol. 68, No. 2, February 1968, pp 341–43.

Wise, Harold, et al.: The family health worker. Amer. J. Public Health, *58*:1823, October, 1968.

The Family History and Progress Record: A Major Practice Tool

The Records System

If asked, most community health nurses could promptly and correctly provide the justification for and the principles of record keeping as given in standard nursing texts. Yet the very word "records" tends to evoke a loud groan from the staff, a despairing gesture from the supervisor, and a caustic remark from the administrator about the disproportionate amount of nursing time spent on "paper work." One might hypothesize that this dichotomy results from some incongruity between what records are expected to do and the ways in which they are in fact designed and used.

Records Serve a Dual Purpose

The family history and progress record is only one part of a total record system that has a dual purpose: (1) to provide the staff member, administrator, or responsible governing body of the enterprise with documentation of the services that have been rendered and with data that are essential for program planning and evaluation (both of which will be discussed later) and (2) to provide the practitioner with data required for the knowing application of professional services for the improvement of family health. It is in the latter area that the family history and progress record is so important. *The family history and progress record can and should serve as a guide to nursing care.*

The purposes of the family history *as it relates to family nursing care* are:

1. To provide facts, intuitive assessments, and shared judgments necessary for evaluating the nursing situation in the family. It should describe the nature and the impact of the health threat. It should delineate the interacting forces of the health condition of the family and of the community as they function in daily life.

2. To afford an opportunity for mutual exploration of the health situation by the nurse and by the family so that they can define their respective concerns, expectations, and probable action.

3. To provide baseline and periodic data from which to estimate the longterm changes in the impact of the health challenge as that challenge is related to the service provided and to the family response.

If the family history and progress record is to fulfill these purposes, it must be more than a faithfully completed form, more than a collection of medical diagnoses and a few scattered remarks about the environment. It should, rather, represent a comprehensive, systematically organized, and perceptive set of data that puts into quickly accessible and assimilated form the information essential to nursing-care decisions.

Record Systems Have Both Prescribed and Optional Components

In most agencies the record system is comprised of a mixture of prescribed or standard forms identical to those of other agencies, and of forms designed to meet the needs of the particular agency. The state health department, for example, may supply prescribed record forms to local agencies, or the local agency may use forms developed by the National League for Nursing. One good example of a standard form is the NLN Assessment and Care Plan Record form shown in Figure 9. The use of common record forms facilitates interagency and interunit comparisons and makes collation of service data easier. These forms may be supplemented or modified to meet the needs of a particular agency and still retain enough similarity to provide a base for comparison.

When the agency is large and is organized to provide several levels and types of service, it may be necessary to have some parts of the family record separately stored. The clinic record for a preschool child may be written and stored in a facility apart from the office where the nurse responsible for the overall guidance of the family operates. When multiple agencies are involved, the fragmentation of the record may be great: a school child's health record may be kept in the school; the record of his father, who has an acute illness, may be kept in the offices of the health department, the visiting nurse association, or his industrial company; and the health record of his infant brother may be in a "comprehensive" maternal and infant care project. Though such dispersion presents obvious difficulties in using record data as a guide to comprehensive nursing care, it does place the record where it is accessible to those providing the special care.

ASSESSMENT AND CARE PLAN RECORD   Page No. _____

Name _____ Sex ____ Birth Date _____ Pt. Record No. _____
Address _____ Phone _____ Soc. Sec. No. _____
Physician _____ Phone _____ Referred by _____
Diagnoses _____

Areas Assessed	Care Status 19___		Findings — Explanation of Condition Requiring Intervention	Care Status 19___	
	Date	Code		Date	Code
Treatments & Meds. (incl. PT)					
Physical—Functional					
Bath, grooming, personal hyg.					
Locomotion					
Elimination, toileting					
Communication, sensory					
Prevention of complications					
Rehabilitation, ADL, rest—activity					
Nutritional					
Therapeutic, supplements					
Fluid balance					
Appetite, eating regimen					
Emotional—Behavioral					
Relationships					
Patterns of growth & devel.					
Adjustment to change					
Reaction to diagnosis, care, etc.					
Other					
X-rays, tests—preven. & diagnostic					
Immunizations					
Accident prevention					
Medical Supervision					
Plan of Care & Expected Outcome:					

Signature of R.N. responsible for patient

CARE STATUS CODES

Care Not Needed	Patient and/or Family Meeting Need	Patient and/or Family Not Meeting Need
00 No need	10 Patient independent	20 Progressing toward goal
01 Discontinued	11 Patient participates with family help	21 Lack information or skill required to move toward goal
02 Not recommended	12 Patient dependent, family has total responsibility	22 Attitudes or customs inconsistent with care required
	13 Under medical and/or other community service	23 Necessary service not available

NLN-PHS Record Form 21-1294. Copyright, 1967, by National League for Nursing.   Printed in U.S.A.

FIGURE 9. NLN assessment and care-plan form. Reverse side of form provides additional space for similar data.

In order to assemble in one place the comprehensive family information needed by the community nurse providing general family care, it may be necessary that the record system include forms that permit quick and easy transfer of information among the care-providing units. The "tear off and stick on" transmittal form is one example; a multiple copy blank that can be positioned to write duplicates when the regular notation is made is another method of efficient record-keeping. Thus, the nurse writing up a home visit in the tuberculosis service may simultaneously make several duplicates of her notation—one for the director of the service, one for the tuberculosis register, and one for the nurse specialist-consultant.

Prescribed and optional components may also exist in individual record notation as well as in the record forms. Record notations may require highly structured approaches, using codes or checking boxes for the description of a health situation and the course of care. This type of notation is increasing as agencies come to rely more on the computer for service analysis. In other agencies, great reliance may be placed on the "free form" type of notation in which the record form consists mostly of blank lines. Notations are usually chronological and sometimes assume massive proportions. This method obviously presents difficulties in the quick location of significant data; but it may serve a useful purpose when records are used to investigate nursing care or when families are served by several nurses, as often occurs when a large student nurse contingent is nearby.

Most practitioners and agencies use a combination of prescribed and optional approaches and allow the nurse practitioner to make the adaptations she finds useful and consistent with her own style.

STANDARD NOTATION PROCEDURES
MUST BE ADAPTED

The individual practitioner must assure adequate record support for her own action. It is the grass-roots practitioner who writes most of the family history and progress record. It is she who has most to gain if these records are comprehensive, available, and relevant to service needs.

Working within the established records system of the agency, the community health nurse can find ways of adapting family history and progress records to her own practice style and informational needs. In so personalizing a record, the nurse may need to clarify her own thinking about the uses to which the record might be put. Her experience with and judgments about records may be a valuable resource when the agency records are being revised or the system reorganized.

It is important to distinguish between data that are useful for the management of the case but are of only *temporary* value and data that have more lasting significance in the present and future evaluation of a family's health status. For families seen over long periods of time or for those infrequently visited, the nurse may need to record some information that is a kind of "memo to self" and which, though helpful to the nurse, is not necessarily justified as part of the official record. Some nurses use a notebook to keep information that is useful only to themselves. Some develop methods of using penciled notations that serve as reminders but are not incorporated into the "official" record. Some develop their own planning sheets or work sheets that can be included in the record or kept apart as a personal guide. For some families, the nurse may wish to use more extensive data collection measures to supplement the official record, such as the interview schedule developed by Schwartz, Henley, and Zeitz for use with the elderly ambulatory patient; this schedule contains information essential for planning nursing care.[1]

The nurse may need to build into the record methods for incorporating information necessary for case planning. If the record provides for chronological recording but not for "quick reference" statements of problems, plans, and action, the nurse may use a system of writing periodic summaries, writing in different colors of ink, or underlining, so that a synoptic reading of long records is possible. Items of general importance, such as the family's pattern of health service utilization, may be located in a specific place on each family record. Such notation procedures can be consistent with the overall records system and meet the particular needs of the nurse.

Criteria for Recording

The criteria for recording should reflect the purpose and the process of community health nursing practice. Perhaps the easiest way to consider the degree to which recording implements purpose and practice is to raise a series of questions.

1. *Does the record focus on the family and community as the object of care?* If nursing practice is geared to a family approach rather than to an individual approach, the record should reflect not only the condition of the members of the family but also the ways in which the family unit is functioning and the impact of the health challenge on the family as a whole. The record should also specify the ways in which a family functions within and with its physical and social environment.

2. *Does the record present the problem in comprehensive, explicit, and dynamic terms?* Records frequently appear to be quite specific about the immediate health deficits in a family: the illnesses, disturbances in development, or the stress conditions that have been diagnosed and that clearly require nursing care. If the record is to serve as a guide for comprehensive care, however, it is important that it also fairly represent those less obvious health threats and health behaviors that have significance for family health. An adequately immunized family is harboring a health threat, as is the family with emotionally immature and impulsive parents. A "well" family may have poor nutritional habits or poor housekeeping practices that invite accidents. A simple medical diagnosis may express a health problem in nondefinitive terms. "Diabetes," for example, does not identify a specific health problem, which may be lack of an adequate educational base for decisions that must be made or an immature or unrealistic attitude toward health care. The problem may be expressed too generally (for example, "poor nutrition") rather than in terms of the basic or contributing factors (such as an absent, working mother or inadequate family skills in the purchase and preparation of foods). The "problem" in most families really represents a complex of many small problems the bits and pieces of which are constantly changing with the passage of time. It is important that the record show the problem *as it develops,* so that change can be readily identified.

3. *Are the goals explicity defined?* Explicit goal statements should clearly indicate the outcomes considered feasible and also the degree to

which these outcomes are agreed upon by the nurse, the referring agent, and the family. For a psychiatric patient returning to his home after lengthy hospitalization, a goal of "providing rehabilitative care" is not sufficiently explicit to be helpful as a guide to nursing practice. The goal of maintaining the prescribed therapeutic regime is explicit and will presumably be one on which all three concerned parties agree. However, the goal of maintaining the family balance in the face of this threat of disruption may create some problems. One family goal may be to keep the patient secluded in order not to embarrass the family's relationship with the neighbors. The desire to secure the maximum progress of the patient in his cure may be equal to or secondary to this limited family goal. The referral agent—the physician or hospital—probably hopes for the best possible treatment of the patient and also for the continued release of the hospital bed. The nurse's goals may be somewhere in-between. She may wish to facilitate the patient's adjustment to the home without prejudice to either patient or family, and to support vulnerable family members whose emotional or physical health may be threatened by the introduction of this source of family stress. The record should indicate this qualified endorsement of goals.

4. *Is the action program explicitly stated?* The record should clearly show what specific action is planned; what activities are actually carried out; and the distribution of responsibility for action among the nurse (or nursing group), the family, and other community resources. The action plan should be in an accessible part of the record so that it can be quickly located.

5. *Is family response to the problem and to subsequent nursing action clearly identifiable?* The family response to problems and to care is indispensable in the planning and the validation of nursing action. The record should indicate family response along four parameters.

Feeling and Value Response: the family's acceptance of the problem, their feelings about the problem's relative importance, their opinion of the adequacy or relevance of available community measures for handling the problem, and their own commitment to the problem's solution.

Therapeutic Response: the family's response to nursing and to other treatment of disease and disability.

Behavioral Response: the action taken—either independently or as an outcome of the care plan—by the family in response to the problem.

Conceptual Response: evidences of the family's understanding or knowledge of the problem.

6. *Is there provision for quick reference to periodic comprehensive assessments?* Community health nursing practice proceeds by a series of revisions. The problem is defined, the action is planned and instituted, and the problem is redefined. This process is continually repeated. The record must show these revisions in the status of the problem and the plan in a way that is quickly accessible to the user. For example, a family may welcome and support the returning psychiatric patient for a while; then, as the newness wears off and the adjustments required begin to chafe, the general movement of family care may deteriorate.

Conversely, the family that was "edgy" about recurrence of disease may gain confidence in the treatment and in their ability to handle a recurrence should it occur. In either case, the change is important for planning care.

Sometimes there is a kind of "time capsule" arrangement in the record: the problem-action-result triad is placed in a conspicuous place and provides for a synopsis of family progress. When the official record does not make specific provision for it, the nurse must find a way to incorporate such summarization into her own recording.

THE RECORD AS A PRACTICE TOOL

Developing the Family History and Progress Record

From the nature of the data required, it is clear that the better the nurse knows and understands the family, the better the record will be as a means for guiding practice. When families are carried over long periods of time and the nurse-family relationship is good and is sustained, the record will be apt to reflect a depth of mutual understanding. For those receiving episodic or limited care, the problem will be more difficult.

THE HISTORY-TAKING INTERVIEW IS BASIC

The history-taking interview is basic to the record development process. It is at this point that nurse and family representatives have an opportunity to sit down together to evaluate the situation as a whole and to explore the areas in which the collaborative effort of family and nurse may be productive. The opportunity this presents should be fully exploited by the nurse. An attitude on her part that recording is merely a troublesome task can effectively block important revelations or inquiries the family might otherwise make. The nurse's task is to elicit and evaluate information, not simply to receive and record it.

An informal and leisurely approach combined with offering second chances for revelation may prove very productive. For example, if asked how she feels about her pregnancy, a young expectant mother may say quite honestly, "I don't know"; she may give a nonresponsive answer such as "OK, I guess"; or she may just giggle as though the question were silly. Through talking about future plans, about the father's attitude toward the pregnancy, or about the things she likes to do, the young woman may be drawn into thinking through for herself how she really does feel.

Initial inquiries about family diet may produce only very generalized or obviously inaccurate responses: "We eat three good meals a day" or "We get plenty of meat." The actual situation becomes clear only as further questioning is used; "What did you have for breakfast today?" or "What do you mean when you say 'plenty' of meat?" may produce an answer of a different quality.

The nurse's nondirective responses, such as listening or reflecting the patient's observations in order to let him think through his problem, rather than overt advisement, may further the family's clarification of their problem and convince them that their ideas and their feelings are of paramount importance.[2]

REASSESSMENT ALLOWS FAMILY-NURSE COLLABORATION

The initial history-taking period is usually quite well defined and requires the participation of an informant in the family. The opportunity for mutual exploration, consequently, always clearly presents itself.

The reassessment period is not so clearly structured. Often the nurse will compose this reassessment statement by herself; she will base her judgments on knowledge and feelings she has shared with the family, but she will not involve the family directly in her stock-taking. This would appear to be a wasteful practice, since at least theoretically, this is an occasion for focusing the combined attention of the family and the nurse on the progress made and the future action indicated. The same care should be given to the development of this periodic statement of status and progress as is given to the original assessment.

GENERAL NURSING SKILLS ARE BASIC TO RECORDING

Recording requires all of the basic skills of nursing itself: communication (including listening), observation, and analysis based on facts, intuition, and interpersonal sensitivity. It takes a willingness to wait for others to think and to speak, to reach out for information that the family may find hard to share even though they would like to do so.

RECORD-READING PROVIDES ADDITIONAL DATA

Information from records of previous services, of other units in the agency, or of related agencies may all be incorporated into the ongoing record. Reading previous or related records may provide clues to matters that should be investigated further; for example, a history of unfounded "cancer scare" might suggest the need to check the present attitudes and early diagnostic efforts of the family.

RECORD-WRITING REQUIRES DISCIPLINE

If the family history and progress record is to serve its purpose, it must be comprehensive without being bulky; objective without being insensitive; and complete without requiring an unreasonable amount of the nurse's or the family's time. To achieve this combination, the nurse developing the record must discipline herself so that two words are not used when one would serve and so that the description of family function is operational rather than discursive and literary. Even more importantly, she must discipline herself to allow an adequate amount of scarce time to develop this important practice tool.

ACCURACY IS ESSENTIAL

Recent studies indicate that the professional worker may have a quite distorted view of the patient's and the family's knowledge and skill with respect to health measures. Recorded family response to casual inquiries about diet may differ considerably from those secured through a systematic inquiry using a 24 hour recall interview schedule.

Nursing has not moved in the direction of medicine, which places great reliance on laboratory tests as a supplement to medical judgment. For example, in the care of diabetic patients at home, the nurse is likely to teach carefully the administration of insulin and the testing of urine, and she will observe the patient in carrying out these procedures until she is satisfied that he can do so correctly. However, systematic pretesting and post-testing, which might be analogous to laboratory procedures, is seldom employed.

It should be possible to put together exactly what information a diabetic patient and his family should have and then to test it systematically for accuracy and completeness. Obviously a knowledge of the nature of the disease process or of the incidence of diabetes is not in this crucial information class. Just as surely, knowledge of how to measure and inject insulin, how to take other prescribed medication, the reasons for exactness, a knowledge of the symptoms of hyperglycemia and hypoglycemia, the exact number to call if help is needed to get to the hospital, and the importance of the careful measurement of foods and of "fair exchange" foods *is* crucial information. Until such specific appraisal is available, records will continue to have a low degree of reliability as a measure of family need and progress. Even a conscientiously compiled "accurate" record will prove inadequate for many purposes unless the quality—*i.e.*, the accuracy and completeness—of the data on which the record is based can be improved.

Using the Family History and Progress Record

Using the family history and progress record is as important as developing it. The notation of pertinent facts, observations, and impressions is only the first step in the utilization of the record as a nursing practice tool. It is only as the record is used to make practice and service decisions that the payoff stage is reached.

First, it is important to analyze the notations to see the *patterning* they reveal. For instance, a notation that a school child who had had several short absences did not report for his conference with the nurse, combined with the notations to the effect that he did not attend school on the day of a screening examination, that he was reported by his history teacher to be jittery and disinterested, and that his grades had gone down despite previously demonstrated ability, has much value as a witness to a recurring threat of trouble. *The flag is up* for checking out possible drug abuse or emotional distress; it might not have been if these things were seen and dealt with one by one. Were the nurse not to seek a pattern in behavior, this might have been one more child on drugs not discovered until the human loss was irremediable. Similar patterning may be revealed by immature parents, the mentally deteriorating elderly patient, or the family that is beginning to shuck its responsibility for a difficult older member currently cared for at home.

Second, when records are fragmented, it is useful to find some way of *putting the family together* again. Perhaps this may be done by encouraging the family, as a help to them when they are asked to supply health information, to keep a health record of all care received from any source. Sometimes a periodic review of all records of the family or case discussions with other members of the health group may fill in the gaps. For instance, in one health department, periodic case reviews by the nurse and epidemiologist were held for all tuberculosis cases under care. Even though the major purpose was to see if the care pattern should be changed and if the follow up was adequate, the nurse frequently made this an occasion for checking the health records (located in various other clinics and in the school) of other members of the family and for reviewing data on the family as a whole.

Third, it is important to take the time to find and to read the record as a basis for planning. Sometimes this is a laborious process of wading through interminable chronological narrative entries with long stretches of "no change."

Fourth, the discipline of a "moment of truth" procedure is sometimes helpful, especially where intuitive free style recording is used. The record is reviewed and the problems noted. The action taken is recorded. Then the two sets of data are reviewed to see to what degree *the problems as indicated in the record* and *the action taken as indicated in the record* correspond. This is very likely to pick up ineffectual recording habits, but it may also pick up failures in planning, in observation, in assessment, or in follow-through on case problems. For example, if the primary problem identified in a young mother was need for social care due to out-of-wedlock status, and the major care provided was in fact identical with that provided other prenatal patients of similar age, the question is whether the problem was poorly defined in the first place or whether this problem was indeed accurately defined and the subsequent nursing intervention inappropriate.

Developing a family history and progress record takes time, thought, and discipline; but when recording is properly done and when the information is properly used, the dividends will be high.

REFERENCES

1. Schwartz, Doris, Henley, Barbara, and Zeitz, Leonard: The Elderly Ambulatory Patient. The Macmillan Company, New York, 1964, p. 299.
2. Rogers, Carl R.: Counselling and Psychotherapy: Newer Concepts in Practice. Houghton Mifflin Company, Boston, 1942, p. 18.

SUGGESTED READINGS

Dunn, Halbert, and Gilbert, Mort: Public health begins in the family. Public Health Rep., *71*:1002, October, 1956.

Granett, C. W. B.: New look in nursing records. Hospital Administration, 8:30, June, 1966.

Schwartz, Doris: Some Thoughts on Quality in Nursing Service. Int. Nurs. Rev., 14:29, March-April, 1967.

Schwartz, Doris: Toward more precise evaluation of patients' needs. In Stewart, Dorothy, and Vincent, Pauline (eds.): Public Health Nursing. William C. Brown Company, Publishers, Dubuque, 1968, Chapter 18.

Schwartz, Doris, Henley, Barbara, and Zeitz, Leonard: The Elderly Ambulatory Patient. The Macmillan Company, New York, 1964, p. 299.

Wright, Doris B.: What's in the record? In Stewart, Dorothy, and Vincent, Pauline: Public Health Nursing. William C. Brown Company, Publishers, Dubuque, 1968, Chapter 20.

CHAPTER
11

Vulnerable
Families

Among the families being served by the community health nurse, there will be some that are more vulnerable than others to health or social disorder. Families that could be classified as one or more of the following should receive particular attention designed to counteract the cause of vulnerability.

1. The very poor family.
2. The multiproblem, crisis-prone family.
3. The incomplete family.
4. The young family with a working mother.
5. The migrant family.
6. The family with genetic risk or handicap.
7. The inadequately functioning family.

Problems unique to the very poor family are discussed elsewhere. In many instances the very poor family will have the same characteristics of vulnerability covered in the following material.

THE MULTIPROBLEM FAMILY

Because early aid helps forestall the worsening of their situation and because they constitute a significant welfare investment, the multiproblem family has been a concern of health and welfare planners for many years. As early as 1952, Buell and associates emphasized the importance of recognizing multiproblem families and of dealing in a coherent way with their needs. They pointed out that this small portion of the population used up the lion's share of health and welfare services.[1] The persistence, as well as the magnitude, of the problems in such families creates a baffling problem for the community as well as for the family itself. Geissmar and LaSorte emphasize the importance of special understanding and attention to multiproblem families if needs are to be properly assessed and dealt with.[2] These families include many that closely resemble those described as "poor copers" by Sir James Spence in his study of families in Newcastle-on-Tyne. They seem unable to deal with the progressively more complex difficulties that beset them, problems that other families in an identical setting are able to handle with reasonable success.[3] Hill and others have pointed out that some families also appear to be "crisis prone": that is, they, more often than their neighbors, tend to meet situations that immobilize them and render them helpless to control, solve, or adjust to the crisis.[4]

Each of these investigating groups was looking at the family from a different viewpoint and thus describing the problem in different terms; but their joint conclusion seems to be simply that some families have many more problems than others and that, moreover, they are less able to handle these problems. If the community health nurse can identify these families and provide intensive care for them, it may be possible to ameliorate their condition.

In dealing with the multiproblem family, assessment of the situation becomes exceptionally important. In the first place, it is important to analyze the situation in terms of its implications for nursing action. In some cases, of course, the nurse has no direct control over the problem and can offer emotional support only. For example, the cause of a family's recurring crises may be the unstable economic base on which it operates and which causes it to vacillate between being dependent on welfare and living in relative ease when work is available. The period of dependence may be accompanied by despair, dejection, stress, and physical manifestations of illness to a degree not present during the "good years." The nurse, realizing that little of lasting benefit may be accomplished, has the responsibility of giving encouragement and support through the crisis period. If, on the other hand, the crises or problems rest on poor use of available facilities, poor habits of problem solving, or failure to resolve the intra-familial competition that prevents adequate mobilization of a family's own resources, the nurse must uncover the specific causes and, at the same time, provide support at the points of stress until the family is strengthened. Assessment is often difficult because the family tends to come under care only during the times of stress, when it is most difficult for its members to communicate in an analytical or projective way.

Timing and content of nursing intervention must also be adjusted. When nursing is judged to be a likely corrective influence, the multiproblem family should be seen as often as possible not only when a crisis is imminent but also between crises. It is at these points that the family's knowledge and skill in dealing with anticipated problems can be developed. Specific, tangible help at the crisis period is, of course, a paramount concern for the nurse. It is the crisis problem that has the highest priority in the family's mind, and it is at this point that they are willing and, indeed, anxious for help that they might reject at other times.

With all vulnerable families, it is important to give more help in direct nursing care than the health situation alone might justify. The nurse's concern and desire to help can be reiterated in many ways by an "extra" telephone call or visit or a more leisurely conference. The nurse may, either alone or in coordination with a social worker or other professional, build the general competence of the family in analyzing and handling its problems and prepare members specifically for anticipated periods of crisis. In her own preoccupation with the specific immediate or expected health crisis, it is crucial that the nurse not lose sight of the importance of developing general family skills, since the multiproblem family is not apt to look beyond the crisis.

Self-help resources for the multiproblem family may reach beyond the immediate family. The enlistment of relatives, neighbors, or institutions such as the church or school is almost always a requirement for providing the support and confidence the family may need. However, the recruitment, briefing, and reinforcement of these volunteer and amateur helpers must be as carefully planned as is the nursing care of the family itself. In working out a local resource for baby minding in an emergency or finding a relative that would be able to help with the housework, it is important to gauge the volunteer's ability, commitment, availability, and reliability. For example, one young mother, who had a growing family and who needed help when she was having each baby, depended upon her mother's assistance. The mother, who lived at some distance, had been a willing helper for the first two babies; and she was a willing, but somewhat less enthusiastic, helper with the third and fourth. For the fifth baby, she was understandably a reluctant source of help, and she came declaring that she was not up to the responsibility and that her daughter should limit the size of her family to the number she could take care of herself. A housekeeper, plus the occasional supervision and help of a nearby younger married sister, supplied a more feasible solution.

For multiproblem families, some of the kinds of help the nurse usually provides may be more effectively supplied by unconventional sources. For example, help with family food management is usually provided by the nurse or by the nutritionist, but it may be that an informal indigenous source could accomplish more. A homemaker whose background closely resembles that of the patient may be a very effective channel for such information. A problem family may feel that the homemaker has "been there" and knows the problems of feeding a family on low income as well as any textbook. If it were possible to organize a small group in which there is a degree of expertise in meal planning, for example, ideas might be transmitted more readily.

In the past, success with changing the status of multiproblem or crisis-prone families has not been outstanding. It is hoped that ingenious and persistent efforts by those involved, including the community health nurse, will change that trend.

THE INCOMPLETE FAMILY

There is a fairly large number of families that might be described as "incomplete": families that are fatherless, motherless, or include widows, widowers, and divorced partners. Such families are often under greater stress than those that have been able to stay intact.

In 1963 it was reported that one family in ten had a woman as head of the family.[5] Although 88 percent of the children in 1965 lived in two-parent families, those children who have only one parent represent a group at special risk. The mounting number of pregnancies among unwed young women and the persistent desertion rate add to the number of fatherless households. In such instances the female head of the family is faced with the double problem of filling the father's role as provider for the household, as well as being responsible for child rearing.

Obviously, there are great individual differences in the impact of this condition on the mother and on the children. In some instances, particularly when the parents are very young, grandparents may take in the child as their own; in such a case the lack of a natural father does not constitute any true deprivation.

In other instances, the unmarried, widowed, or divorced mother may face the problem of supporting herself and her children while at the same time providing for their adequate nurture. When there are available, willing, and able family members to take on the child care responsibility, the situation may be mitigated. In the absence of such family support, however, the situation may be extremely difficult, especially in highly industrialized countries where the low status and low pay accorded housework has created an acute shortage of such home helpers. At the same time, in the United States at least, there has been no adequate growth of group facilities such as day care centers or nurseries. Thus the mother-and-head-of-household may be faced with the choice of accepting either patently inadequate child care facilities or dependency on state aid. Her choice is not an easy one, especially since recent welfare policy emphasizes the need for an individual's financial independence. Even with reasonably good child care facilities, parents who have delegated this responsibility for a substantial part of the day are apt to feel guilty over their inability to personally care for their child. When care is inadequate, this stress becomes even greater; and for the unwed mother, social or family disapproval may add to the strain.

The motherless family is fortunately a less frequent phenomenon, but the difficulties presented are great when the father is trying to assume both the paternal and the maternal roles. Whether the absence of the mother is due to longterm illness, divorce, or death, those functions that she would ordinarily perform must be filled by someone. When the someone is a trusted and willing relative or when it is possible to employ a suitable mother substitute, the situation may not be too complex. However, even with the best possible solution, the healthy situation in which parents share the responsibility of child rearing cannot help but be distorted.

When the one-parent family is the outcome of divorce, emotional deprivation of the spouse may cause severe physical or emotional symptoms—insomnia, depression, cynicism, and hostility—that spill over to the children, who may become legal or emotional pawns.

When the death of a spouse depletes the family, the likelihood that the children are grown and away is greater; in general widows are 50 years old or older, whereas divorcees tend to be under that age. Thus the remaining family may be a "family of one" who lives either alone or with children and all the intra-family problems associated with the generation gap.

Whether living alone or "in another woman's house," the acute loneliness immediately following the death of a spouse is frequently replaced by sustained loneliness. Health tends to be neglected; there is no one to urge a visit to the clinic; there is no one for whom to prepare meals. Emotional deprivation adds to the burden. The result may be poor eating habits and symptoms of distress such as gastrointestinal discomfort, choking, and sleeplessness.

In some communities, efforts are made to help meet the needs of these incomplete families. In one community in England, a "widow's counselling service," staffed by health professionals (including nurses), was organized to try to locate and help deal with health problems arising from the crisis of widowhood.[6] "Parents Without Partners" associations exist in many localities in the United States. Divorcees' and widows' clubs are developing; and for the older person, membership in the Association of Retired People may provide a social outlet.

THE YOUNG FAMILY WITH A WORKING MOTHER

Among the nearly 27 million women workers in the United States in March 1966, there were 9.9 million mothers with children under 18 years of age; this constitutes 36 percent of all of the mothers in the population. Almost 2 out of 3 of these working mothers had children under 6 years of age.[7]

There are, of course, many reasons that mothers work. For some, especially those with special or professional preparation, work may provide a welcome respite from the tedium of housework and child care, especially when the children are older. For others it may be a means of earning money to meet what the family sees as an important goal, such as providing the down payment on a house or helping to pay for the education of the children. The great majority of working women with small children must work out of economic need. About one in seven of the working mothers in the United States in 1966 came from families in which the income was less than $3,000.

The family of the working mother may in some instances be able to make adequate provision for child care and for assistance with household tasks. The mother substitute may be trustworthy and warm. However, this often is not the case.

One overriding problem is the health hazard to children left behind with inadequate child care. In the absence of community child care facilities or services, parents must make their own arrangements. A low family income means that they can in turn afford only low-priced child tending services. The result may be that the child is left in the care of a nonworking family member who may be grossly unsuited to the task: an aged and crippled uncle or a kind but sometimes disoriented grandmother. Children may be left untended for long periods of the day with all the hazards that come with lack of adult supervision; and obviously, the likelihood of accidents is increased. Older children, especially young girls, may be given more responsibility than they should be expected to carry at their age; this may, in turn, deprive them of social opportunities that are open to their peers.

The mother, too, may suffer from feelings of conflict and guilt as she finds herself torn between what she sees as "necessities" for the children and the evidences of lack of adequate care in her absence. She may suffer from simple fatigue. The strain of maintaining two full-time jobs (as homemaker and worker) takes much more than the usual level of energy; and if, as is often the case, she comes from an impoverished setting to begin with, there may be little reserve energy to call on. Children may react to the mother's fatigue and irritability or to the chaotic situation in her absence by tension, anxiety, and a host of trivial complaints.

For the community health nurse there are several imperatives in her care of this type of family. She must:

1. Assess and improve the adequacy of the child care that takes place in the mother's absence. This may involve supporting the individual who is inadequate by making more frequent nursing visits in order to encourage and assist with the immediate care problems. It may involve meetings with actual or potential "babysitters" for the purpose of teaching them the simple elements of well-child care and equipping them to recognize the need for help and to seek help in emergencies.

2. Check to see if the ordinary environmental hazards to health are increased by the absence or inadequacy of adult supervision and take action to reduce the risk if possible. For example, the use of a gas heater is normally quite safe in the hands of an adult, but this situation is not at all safe if young children are nearby and inadequately controlled.

3. Evaluate the distribution of responsibility for homemaking activities among the various members of the family and where possible encourage sharing of responsibility to relieve the mother. Of the working mothers in 1967, 83 percent had husbands in the home.[8] However, winning the assistance of those husbands may not be an easy task when family roles are rigidly perceived.

4. Evaluate the need for available outside assistance that would free more of the mother's time for child guidance. For example, if community housekeeper services are available, could this family qualify for such assistance? Is there a family member who might help on a regular basis?

5. Help the mother to deal with her present health problems in order to minimize any strain arising from untended incipient illness. For example, anemia is frequently found among low-income groups, and its likelihood may be enhanced by irregular eating habits. Nonemergency health problems, such as the need for elective gynecologic surgery, may go untreated and add to the energy drain.

6. Help the mother with the control of fatigue, especially with respect to management of time, and establish home responsibilities in terms of their priority. For example, "time for the children" may have been neglected in favor of freshly washed kitchen walls; reconsideration of what really matters most in the long run may reverse this emphasis.

Even though in many instances the nurse is not dealing with "illness" problems, she is in fact dealing with health problems that are of great importance to the welfare of the family and its members.

THE MIGRANT FAMILY

Families that are required to move frequently because of job or social requirements face additional strain. The family must accustom itself to new communities and the attendant new health problems, facilities, and habits of utilization. For example, a family moving from New England to the South faces many new cultural and health conditions. Relationships with neighbors must be re-established, sometimes under different patterns. Facilities for health care may vary in sponsorship, in content of program, and in the type of help available. Migrant agricultural laborers are unusually vulnerable families. Their problems are discussed in Chapter 21.

The nurse can help establish health ties in the new location, for instance, by writing ahead to the nursing service director if the family has been receiving intensive nursing help. She may suggest to the family that they get in touch with local health agencies—by calling the health department about available services or by asking the local medical association for names of reputable family physicians—before the need for care is urgent.

She can also help parents to anticipate the stress that the move will place on them and on their children, and she should discuss with them ways of dealing with it. Sometimes referral to a church in the new community may provide a useful link. When the nurse knows that the new community has health hazards different from those of the present community, specific instruction regarding preventive action may be given.

THE FAMILY WITH A GENETIC HANDICAP

It has long been known that each family represents a collection of genetic forces that significantly influence health and development. The current rapid expansion of knowledge about the nature of genetic materials and about the process by which genetic traits are transmitted is increasing medical understanding of genetically influenced disease. It is also producing new opportunities for preventive health care. It is reasonable to expect that the community health nurse will be involved in many ways with the application of this new knowledge to health care.

For example, more precise estimates of the risk of transmitting undesirable traits make it possible to provide prospective parents with information that will enable them to make decisions about childbearing and to clear up misconceptions that may have occasioned unreasonable guilt and anxiety. Early knowledge of genetic risk may make it possible to anticipate and counteract natural genetic outcomes, as, for instance, when knowledge of incompatible Rh factors in the paternal genes enables the medical team to prepare for necessary therapeutic intervention.

Recent breakthroughs in the chemical identification of genes makes the possibility of modifying genes "not impossible."[9] Such capability would, of course, increase immeasurably the opportunity for control of a genetically determined defect. In the meantime, genetic research and interpretation of what is known is a "here and now" demand upon health workers as well as on scientific investigators.

The community health nurse, unless she is also trained as a geneticist, cannot undertake independent counseling in this complex and rapidly changing field. She can, however, support and extend the efforts of the specialists. The nurse should be alert to clues suggesting the need for genetic assessment and counseling; a history of diabetes in the family or the mention of symptoms in a relative that are suggestive of Huntington's chorea are examples. Genetic counseling centers have been established in many communities. These centers are directed by geneticists who usually depend heavily upon other health workers to interpret the genetic findings and to support families who must make decisions based on the results of genetic studies. With the backstopping of the genetic counselor or physician, the nurse participates in the family counseling. She might be called upon to explain the estimate of genetic risk—that is, the likelihood that an undesirable trait may be transmitted to the offspring. She may prepare the family for genetic counseling, pointing out the kinds of help that can and cannot be provided. She may reinforce the philosophy of most genetic counseling services: the geneticist can estimate the risk, but only the family can decide what to do about it.

The nurse should also help support the family in the decision they have made. For example, should a couple decide on the basis of genetic advice that they will not have children, there is almost inevitably some inner conflict. Related decisions about contraception, sterilization, adoption of children, feelings of inadequacy, or feelings of unfulfillment may take their emotional toll. The couple's primary need is likely to be for help in accepting their decision; counseling relative to available means of contraception is secondary. Through direct support or referral, the nurse can strengthen the couple's ability to cope with their problem.

The community health nurse may be a valuable aid in the diagnosis of genetic risk through her participation in eliciting the family pedigree. This requires patient and persistent searching for relevant family data. The accuracy and usefulness of the pedigree depends upon the ingenuity of the nurse and on her ability to win the confidence of the informant.

For some disease entities, there appears to be a definite familial genetic linkage, but the genetic consequences vary according to one's overall resistance to disease. Effects detrimental to the health of an individual carrying a harmful or lethal gene may not appear unless the patient's health environment is appropriately poor. For example, the likelihood of diabetes is greater in families where there is known to be a genetic risk of the disease. However, the occurrence of diabetes may also be related to overweight, so the genetic influence can in some instances be mitigated by good nutritional practices. When genetic disposition to disease may be mediated or worsened by environmental influences, the nurse can encourage health behavior designed to forestall possible genetic consequences. Thus the nurse in the community becomes integrally involved in the processes of dealing with health problems related to genetic risk.

THE INADEQUATELY FUNCTIONING FAMILY

In a few families all the elements are present for effective family interaction, but for some reason family function is inadequate. The causes for this failure may rest in immature or inappropriate attitudes toward family responsibility, a failure to develop family goals and identity, or a lack of homemaking and family living skills.

Immature Attitudes

Immature or inappropriate attitudes toward family responsibility are reflected in health practices. The average age of marriage in the United States at present is just under 20 years. For many, the age is considerably lower. When the marriage partners are very young, it may be difficult for them to assume family responsibilities when they go counter to those things that are felt to be important in their chronological age group. In many instances the bride is already pregnant at the time of marriage; her pregnancy sets higher demands on the marriage from the start.[10] Also, early marriages may precede the completion of the young husband's job training, and the continuing parental support of married offspring is increasingly frequent. This maintenance of parental support may strengthen family bonds along generational lines, but on the other hand it may make it difficult for the new family to establish its separate identity. When the help comes from one or the other family rather than from both, tensions may erupt between the young marrieds themselves; too, there may be resentment of the need for help.[11]

Sometimes immature attitudes toward marriage and the family reflect the personal developmental problems of individuals; the woman who uses blackmail tactics to satsify her demands for a fur coat or a new range and the father who courts the admiration of his sons by relinquishing his responsibility as an adult in favor of an "all boys together" relationship are examples. These attitudes hamstring both the father who is trying to offer guidance to his son on the health hazards of smoking and the mother who is asked to meet a crisis that demands some personal sacrifice on her part. Furthermore, parental immature attitudes are frequently reflected in the parents' own health practices such as excessive smoking and ignoring demands for adequate sleep.

Group functioning—the character of the whole network of reciprocal relationships within the family—as well as individual functioning, affects the family. Dominance of one member of the family, favoring one child above the others, or a lack of intra-family communication may hamper required health action.

Failure To Develop Family Identity

The failure to develop family identity and goals makes concerted family efforts difficult. Some families appear to be always a collection of individuals rather than an integrated, functioning group. They may be polite and considerate without really sharing their thoughts and ideas. They may respect each other's individual rights to the extent that there is little feeling of any constraints imposed by being one of a group; the problem of any member is seen primarily as *his own* problem. For example, if the tasks of the family have been divided in such a way that the mother of the family is responsible for matters relating to child rearing and health care of the children, the father may feel that it is not his responsibility to interfere, to back her up, or in any way to get involved with her problem. The mother may, on the same basis, exert considerable effort toward the health care of the young children; but as soon as they reach the age where they can reason, she will leave all decisions up to them, saying, "It's your life."

This lack of any central sense of identity or goal may leave youngsters feeling quite isolated. It deprives the individual members both of the support that is needed at times of decision or crisis and of the human experience of surrendering one's own immediate wish in favor of another's.

Often this attitude appearing early in a marriage changes as the family grows and matures and as greater mutuality of interests and concerns develops. Time takes care of the situation. In other families, however, this attitude may persist as a durable family characteristic. There is usually little that the nurse can do to remedy such a situation. She can appeal for support when it appears to be indicated. For the most part, however, she must work within the constraints that this sort of family functioning imposes.

Lack of Housekeeping Skills

Despite the recent proliferation of family-life courses, there is in fact only very casual preparation of young people for married family life and homemaking. Many of the young find the point of view and content of these formal classes irrelevant. For the most part girls and boys receive the same formal educational preparation, yet they are expected to undertake very different roles when they establish a family.

But family education for family life may be equally inadequate. Young people who come from families where housekeeping patterns are poor, child management casual and chaotic, and money management unrealistic have little preparation for participation as family partners.

The nurse may identify pressure points where poor household management endangers the family's health, and she may help them to develop a sounder base of operations. For example, reckless handling of money can mean an erratic diet, which is a true health hazard to the small child. Likewise, careless housekeeping is a large factor in home accidents; a failure to pick up toys, or to repair a lamp with a frayed cord may lead to serious consequences.

The nurse should acquaint herself with the community resources that exist for the improvement of housekeeping skills. In housing developments, community action centers, agricultural extension groups, or voluntary organizations, there may be classes in homemaking. Such courses usually include content on food preparation, clothing repair, and purchasing problems.

It may seem that little mention has been made of the health facets of care in these discussions of vulnerable families, but the cause of the health problem may often lie in the family itself; and the method of dealing with the health problems may be by bringing pressure to bear on the family situation as a whole.

The goal in working with vulnerable families is change rather than adjustment. The approach is the positive one of using the capacities of the family and the nurse to modify a situation, thereby raising the threshold of vulnerability.

REFERENCES

1. Buell, Bradley, *et al.*: Community Planning for Human Services. Columbia University Press, New York, 1952, p. 1.
2. Geissmar, Ludwig, and LaSorte, Michael: The Multiproblem Family. Association Press, New York, 1964.
3. Spence. Sir James. *et al.*: A Thousand Families in Newcastle-on-Tyne. Oxford University Press, Oxford; 1954, p. 120.
4. Hill, Reuben: Generic features of families under stress. *In* Parad, Howard (ed.): Crisis Intervention. Family Association of America, New York, 1965, p. 40.
5. American Women: Report of the President's Commission on the Status of Women, U.S. Government Printing Office, Washington, D.C., 1963, p. 4.
6. Gunn, Alexander: Vulnerable Groups—1. Lives of loneliness: the medical-social problems of divorce and widowhood. Nurs. Times, *64:*391, March, 1968.
7. Who are the Working Mothers? U.S. Department of Labor, Leaflet 37, 1967.
8. *Ibid.*
9. Haskins, Dr. Caryl: *In* The New York Times, January 30, 1969.
10. Blood, Robert: Trends of change in American life. *In* Comprehensive Health Care for Children and Families: Report of a Conference, Dearborn, Michigan, 1967. University of Michigan School of Public Health, Ann Arbor, 1967, p. 1.
11. Sussman, M., and Burchinal, Lee: Parental aid to married children: implications for family functioning. Marriage and Family Living, *24:*320, November, 1962.

SUGGESTED READINGS

Brantl, Virginia, and Essingler, Phyllis: Genetics: implications for the nursing curriculum. Nurs. Forum, *1:*90, Spring, 1962.
Geissmar, Ludwig, and LaSorte, Michael: The multiproblem family. Association Press, New York, 1964.
Gunn, Alexander: Vulnerable groups—1. Lives of loneliness: the medical-social problems of divorce and widowhood. Nurs. Times, *64:*391, March, 1968.
Hillsman, Gladys M.: Genetics and the nurse. *In* Stewart, Dorothy, and Vincent, Pauline (eds.): Public Health Nursing. William C. Brown Company, Publishers, Dubuque, 1968, Chapter 24.
Jolly. Elizabeth, and Blum, Henrik: The role of public health in genetic counseling. Amer. J. Public Health, *56:*186, February, 1966.
Sussman, M., and Burchinal, Lee: Parental aid to married children: implications for family functioning. Marriage and Family Living, *24:*320, November, 1962.
Tips, R. L, and Lynch, H. T.: Impact of genetic counseling upon the family milieu. J. A. M. A., *184:*183, April, 1963.
Who Are the Working Mothers? U.S. Department of Labor, U.S. Government Printing Office, Washington, D.C., 1967.

The Growing Family: Reduction of Risk in Childbearing and Infancy

THE GROWING FAMILY

The growing family is considered a valuable national resource, and the health of the family — especially of mother and child — has been a traditional community concern. Throughout the world, nursing and nurse midwifery have played a key role in the important task of safeguarding family health.

The growing family represents a large segment of the population. In 1965 there were in the United States 28.3 million families with children under 18 years of age. The 70,432,000 children under 18 constituted 36 percent of the population. Most of these children (88 percent) were living with their parents.[1]

The people of the United States have given many tangible evidences of their concern for the growing family. In 1910 President Theodore Roosevelt approved the first White House Conference on Children; and since then, these conferences have been convened each decade to bring together experts in the field to study and make recommendations on the problems faced by the nation's children. The Children's Bureau, established within the framework of the national government, was organized two years later in 1912 to "investigate and report on all matters pertaining to the welfare of children and child life among all classes of our people." Typical (but by no means inclusive) activities included massive grant programs to state and local government and voluntary agencies to expand services to disadvantaged groups, model legislation for the protection of children (battered children, for example) as a guide for states, support of clinical and basic research into causes and care of mental retardation and other interferences with development, consultation services for crippled children, and studies of life styles of low-income families.[2] The functions of this bureau have recently been distributed throughout other government units that continue in similar ways to exert national leadership on behalf of mothers and children. Now, every state and local government in the United States has some program in maternal and child care.

Professional associations have also shown their special concern. As early as 1873 the American Medical Association organized a department on obstetrics and diseases of women and children;[3] in 1921 the American Public Health Association created a section on maternal and child health; and in 1930 the National Academy of Pediatrics was formed.

Voluntary groups, too, have been persistently busy: their activities have ranged from the "milk stations," organized in the 1920's in New York City to provide safe milk for infants and to combat the scourge of infant diarrhea, to the Citizens Committee on Children and Youth, formed as an outgrowth of the 1960 White House Conference.

Health care of the growing family must be viewed as more than maternal and infant care. The health challenge implicit in childbearing and child rearing affects every member of the family as well as the community at large. The addition of a child to the family may create problems of emotional security for the siblings, economic concern for the father, and physical and management problems for the mother. The additive effect of family size may create serious economic developmental problems for a community or for a country.

There are three general problem areas with which the community health nurse must deal in providing nursing care to the growing family:
1. Problems associated with childbearing and early infancy.
2. Problems associated with child development and child rearing.
3. Problems associated with prevention and care of childhood illness or injury.

The first of these problem areas is the concern of this chapter; the two remaining areas will be discussed in Chapter 13.

THE RISK TO MOTHER AND INFANT

Childbearing and early infancy are inevitably accompanied by some degree of stress, especially for the mother and infant. For the family, this is usually the time at which they feel a need for some additional help or emotional support. For the community, there is need to reduce maternal risk in order to maintain an intact healthy family that is able to take its place in society and to fulfill its societal obligations.

Between 1940 and 1964 the rate of maternal deaths in the United States dropped from 376 deaths per 100,000 live births to 33.3 per 100,000 live births. During that same period, deaths of infants under one year of age fell from 47 per 1000 live births to 24.8.[4] However, infant mortality in the United States ranked tenth among advanced countries

Table 3.   Maternal and Infant Deaths, 1940 and 1964, for White and Nonwhite Populations. (From *Statistical Abstract of the U.S.*, 87th ed. U.S. Government Printing Office, Washington, D.C., 1966, p. 55.)

	Maternal Deaths per 100,000 Live Births			*Infant Deaths per 1,000 Live Births*		
	White	*Nonwhite*	*Total*	*White*	*Nonwhite*	*Total*
1940	319.8	773.5	376.0	43.2	73.8	47.0
1964	22.3	89.9	33.3	21.6	41.1	24.8

(From *Statistical Abstract of the U.S.*, 87th ed. U.S. Government Printing Office, Washington, D.C., 1966, p. 55.)

during the years 1961 to 1963; the United States' rate of 25.6 deaths in children under one year per 1000 infants is compared to a rate well under 16 deaths per 1000 infants in the Netherlands and Sweden.[5]

Furthermore, substantial differences in rates continue to characterize certain subgroups in the population. For example, as shown in Tables 3 and 4, the nonwhite population continues to have a greater risk than does the white population. Similar differences can be observed in different socioeconomic levels.[6]

In a recent conference concerned with the education of professional health workers, it was felt that a reasonable goal would be a reduction to 10 maternal deaths per 100,000 live births, a decrease to approximately one third of our present rate.[7] In 1959 McMahon suggested that a realistic minimum for infant mortality (deaths under one year of age) is about 12 deaths per 100,000 live births; he set the possible lower limit at approximately 8.[8]

Even though the causes of some conditions, such as prematurity, are not fully understood and even though truly effective treatment must await further research, most professional health workers feel it would still be possible to reduce these mortality rates. Recently inaugurated massive programs to provide comprehensive care to mothers and children in low-income, high-risk groups are designed to bring what is

Table 4.   Fetal and Neonatal Deaths, 1945 and 1964, for White and Nonwhite Populations. (From *Statistical Abstract of the U.S.*, 87th ed. U.S. Government Printing Office, Washington, D.C., 1966, p. 55.)

	Fetal Deaths per 1000 Live Births[1]			*Neonatal Deaths per 1000 Live Births*[2]		
	White	*Nonwhite*	*Total*	*White*	*Nonwhite*	*Total*
1945	21.4	42.0	23.9	23.3	32.0	24.3
1964	14.1	28.2	16.4	16.2	26.5	17.9

[1]Fetal deaths gestation of 20 weeks or more or not stated.
[2]Deaths of infants under 28 days old, exclusive of fetal deaths.

already known to bear on the care of this population; it is hoped that the gap between different groups in the population can be narrowed.

The community health nurse contributes to the reduction of avoidable risk in three ways:

1. By identifying and providing intensified care to high-risk groups.
2. By providing supervision and support throughout the maternity cycle in order to recognize or avert unanticipated risk.
3. By providing prepregnancy and interpregnancy care, which adds to the family's physical and emotional capability for coping with the problems attendant on childbearing.

IDENTIFICATION AND INTENSIFIED CARE OF HIGH-RISK GROUPS

High-risk groups include:
1. All vulnerable families with members of childbearing age. (These groups are described in Chapter 11.)
   a. Low-income groups.
   b. Immature or incomplete families.
   c. Genetically disadvantaged families.
2. Families in which the mother is subject to special obstetric risk. Mothers who are especially vulnerable include the following.
   a. Those under 16 or over 35 years of age.
   b. Those having poor nutritional status or poor food habits, particularly those women who have anemia, who are substantially overweight or underweight, and who report an inadequate diet.
   c. Those with a history of systemic or metabolic disorders, especially hypertensive disease or genetic risk.
   d. Those undergoing a first or fifth (or more) pregnancy.
   e. Those with a history of previous obstetric complication: difficult labor, premature labor, or fetal loss.
3. Families in which the infant is at special risk. Special risk infants include the following.
   a. Those premature or low weight for age—2500 grams or less at birth.
   b. Those showing poor progress in hospital, especially infants who have a low Apgar score, a prolonged hospital stay, or who have undergone difficult maternal labor.
   c. The child who is failing to thrive.
   d. The damaged child.
   e. The child with a very poorly nourished mother.
   f. The child of a mother who suffered viral disease, especially rubella, during pregnancy.
4. Families in which deleterious emotional or social factors are operative.
   a. Those in which the baby is unwanted, especially those families in which efforts have been made to interrupt the pregnancy.
   b. Those in which pregnancy has been undertaken for secondary reasons such as to hold together a shaky marriage or to force a marriage.

   c. Those which display grossly inadequate family functioning such
      as irresponsibility, alcoholism, or a history of child neglect.
   d. Those in which the mother is unmarried.

Early Identification Is Important

The health of the infant is very much affected by the conditions which
pertain during the intra-uterine period of his life, and these in turn are
dependent upon the nutrition and general health of the mother. Furthermore, both the growth and development of the child after birth are
dependent in large measure upon the quality of nurturing the family is
able to provide. Parents, in turn, must derive satisfaction from their
family roles and be enabled to meet their parental obligations. If the
mother is grossly malnourished, whatever the reason, or if her ability to
mother (or the father's ability to assume the fatherhood role) is endan-
gered by emotional or social inadequacies or stress within the family,
both the parents and the child will be jeopardized.

Out-of-wedlock births have increased from 7 births per 1000 unmarried women between the ages of 15 and 44 in 1939, to 23.4 births in
1964 when there were 275,000 out-of-wedlock births in the United
States. Risks to mother and baby are usually increased in this circumstance; in one New York City study, infant mortality was much higher,
and premature birth was about doubled, in the out-of-wedlock group.[9]

MULTIPLE APPROACHES REQUIRED

The early identification of high-risk pregnant groups is not always a
simple problem, inasmuch as the family itself must most often take the
initiative in reporting early pregnancy and in seeking care.

It would be desirable to identify high-risk groups in the prepregnancy
period in order to encourage early and comprehensive use of the services available. When the incidence of multiple adverse conditions is
known to be high, it may be best to consider whole populations in
certain low-income areas as operating at special risk.

The importance of a careful and probing nursing history in identifying
undisclosed or covert risk factors cannot be overemphasized. The informal setting of the home visit and the one-to-one and usually close nurse-
family relationship, combined with the opportunity for observation of
the family in its own setting, give the community health nurse an unusual
advantage in seeking out these important data.

Records of high-risk mothers should be clearly identified, both during
the period they are in the active case load and after they are put in the
closed or inactive file; a notation in red ink in an obvious place of the
record, a tab, a special sticker, or any other device that will make the
record stand out from the others will serve. In this way the family does
not get "lost" in the file or fail to be identified as a high-risk family
immediately upon readmission to service.

Prepregnant groups may be reached through health and education
programs in schools, through community action centers, or through
other community health educational activities. Some nurses have used
the "every one teach one" approach, asking pregnant mothers who come

under care to serve as emissaries of the health services: to help locate others who should receive care and to talk with prepregnant friends. In some settings, indigenous short-trained paid or volunteer workers may be used to inform people of the urgency of early care and to explain the availability of health services to the community.

Intensified Care of Mother and Family

For the most part, high-risk mothers need just what other mothers need, but they need it more acutely. In only a few instances will there be special medications, diets, or treatments that create unusual care patterns. The intensity of the care required is the main difference in caring for high-risk mothers.

More frequent nurse-family visits are usually needed to provide for intensive monitoring of the mother's condition and to assure concentrated and inclusive teaching, support, and referral. The crucial need for mustering the support and assistance of the patient's husband, mother, or "important others" may require special efforts on the part of the nurse. Furthermore, increased risk in childbearing is frequently accompanied by other adverse conditions in the family as a whole, including a low level of family functioning. These related problems must be equally the responsibility of the community health nurse. For these reasons, families designated "high risk" may require from a third to a half more nursing time than that needed for a family hailing from a low-risk population.

The identification and intensified care of high-risk groups is an area of community nursing care peculiarly dependent upon the efforts of those in the community for the effective administration of the nursing program. Thus the nurse must plan for the education of volunteer or paid aides; for general educational efforts in school, industry, and other ready-made groups; and for constant liaison with health, welfare, and social organizations that are likely to be in contact with those who should know about the need for and availability of care services. This is one nursing task that "can't be done by one"!

NURSING SUPERVISION DURING THE MATERNITY CYCLE: MONITORING

Community health nursing operates in two ways to maintain or improve health during the maternity cycle:

1. Monitoring: continually evaluating the condition or environment of the patient and her family for evidence of need for special care.

2. Conditioning: preparing the family to deal with the physical, emotional, and social changes incident to childbearing.

Monitoring Is Shared with the Entire Care Group

Monitoring is a task shared with the physician, other nurses, and the family. Early and continuing medical supervision is an essential element in prenatal care. It has been shown to be associated with favorable obstetric outcomes. The physician's observations and evaluations are supplemented by the observations of others, particularly the nurse and the family. Unless these additional observations can be communicated to the physician, he may miss many important clues, either because his time with the patient is so limited or because the patient may not be able to recognize her problems or verbalize her concerns during the visit to the physician.

The ways in which the community health nurse will share responsibility with the physician and with nurses in other settings will differ. Nurse midwives or obstetric nurse specialists may take great responsibility in case management, as may the community health nurse working in isolated areas where there are few physicians available and the distances to medical care are great. Some physicians will take the major responsibility for counseling the expectant mother and leave little for the community health nurse to do other than support his instruction and perhaps concern herself with other family members who may be affected by the pregnancy but who are not seen by the physician. When comprehensive maternal and infant projects extend into home care as well as clinic care, new patterns of coordination may be required of the community health nurse.

Most often neglected is the support of the private family physician, who often works without the social work, nutrition nursing, and other technical support the clinic physician takes for granted. The community health nurse may work directly with the private physician's patients (either singly or in groups), or she may work through the physician's office nurse or receptionist. It is important that there be plenty of opportunity for communication among the various individuals or groups caring for a particular family in order to ensure continuing relevant and coordinated care.

Monitoring must involve the family, too. The nurse cannot expect to be present when changes occur that suggest a need for immediate care or for further study. Therefore she must depend upon the family's ability and willingness to recognize and report symptoms or concerns that have health significance. In some instances the expectant mother herself may take most of the responsibility; in other situations she may seek the help of her husband, of her mother, or of a friend who has had childbearing experience. For example, the husband may help monitor his wife's food intake or a trusted friend may check with the patient who has missed a clinic appointment.

The Monitoring Process

The frequency of direct contact with the family and the actual content of the monitoring will vary considerably with the style of medical practice, the capability of the family, and the condition of the patient.

PROVISION OF EARLY MEDICAL SUPERVISION

Assuring early and adequate medical supervision is the first and basic step in the monitoring process. The proportion of women who receive medical care early in pregnancy has gone up. Of all those who saw a physician at least once in 1953, 65 percent saw the physician by the end of the third month of pregnancy, and 38 percent saw him during the first or second month. By 1963 the proportion of those seeing the physician by the end of the third month had risen to 78 percent, and those seeing him during the first or second month rose to 52 percent.

However, the proportion seeking early medical care was lower among low-income families. In 1953 only 42 percent of those in low-income families saw a physician by the end of the third month, compared to 89 percent in the high-income group, and in 1963 the rates were 58 percent and 88 percent, respectively.[10]

The community health nurse can do much to impress on the public the urgency of early prenatal care and to identify and deal with the barriers of obtaining care. "Red tape"; difficulties of transportation or of securing a baby-sitter; a lack of confidence in, or a failure to recognize the need for, required care; or intervening work or family demands may all lead to delay. Yet such care is crucial during the first trimester of pregnancy when the fetus is so susceptible to damage.

RECOGNITION OF ADVERSE CONDITIONS IN MOTHER OR BABY

Obviously, the focal concern in the monitoring task is the early recognition of adverse conditions in the mother: finger or ankle swelling; excessive weight gain before 30 weeks' gestation, which may presage hypertension; too nonchalant an acceptance of an unplanned pregnancy, which might indicate mental distress or contemplated abortion; listlessness or apathy; or undue prolongation of prenatal nausea and vomiting. These are areas in which the physician takes the major monitorial responsibility.

EVALUATION OF "NORMAL" DISCOMFORTS

Because such discomforts as backache, nausea, vomiting, and occasional depression are so common during pregnancy, they may tend to be discounted by the patient. As a consequence, she may suffer unnecessary discomfort; or even worse, she may not realize the importance of reporting when these conditions are persistent or unusually severe. The physician, too, may tend to minimize the discomforts, especially when the patient is shy and takes a rather fatalistic attitude about her own well-being. The nurse may need to interpret the patient's responses to the physician. She must remember that one mother will discount or disregard her symptoms, whereas another will tend to overreact. The community health nurse serves as the link between family and doctor: she can alert the family concerning those things to watch for, and she can aid the busy doctor in diagnosing and treating the patient who seeks treatment.

ATTENTION TO OTHER HEALTH THREATS

Exposure to rubella or other infectious diseases or to roentgenography in early pregnancy, contact with a family member who has tuberculosis, or the history of genetic fault are all important indices of need for more intensive medical surveillance and study.

Deleterious health practices, such as grossly inadequate diet, exercise or recreational habits that require great physical effort or interfere with sleep, or unsuccessful attempts to terminate the pregnancy, represent another important area of monitoring.

Unusual Stress—the death of a family member, marital difficulties, economic problems, or an overanxious and ubiquitous interfering mother or mother-in-law—may start a series of reactions that can be harmful to mother and baby.

Adverse effects of the situation on other family members may pose a health threat. The embarrassed adolescent whose mother is having a "menopause baby," the somewhat resentful, ambitious husband who believes the pregnancy could and should have been averted, the about-to-be displaced sibling who has mixed feelings about "this little brother or sister," and the parents of an unmarried mother who feel "disgraced," all have very real problems and may need help. Failure to effectively handle these problems may lead to more serious manifestations and present a threat not only to the individual who undergoes them but to others in the family as well.

PREPREGNANCY AND INTERPREGNANCY CARE: CONDITIONING

As noted previously, the term *conditioning* refers to the preparation of the family to deal with the physical, emotional, and social changes incident to childbearing.

Preparation for childbearing and for parenthood begins long before a baby is born. Ideally, the expectant parents should have experienced a satisfying relationship with their own parents, should have achieved good physical and emotional health, should have benefited from family-life education during their school years, and should have had adequate counseling before marriage about childbearing. The couple should have received adequate education about methods of controlling family size and taken steps to correct any reproductive disorders before marriage. When the wife becomes pregnant, they should ideally seek early and continuous medical supervision throughout the period of pregnancy and early infancy. The community nursing care provided throughout childhood may serve to improve maternal and infant care to a degree not now possible.

Preconceptional and interconceptional care is the look of the future. Even though now there is little in the way of an organized program for preconceptional and interconceptional care, the community health nurse may find many ways of interjecting such care: for instance, prolonging the supervision of high-risk patients and their families (including those particularly susceptible to crisis) beyond the usual postpartum period or integrating material into the ongoing programs of health education provided to parent discussion groups.

Preconceptional and interconceptional care might include the following content:
1. Instruction in reproductive processes.
2. Training in child care.
3. Orientation to family planning and family planning resources.
4. Discussion of the effect of parental attitudes on child development.
5. Marriage counseling services (nurse would refer applicants).
6. Growth and development and anticipatory guidance.
7. Effect of physical and social environment on health and development.
8. The nature and importance of health maintenance.
9. The nature and services of the health-care system and the problems in utilization.
10. The importance of correcting "small" defects.

Obviously, this would not all be the responsibility of the community health nurse, nor is it likely that this content can be offered in formal courses to individuals or groups; but the community health nurse may work to enrich the services she affords to those presently in her case load and to reinforce the care provided by other individuals.

The Nurse's Responsibility

During the months before delivery, there is an opportunity to help the mother and her family safeguard the mother's health and that of the infant *in utero,* to prepare the parents to be intelligent collaborators in the birth process, to anticipate the period of physical and mental readjustment following delivery, and to plan for the responsibilities of caring for the new baby.

This "nine months to get ready" is valuable, since it is a time in which there is unusual motivation in general matters relating to family health. The nurse's help is directed toward enabling the family to:
1. Provide any special care that has been ordered by the physician.
2. Learn their role in the maternity health-care program.
3. Develop skills required in childbearing and child rearing.
4. Improve general health practices in order to assure a better maternity experience and also to provide a long-term investment in better health care.

PROVIDING SPECIAL CARE

For some mothers—those with anticipated complications or those at special risk in other ways—treatments, medications, exercises, periodic tests or measurements, or special rest may be prescribed to relieve an existing condition or to prevent later difficulties. The nurse may be responsible for carrying out certain tests—blood pressure and urine determinations, for example—in intervals between clinic visits. Sometimes the actions required of the family, such as taking iron pills or vitamins daily, are in themselves simple but are hard to maintain because they require regular and continuing attention. At other times conformity to the regimen ordered may be much more difficult, as when the woman with an irritable uterus and a history of miscarriage or premature birth must spend much of her time in bed. Here the nurse's responsibility is to be sure that the patient and the family understand the reason for the recommended action, that they know how to carry it out, and that they are sufficiently convinced of its importance. It may take constant encouragement by the nurse and her coworkers to help the family make the necessary effort.

There is need, also, to suggest the simple homely aids to combat the discomforts of pregnancy: the dry cracker in the morning, the small frequent meals for nausea, the changes in posture to help relieve backache. The patient needs the assurance that the nurse does indeed know of these measures and is aware of their importance.

HELPING FAMILY MEMBERS REALIZE ROLES AND SKILLS

Because childbearing requires a considerable amount of adjustment and change, it may leave prospective parents vulnerable to anxiety and self-doubt, and lacking in adaptive mechanisms with respect to their new role. The nurse can be very helpful with these problems, providing both tangible help and what Stone calls "a womanly empathy."[11] For the most part, the problems are fleeting and yield well to what might be called "common-sense" measures.

The objective of family monitoring (that is, early recognition of conditions adverse to health of mother or child) has already been discussed. To be effective at their task, however, a family must have at their disposal the authority and the knowledge required.

Development of Confidence. First, the parents are expected to develop commitment to and confidence in their ability to handle parental tasks. Fathers as well as mothers may have serious doubts about their ability to fulfill this role. They may remember their own resentment toward inadequate parents, and they may fear being the same to their own children; they may worry about the financial obligations entailed in parenthood; or they may fear that a happy marital relationship will end with these new responsibilities. These anxieties can be heightened by the wife's adaptive mechanisms — her retreat to her own mother for advice and support — which seem to separate her from her husband. She may be depressed. Although usually very independent she may suddenly take a highly dependent stance, especially if the pregnancy was unplanned or requires a sharp change in her usual mode of living (such as leaving her job). She, too, may worry about whether she can be a "good" mother. An understanding of the interrelated physical, emotional, and psychological changes that occur with pregnancy can help the young family to deal with them effectively.

Alternatively, parents, especially teenage parents, may seem to be totally uncomprehending as to the responsibilities they will actually be expected to face. The young expectant mother may croon about the "living doll" she will have, without realizing that this doll will take much more care than the inanimate variety; or parents may feel there is no need to adapt highly unsuitable living conditions to the baby's needs and will expect to continue with such habits as the late dance and drinking parties. Siblings, too, will need help in getting ready for the new baby.

Marital Sharing.   The habit of marital sharing may be developed or strengthened during the childbearing period. The wife's tendency to withhold information from the husband (the I-don't-want-him-to-worry or I-don't-want-him-to-think-I'm-a-baby attitude) or the husband's possible guilt about the pregnancy or his probable shyness about discussing it (the it's-your-problem-so-you-handle-it attitude) may lead to later, more serious breaks in marital communication. The community health nurse can do much to help avoid this by her own planning, being sure to make some visits at a time the father can be present, talking with the mother about discussing certain aspects of care with her husband, or encouraging the wife to include little details when she writes to a husband on military duty. The couple must realize that the wife's tendency to go back to her own mother at this period may put a strain on the husband-wife relationship, and they must learn to deal wisely with the wife's need for this security.

The nurse may act directly or indirectly in dealing with these problems of support. By being available and visible to the prospective parents and by her listening and interested attitude, she can encourage the family's ability to express their concerns, which is, after all, the first step in dealing with problems. Sometimes these expressions can be coaxed out by leading comments such as "Lots of times after starting a pregnancy, mothers wonder if they did the right thing . . . " or "I guess we all worry about things like this; it's such a big step to take! . . ."

Enlist the Help of Others.   It may be helpful to enlist others in the job of support. A wise older neighbor, the grandmother-to-be, the physician, the aide in the agency, and the school counselor are possible helpers.

It is essential that parents understand that they will still be themselves in addition to being parents — that as parents they will still be expected to "do their own thing." There are many parental styles; not every mother looks like the Whistler portrait!

Sharing in the Birth Process.   The ability to be an intelligent participant in the birth process requires that the patients have an understanding of the process of labor and delivery and of the part played by the physician, drugs, and themselves in this process. "Understanding," in this context, is more than knowing about the process; the young mother who knows the physiologic facts about delivery may still have little confidence in her own ability to deal with the phenomenon. She may be afraid of "making a fool" of herself, or she may have great fears about the actual process of birth. Husband and wife need to know about the conditions that will influence the doctor's decision to intervene in the birth process or to use or not to use drugs; they must, in short, learn to have trust in the medical system. If the husband is encouraged by the hospital to be with his wife during labor, he should understand his role as supporter. Knowledge of the hospital's policies and regulations helps the young father know how he can best support his wife during her hospital stay and permits the couple to facilitate matters by bringing the right records, information, clothes, and equipment to the hospital.

Skills Practice.   Skills practice may also increase parents' confidence and make it easier for them to assume their new roles. Practicing how to bathe a small baby and how to deal with simple emergencies is valuable preparation for the expectant mother and, in some instances, for other prospective child care agents as well.

Such skills practice may also provide an opportunity for mothers to benefit from peers who have had the experience they now anticipate. Young mothers may bring their own babies to a prenatal study group and demonstrate how to handle the infant while the inexperienced mother-to-be practices with the model. Mothers may come into parents' classes to discuss what is expected of one at the hospital and during the delivery process.

Special Problems of the Unmarried Mother.   The unmarried mother starts pregnancy with the handicap of not having a marital partner with whom to share responsibility. In addition she may face the hazard of social disapproval, family rejection, or ego diminishment resulting from a sense of guilt. When the expectant unwed mother is an adolescent, she has the problem of the crisis of adolescence to which is added the maturational crisis of a first pregnancy—rather a hard load for a young girl to handle. The problem may loom especially large in an upwardly mobile family.

However, as with any nursing situation, there is no formula for diagnosing and dealing with the problems of out-of-wedlock pregnancy. The situation is highly individual and highly personal in its manifestations.

If the pregnancy occurs in a cultural group that places a high value on children, concern for and delight in the child may override all other considerations; and the marital condition may represent only a nuisance or a temporary disappointment rather than a calamity.

The problem is seldom that simple, however. The pregnancy may be a manifestation of other problems, such as loneliness, isolation, low self-esteem, or even a desire for revenge, and these situations can be dealt with only through the most sophisticated of case work techniques. Of course, the reason for pregnancy may be that the girl "just fell in love" and reacted in a simple and natural way. There may be no deep feelings of guilt or embarrassment attendant on this situation but only a satisfaction of demonstrated "womanliness" and of having someone to love. Also, sex may have been experienced as fun, with a cost tag attached that may or may not be considered unreasonable for the satisfaction achieved. Individual reaction to the situation also varies widely, from happy acceptance—"I'd like to have a cute little baby of my own"—to rejection, guilt, and shame. The lack of a husband's support may be compensated for by the strong support of the girl's own parents; sometimes this parental support extends to the point that the baby becomes the charge of the maternal grandmother and the new mother goes back to being a child in the family again. It is important for parents to realize their daughter's need for understanding; their successful empathy can make a tremendous contribution to the mental and physical health of their daughter and her child.

The health problems engendered by out-of-wedlock pregnancy include:

1. Physical inadequacy or risk attendant on the age or physical condition of the mother. (In this, the unmarried mother does not have any greater risk than does the married mother of the same age.)

2. Risks incident to the results of poor handling of the health problem: seeking abortion, attempting to "lose the baby" by excessive physical activity or the use of purgatives or other drugs, concealing pregnancy, failing to seek early care, and a rejection of the care and advice provided.

Since illegitimacy tends to be higher among low-income groups, the unmarried mother, more often than the married mother, may share the risks of all low-income groups. In other words, the risk level of the unmarried mother may be more the result of her social milieu and psychological response to the situation than to the physical hazard. When the statistics of pregnancy experience and outcome for married and unmarried mothers are looked at separately by age and socioeconomic status of the mother, the physical differences appear to be sharply reduced; and nursing intervention required with respect to maternity care will for the most part be identical with that required by all expectant mothers.

It is in the area of preventive care and the development of self-help potentials that nursing can have a larger part. The school nurse may have an important role before pregnancy occurs by working with young people and their parents, and interpreting the hazards and problems that out-of-wedlock pregnancies entail. In some areas, there are special programs aimed at girls known to be sexually active; these programs are planned on the premise that it is exceedingly difficult to change such patterns and that planning must be done realistically. Programs for continuing the education of young unmarried mothers and for combining this education with intensive social and health counseling have been established in many cities. McMurray describes a typical special program developed to serve the needs of pregnant, unmarried teenagers.[12] In general these programs are designed to combine and coordinate the efforts of several educational and health agencies and to provide such services as medical and nursing care, personal counseling, health counseling, and training in homemaking or job skills.

Although little concern is expressed for the fathers of these out-of-wedlock babies, they often need help. Usually the help required comes under the heading of social work rather than nursing and encompasses efforts to build intergeneration bridges in the family and to develop responsibility and alternative life satisfactions.

The decision to keep or not keep the baby may be made simply and unquestionably when the grandmother takes the child as her own. But more often it is a difficult decision in which the young mother and her parents may need help. The reasons for wanting to keep the baby are not always obvious. The young mother may consider this child her most precious possession, someone who provides unquestioning love and can be loved in return and who provides or reinforces a sense of identity and achievement. Perhaps her friends are keeping their babies, or perhaps her parents want the baby to stay. Keeping the baby may serve extraneous purposes: keeping a hold on the baby's father or defying or punishing the family or social group. These, too, are problems for the social worker, who will profit from the observations and judgments of the nurse.

One problem the nurse herself must face is the need not to overact in this situation. The patient and family in many instances will need time to get to know the nurse and to learn what help they might expect from her. Too early or too definite advice may shatter a budding nurse-patient relationship. Furthermore, the nurse may find it hard to deal with what seems to her unrealistic or irresponsible behavior. For example, it may seem to the nurse that the plan to keep the baby in the face of a low income, the lack of job skills on the part of the mother, and no likelihood of any responsibility being assumed by the father doesn't make sense. She may not see the capacity for warmth and love that exists in the situation. Also, the young nurse may balk because she feels "this could happen to me."

There may already be too much available advice: a school counselor, a school nurse, an interested teacher, a district nurse, and a minister may all be involved in "helping Bess to solve her problem"; but often each has a different idea of what it would take to do so. Perhaps what Bess most needs is a chance to think for herself.

Since illegitimacy tends to be repeated, a major problem is prevention; and this is a long and difficult road. It may not be possible to reverse the pattern for many of those already pregnant, although some intensive special programs are showing encouraging results. The real prevention would seem to lie in strengthening the family itself so that the child will grow up in an environment in which warmth and affection are tempered with internal discipline and training in responsible action.

THE DEVELOPMENT OF BETTER FAMILY HEALTH PRACTICES

The most significant and lasting conditioning is the development of better general family health practices. Improving general physical capability is an important aspect of the preparation for childbearing. An early general medical appraisal is a vital first step in this process. It permits the correction of handicapping conditions that may threaten mother or baby or that may contribute to unnecessary discomfort during the childbearing period. It also contributes to the mother's general health and hopefully to her understanding of the need for preventive health care for herself and her family.

Supplementation of the diet with medications is frequently desirable, and the nurse can do much to assure that the family follows the advice given. However, the most lasting result is achieved when this instruction is accompanied by education directed toward changing the food habits of the family, thereby building up the general nutritional status not only of the mother but of the family as a whole. Of particular importance to low-income populations is the provision of an adequate protein intake. Pamphlets developed by the Children's Bureau, the Department of Agriculture, or state or local health departments may prove useful aids in teaching family nutrition.*

---

*The list of suggested readings for Chapter 12 is combined with that for Chapter 13 on page 204.

REFERENCES

1. Some Facts and Figures About Children and Youth. U.S. Department of Health, Education and Welfare, Children's Bureau, U.S. Government Printing Office, Washington, D.C., 1967.
2. Goals for Children, Ten Year Objectives for the Children's Bureau, 1960-1970 and Facts About Children's Bureau Program, 1966. U.S. Department of Health, Education and Welfare, Children's Bureau, U.S. Government Printing Office, Washington, D.C.
3. Wallace, Helen: History of development of health services for mothers and children. *In* Health Services for Mothers and Children. W.B. Saunders Company, Philadelphia, 1962, pp. 3-8.
4. Statistical Abstract of the United States. 87th ed., U.S. Government Printing Office, Washington, D.C., 1966, p. 55.
5. Some Facts and Figures About Children and Youth. U.S. Department of Health, Education and Welfare, Children's Bureau, U.S. Government Printing Office, Washington, D.C., 1967.
6. Recent Demographic Trends and Their Effects on Maternal and Child Health Needs and Services. U.S. Department of Health, Education and Welfare, Children's Bureau, U.S. Government Printing Office, Washington, D.C., 1966. pp. 12, 13.
7. Professional Education for Maternal and Child Health: Report of a Conference. American Public Health Association, New York, 1962, pp. 3-4.
8. McMahon, Brian: The Lower Limit of Infant Mortality. Milbank Memorial Fund Quarterly, 1959, pp. 37, 337.
9. Pakter, Jean, Rosner, Henry J., Jacobziner, Harold, and Greenstein, Freida: Out-of-wedlock births in New York City. Amer. J. Public Health, *61*:683, May, 1961 and *61*:846, June, 1968.
10. Progress in Health Services. Health Information Foundation, vol. 15, no. 2, March/-April, 1966, p. 1.
11. Stone, A. R.: Cues to interpersonal distress due to pregnancy. Amer. J. Nurs., *65*:88, November, 1965.
12. McMurray, Georgia A.: Project teen aid: a community action approach to services for pregnant unmarried teen agers. Amer. J. Public Health, *58*:1848, October, 1968.

CHAPTER

13

The Growing Family: Child Development and Childhood Illness

THE ROLE OF THE COMMUNITY NURSE IN CHILD DEVELOPMENT

Parental Skills

Mothering and fathering are important social skills. The quality of mothering and fathering and of the parents' child rearing practices is increasingly recognized as crucial to the physical and social development of children. The deleterious effects of *maternal deprivation* were described by Bowlby in 1951; in 1962, a World Health Organization report reiterated the seriousness of such deprivation for the child and indicated that the quality of the deprivation was also a factor to be considered when predicting the damage maternal deprivation might produce.[1, 2] Though it receives less public attention, *paternal deprivation*— the absence of the father or of a satisfactory father-child relationship— has been implicated in some of the problems of identity experienced by boys in very low-income areas. *Sensory deprivation,* which has been implicated in abnormal or retarded development or learning,[3] may also result from a lack of parental skills. Public health action directed toward preventing parental deprivation in its varied forms is thus a fundamental part of the program for protecting the health of the growing family.

Although the needs of children must entail community action in terms of the provision of adequate family incomes, decent housing, preventive and illness care, and a sound education, social action will be less than successful if the parents, as the leaders in family development, are incapable of assuming or are unwilling to assume their parental responsibilities; and if the family is to carry its share of this responsibility, there is need for the systematic preparation for parenthood and family living.

Jointly, the family and the community should assure each child of:
1. A secure and stimulating environment in which to grow.
2. Protection from avoidable disease or disability.
3. Assistance in the recognition of his own individuality and an appreciation of the rights of others.
4. Prompt and adequate care when he is ill or injured.

In order to carry out these responsibilities in child rearing, the parents will need:
1. Knowledge of what to expect as children grow and develop.
2. A relaxed confidence in their ability to fill the parental role.
3. Proficiency in the homemaking skills required for the daily management and care of children.
4. Confidence and judgment in the use of available health resources.
5. The ability to understand and control their own behavior.

MONITORING THE CARE PLAN IS A SHARED RESPONSIBILITY

The needs of children are unlikely to be met by chance. It takes persistent and planned action on several fronts to achieve proper care. The *family* must take the primary responsibility of planning for child rearing. The parents, especially the mother, are expected to take appropriate action when it is time for a preschool medical checkup, or for immunization. Fulfillment of the immunization schedule is one job that is often undertaken rather haphazardly: immunization during infancy is usually secured because it is an integral part of the infant care program; booster shots, on the other hand, may be forgotten, especially if they are not tied to requirements for going to school. There is need for some practical systematic approach for families planning for health care and also for someone to monitor the overall care plan to be sure that the various parts are carried through at the right time and by the right methods.

The use of a family health record, kept with the other family records such as birth certificates, may prove invaluable in completing history forms or in checking the date of (for instance) the last smallpox immunization. If it were possible to encourage every family to keep such a record, it would provide a guide for family health planning, supply needed information in time of emergency, and encourage positive health action.

Monitoring responsibility may be assumed by the family physician, who reminds the families under his care when certain procedures are due and who, either singly or in coordination with his office staff, develops a systematic assessment and counseling program. The physician in the well-child center may assume the same kind of responsibility, with the nurse in the center or in another community health agency supporting his activities; or the nurse may be the principal monitor, referring the family to the physician as necessary. Sometimes the community health nurse is the principal monitoring force; and through systematic recording and case management, she guides the family in securing the necessary care.

Unfortunately, the community health nurse's case load is developed for the most part not on a population base but rather on a selected group of families or individual patients requiring specific care. As a result, family health planning surveillance for the population as a whole would require substantive restructuring of the organizational patterns under which nursing is provided; moreover, this program of health surveillance would probably be beyond our present nurse manpower capability.

The responsibility of the community nurse, then, must not be to personally monitor the general health-care plan of every family but rather to try to see that every family has some provision for such systematic, sequential, and continuing health action on behalf of children.

KNOWING WHAT TO EXPECT AS CHILDREN GROW

The community health nurse improves the family's capacity to make meaningful observations of their children by *teaching parents what to look for* at given developmental points and how to recognize deviation from expected behavior. The instruction may be bolstered by printed guides or informational pamphlets to which the family may refer. If it is possible to prepare for developments slightly in advance of their probable occurrence, parents feel more comfortable in asking questions about the developmental phenomena now included in the "legitimate content" area and are consequently better prepared to take more effective action to support their children.

In some communities a series of letters is prepared and sent to new parents at intervals after a baby's birth; these letters give information about growth milestones and suggest methods of managing them. Gentry and Paris[4] and Leavitt et al.[5] have developed tools that serve as a guide to the nurse in teaching parents what to expect. The Children's Bureau pamphlet series provides a simple source of information on development, and serves as a guide for parents of children at different ages. Similar materials are frequently developed and distributed by state or local health agencies.

It is important for parents to realize that despite the fact that there are developmental landmarks, each child will grow in his own way. Anticipatory guidance should not lead to a kind of scoring system in which the game is to keep the child at or ahead of the scientists' schedules.

Harper points out that there are predictable problems of growth or behavior for which the parent and professional worker may be prepared.[6] For example, most very young babies will experience some difficulty with eating and sleeping, which they show by crying or wakefulness. The danger of accident or poisoning that comes as a result of the preschool child's characteristic exploration and testing may also be expected and, hopefully, circumvented. Going to school is another predictable maturational crisis for many children.

To observe accurately, the parents must recognize and evaluate the cues the child is giving them; they must learn to communicate despite a semantic gap that arises from age difference. This communication difficulty is quite clear to parents of infants who have not yet learned to speak. They can appreciate the need to try to understand the meaning of the infant's crying — whether it denotes anger, pain, or just a healthy desire for exercise. It is sometimes more difficult for parents to realize that communication with children who *can* verbalize may also be difficult; the child who "lies" when asked about a broken or lost toy may be saying he has learned that honesty brings punishment. Similarly, they may not be aware that the child who "does not obey" may in fact have missed the parents' direction either because of a short interest span or of absorption in another task. Frequently the nurse will be required to do little but bolster the parents' sensitivity to clues and to specific danger signals.

However, in the case of the child at special risk — for instance, when a child is failing to thrive or when parents appear inadequate to their task — the observation of the nurse may become more direct. In these instances the nature of the observation involves evaluation of complex psychosocial aspects, as well as physical aspects, that are beyond the capacities of most parents. Moreover, the attitudes and practices of the parents themselves may be implicated in the etiology of the situation, and their interest in the child's welfare may be low.

CONFIDENCE IN PARENTAL CAPABILITY

Parents as well as children have their own developmental styles. The patterns of mothering (and of fathering) will differ widely among subcultures in the population and, of course, also from family to family. The parental style may be one of stern control or of easy participation, of tightly organized action or of highly casual action. There is no one style that is good or bad. Each couple must learn for themselves how best to meet their responsibilities. The nurse providing guidance in the development of parental skills must be careful not to be influenced by her own experience as a child or as a parent or by her theoretical concept of what "good" parents are like. Rather she should be sure that parents are helped to recognize the importance and the nature of their role and that they are aided in gaining confidence in the skills and techniques required in child care.

Confidence in parental competence (or capability) depends upon the dual pillars of a sense of personal worth and an assurance of technical skill. If parents are to be relaxed and confident in the care of their children, technique alone is not a sufficient guarantee. Each parent must feel he is important to his children and to his spouse and that what he does as a person and as a parent is important to his family and to the community.

In some situations the lack of a sense of personal worth may be the primary barrier. The unmarried mother may feel she does not merit marriage and the respect of others, and she may expect she can not be a good parent because she is not a "good" person. The unemployed or alcoholic father may feel inadequate because he has lost the provider role in the family and as a consequence may feel that his contribution to child development is worthless; he may feel, as one man poignantly stated, "You think he'd want to be like ME?" or he may vent his frustration through child abuse. Obviously the community health nurse cannot expect to remold personalities formed over many years. However, she can use every nursing contact to help support self-esteem in family members, and she can be alert to the effect of personality problems upon parental functioning. Thus one arm of the program of building parental confidence must be sustaining and strengthening a self-image that is consistent with the parental role.

The second facet of parental confidence lies in a feeling of control over the skills and knowledge required, knowing where help and advice may be secured if they are needed. For that reason, whether undertaken by the community health nurse herself or by other groups, the nurse should encourage a systematic educational program reaching both parents and providing them with the essential knowledge needed to make wise decisions. This might take the form of seeing that the content of the family life course in the local high school supplies the needed information, of teaching individual families directly in their own homes, or of arranging for adult classes in child care and management.

THE "QUIET" NEED FOR SKILLS AND REASSURANCE

The daily tasks of child care perplex many parents, especially those of a first child, those of a "caboose baby" who puts in an appearance long after the previous sibling, or those mothers and fathers who are considerably younger or older than most parents.

When mothers are asked what help they want from well-baby care, the most frequent request is reassurance in the simple aspects of care. The nurse can provide some instruction in child care during the prenatal period, either at parents' classes or through individual visits to the home or office. In such a setting there is an opportunity for leisurely practice in skills and, in the case of group work, for sharing ideas and worries with other expectant parents. In the hospital, instruction may be provided relating in particular to bathing and feeding the new baby and to the mother's need for safeguarding her own health. However, the hospital setting and the very short hospital stay limit what can be done. As the child develops, many mothers will feel the need for continued instruction in such simple matters as bathing the baby, when to stop sterilizing bottles, or how to handle crying.

The decision to breast-feed the infant is one in which the mother may need considerable help and support. If the mother elects to breast-feed, she will usually have many questions about leakage, diet, the mechanics of positioning the baby, and the problems of reconciling breast-feeding with social obligations.[7]

Obviously, families will differ greatly in the amount and type of support they need and want. Nurses, too, will differ in the amount of help they are able to give because of either a lack of time or a lack of confidence in this aspect of nursing practice. It will be necessary for the community health nurse to find new and ingenious means to meet this "quiet" need. She can find ways to interject instructional components into the usual well-baby clinics or in the visit to the doctor's office; she may restrict home visiting to those families whose problems seem most overwhelming and use telephone conferences for those whose needs are not so great. She may mobilize volunteer instructors under the Red

Cross teaching program or in the adult health activity sections of the public schools. She can work through individuals, such as the experienced mother in the same block who may become a source of reference, the school nurse, or the nurse in the physician's office.

Because it is not a spectacular need, this need for reassurance and skill may be considered "frosting on the cake." Actually, it is an important factor in increasing the mother's satisfaction in her role and the father's ability to provide support to his wife in many areas other than that of child care. It improves the parent-child relationship, and it is an important arm of prevention.

CONFIDENCE IN THE USE OF HEALTH RESOURCES

Despite the availability of resources for care directed toward health promotion and prevention, many facilities are underused. In a recent study of 375 infants in a North Carolina rural county, only 10 percent received the usually recommended well-child care in the first 14 months of life, and only 41 percent had been fully immunized against diphtheria, pertussis, poliomyelitis, and smallpox.[8] Although distance to the facility may have been a factor, the researchers felt the most important deterrent was a low level of health awareness. The lack of urgency in securing care for well children, particularly after the first year, doubtless contributed.

The community health nurse can do much to encourage adequate use of available services. She may organize the nursing effort in the clinic to provide reminders, to make the clinic experience a pleasant one, and to build up the parents' sense of pride and accomplishment in child care. She can also study and act on the barriers to care. She can use volunteer or short-trained paid workers to supplement her efforts. She can call to the attention of planners the need for extended or different kinds of facilities, so the facilities and the needs and the expectations of the users are congruent. Most important, the community health nurse can communicate her own conviction that the quality of early child care is an important factor in the child's future development.

Child Care Outside the Home

Child care in settings other than the home is increasing and presents special problems. Day care centers, foster homes, extended school care, and all types of informal arrangements are being used to provide care for children whose mothers work or who need an antidote or supplement for an inadequate home environment. Recent government and voluntary efforts have been directed toward replacing haphazard and dangerous child care arrangements with more controlled care. In 1963, 41 states had day care centers using federal and state funds.

Although this kind of care is immeasurably better than the frankly inadequate and expedient arrangements that too often prevail, it is not without problems. There is, of course, the obvious problem of assuring that the out-of-home environment is indeed safe and conducive to the health and development of the child. Nursing activities directed toward such institutions are similar to those involved in providing services to nursing homes (see Chapter 22). Parents may need substantial support when children are placed outside the home. Out-of-home care is often associated with the inadequate or incomplete family, so that the responsible parent may be troubled with loneliness arising from lack of a partner, a sense of bereavement or helplessness at not being able to stay close to the children, or of guilt and anger that the children "have been taken away from me."

Informal sources of substitute care for children require careful evaluation. It is important to know just where and under what conditions children are cared for in the absence of their parents. Often a grandmother or unemployable male, with little motivation and less ability to provide the kind of care so badly needed, may be left to "mind" the children. The community health nurse should attempt to set up a supportive and educational program to be sure that the child is properly protected and that he is receiving the best care possible. Nursing plans for the substitute child care agent or agency should be as carefully and as comprehensively planned as would be the program for the natural mother.

The improvement of parental competence is certainly a powerful factor in assuring adequate protection for children, and the community health nurse is in an exceptionally favorable position to contribute to the development of this competence. However, it is well to remember the observation recently reported by the Newsons to the effect that often parents will develop their own way despite what is taught by "outsiders," such as health professionals, and that parents will indeed have the final word![9]

THE ROLE OF THE COMMUNITY NURSE IN CHILDHOOD ILLNESS AND DISABILITY

The nature of the community health nursing required to deal with the prevention and care of illness and disability in children will depend on the causes of death and disability in one's assigned population and on the degree to which these conditions may be averted or their progress modified by community nursing action.

Some of the most important causes of death or disability may be little affected by community nursing action, or they may require nonspecific action such as improvement of the general health and health awareness of families; for other childhood illnesses, specific community nursing may be a major factor in prevention or care.

The overriding causes of death among infants are due to prenatal or natal conditions; these account for about 60 percent of the neonatal deaths (death in the first 28 days of life). Low birth weight increases the risk enormously. Pneumonia and accidents are also among the leading causes of death in infants.

For children one to four years of age, accidents are the leading cause of death, and pneumonia and congenital malformations are the second most frequent. For school children 5 to 14 years of age, accidents, malignant neoplasms, and congenital malformations head the list.[9a] However, since death rates in the group aged one to fifteen are low, illness estimates may have more significance as an indicator of required nursing action.

Studies on the illness patterns of children, conducted by the National Center for Health Statistics as part of their program for a continuing national health survey, provide much information that has significance for planning community health nursing. The most striking fact to emerge from a recent study was the great frequency of illness among children. The survey revealed that in the year ending June 1961, there were about 291 episodes of acute illness severe enough to require medical attention or to restrict activity for each 100 children; this amounts to almost 3 episodes of illness per child per year. The rate was higher among children under 5 than in children between 5 and 14.[10] This rate is much higher than it is for other age groups in the same population.

Among the acute illnesses, respiratory disease accounted for more than half of the reported episodes, whereas injuries accounted for about 11 percent. (See Fig. 10.)

Longterm illness was also very prevalent among children. In the two year period between July 1959 and June 1961, a survey revealed that there were about 226 chronic illnesses for each 1000 children under 17 years and that 18 percent of the population under 17 years of age had at least one chronic condition.[11] The proportion of those reporting chronic conditions rose with increased age and among those in higher income

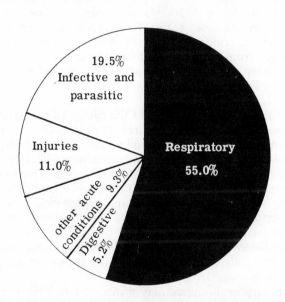

Based on U. S. National Health Survey data for year ending June 30, 1961.

FIGURE 10.   Distribution of acute illnesses among children under 15 years of age. (From Schiffer, Clara G., and Hunt, Eleanor P.: *Illness Among Children.* Children's Bureau Publication 405, U.S. Government Printing Office, Washington, D.C., 1963, p. 4.)

groups. Hay fever and other allergies were responsible for almost 33 percent of these illnesses, and bronchitis and other respiratory diseases accounted for another 15 percent. Of those reporting a chronic disease in children, 61.9 percent had had medical care within a year; but almost 29 percent had had *no* medical care within a year, and 10 percent had neither seen nor talked to a doctor about their condition.[12]

The Major Areas of Community Health Nursing Effort

There will be differences in the programs of community health nurses; these differences will depend on the availability of resources, the programs of related agencies, and the adequacy of each community health nursing staff. However, certain areas may be identified as likely to engage any community health nurses' attention. These include efforts directed toward:

1. Preventing prematurity and caring for the premature.
2. Contributing to the reduction of congenital defects.
3. Preventing, and caring for victims of, accidents and injury.
4. Recognizing and caring for illness.
5. Preventing or controlling communicable disease.
6. Securing early and continuing care for handicapping conditions.

PREMATURITY CARE

In 1963, 8.2 percent of the live births were "low birth weight" infants, who weighed less than 2500 grams. This represented an increase of nearly 25 percent since 1950.[13] These babies operate at a handicap because they are physiologically ill-equipped to stand the rigors of adapting to extra-uterine life. They are much more likely than full term babies to suffer from congenital defect, retardation, and neurologic defect. Harper estimates that the risk of neurologic defect is fifteen times as great among low birth weight babies than it is for normal birth weight infants.[14]

There is still too little known about the causes of prematurity to allow for highly specific preventive measures. Harper estimates about half of the premature births are due to "unknown causes."[15] However, it is possible to identify many of those mothers who are likely to be at higher risk of premature delivery and for whom intensified prenatal care may help lengthen the gestation period. Prematurity tends to occur more often among women who have multiple pregnancies, who have experienced previous fetal loss or obstetric complications, who suffer from chronic hypertension, or who are poorly nourished. Low-income groups must be considered as at special risk. There is some indication that prematurity may also be associated with heavy smoking in multigravidas.[16]

The community health nurse may provide more intensive supervision and anticipatory guidance to this high-risk group in an effort to take preventive action for those who can be helped. Although premature care in the critical early days is usually provided in the hospital, the community health nurse may do much to help the parents in caring for the baby after his return from the hospital. The mother's separation from the baby at the critical period immediately after birth may cause some estrangement, and the size and appearance of the baby may add to her uneasiness. Because she is starting her maternal responsibilities a little later than other mothers, she may need far more than the usual encouragement and reassurance. Additionally, the mother must take greater care in avoding exposure of the baby to infectious disease, and she may expect more feeding problems than usual. For these reasons, families with low birth weight babies may require extra nursing effort in the early infancy period.

REDUCTION OF CONGENITAL DEFECTS

The causes of congenital defect lie in the alteration of the genes or of the chromosomal structure and in the uterine environment of the developing fetus. Preventive measures to be taken against congenital anomalies must then be directed toward genetic controls and the avoidance of conditions that might impair the uterine environment.

For the community health nurse, this two-fold plan requires, primarily, an intensification of the maternal health supervision that is needed by all mothers. A careful history is essential and should include a record of exposure to x-ray or to infectious disease in early pregnancy; possible familial genetic defect; an estimation of the probable nutritional state of the mother as revealed by a history of food intake; careful observations and any unexpected occurrence during pregnancy; and reported use of drugs of which the effects are not fully known. It also involves encouraging and supporting parents in securing prompt and adequate medical appraisal, ideally before conception but certainly early in pregnancy, interpreting medical findings, and helping to implement medical recommendations.

PREVENTION AND CARE OF ACCIDENTS

An occasional home "safety check" or lecture on street and school safety may be a good opener for the kind of instruction required to prevent accidents, but the real pay-off comes only when the family has developed ingrained habits of safe behavior. Storing dangerous household substances such as ammonia or other cleaning agents under the sink is common, since the materials are then handy for use when they are needed. For an all-adult family this is not a dangerous situation; but in a family with a toddler, it may be fatal. The habit of locking the medicine cabinet, replacing medicines out of the reach of children immediately after use, keeping floors and stairways free from articles that may trip someone, or the proper storage of guns and ammunition may also require new housekeeping habits.

The establishment of safe play areas for children, both in and out of the home, may likewise require specific family effort. A grandmother caring for the child of a working mother may find it easier for the child to play in the street where he is certain to find playmates than to take him to the safe play area in a nearby park. It may be difficult to provide in the home a "fenced in" area that will keep small children in sight and protected from stoves or open heaters.

The suburban father driving to the supermarket on a sunny morning when he'd rather be playing golf must have the *habit* of checking the area behind the car and backing out slowly. Children who are cycling need to learn the habit of riding carefully and only on the proper side of the street. Family members must have the habit of fastening seat belts in the car and of being sure small children or dogs riding in the car are properly restrained.

The care of accidental injury must be immediate. Ideally, one member of every family should be prepared — through a Red Cross or other first-aid course — to deal with emergencies. In any event, the mother or other child care person should be familiarized with care of common emergencies. It is wise to post in a conspicuous and readily available place directions for first-aid care of accidents or other emergencies. In many communities there is a poison control center that operates on a round-the-clock basis. All families in which there are small children should know about this resource and learn to keep this telephone number, along with the number of the physician or other emergency medical source of care, in a prominent and convenient place near the telephone.

Every child care agent, including baby-sitters and part-time care agents, should know:

1. The importance of knowing *exactly where* a small child is at all times.
2. Who and how to call for immediate help in case of accident or emergency.
3. Methods of "child proofing" home and yard for prevention of accidents.
4. The importance of defensive action against accidents: for example, defensive driving; defensive organization of home, school, and play areas; and teaching children to handle equipment properly *before* there is an accident.
5. The importance of continuing, automatic application of the known safety rules, including the use of "reminders," such as a red "twister" on all poison bottles.
6. Exactly where to find immediate instructions of what to do before the doctor can get there.

This information should be routinely included in community health nursing service rendered to *any* growing family. One mother suggested that the nurse distribute gummed labels containing space for the telephone number of the doctor, poison center, fire department, and public health nurse. The nurse should also be sure her own knowledge of first-aid and emergency care is up-to-date!

CARE OF ACUTE ILLNESSES

For the most part, the acute illnesses of children will be minor and can be cared for by some family member. Thus, in planning for community nursing care to families, it must be recognized that someone in each family should be educated as a primary care giver. This individual is the one who will recognize any deviation from usual behavior, who will be able to take the initiative in seeking such care, who will be able to use the care wisely, and who can herself administer the simple nursing required, with or without the help of a community health nurse.

To achieve care for acute illnesses, the mother or other child care agent will need to know:

1. How to tell whether the child is ill.
2. How and where to go for help if illness is present.
3. How to give simple care to the sick child at home.

Systematic instruction such as that provided in Red Cross or adult education classes has many advantages but does not reach all who need it. The community health nurse must find other ways of reaching individuals or small groups. Much is done in this respect when the nurse is called in to provide care to a sick child and, in the course of care, teaches the whole family. However, the number of illnesses attended by the community health nurse is known to be small, and this, too, is at best a haphazard approach to meeting the need. Much ingenuity and resourcefulness is required to find alternate ways; volunteer teachers, short-trained workers, school or other agency-sponsored courses, and the everyone-teach-one approach are some of the methods that have been tried.

CONTROL OF COMMUNICABLE
DISEASES

Although deaths from, and the incidence of, communicable diseases in children have dropped to very low levels, unless immunization measures are fully maintained there is always the threat of new outbreaks. The American Public Health Association recommends that children should be immunized against smallpox, pertussis, poliomyelitis, diphtheria, measles, and tetanus.[17] Each health department will have its own recommended schedule for these immunizations; and schedules may also be found in most public health or pediatric textbooks, in reports of the American Academy of Pediatrics, and in the American Public Health Association's publication "Control of Communicable Diseases in Man."

The American Academy of Pediatrics recommends the following schedule:[18]

Primary inoculation of all infants against: diphtheria, pertussis, and tetanus starting at 2 months; polio at 3 to 4 months; measles at 9 months; and smallpox toward the end of the first year.

Re-inoculations against diphtheria-pertussis-tetanus at 15 months, 4 years, and 8 years; re-inoculation against tetanus should be repeated at 10 to 12 years, and re-inoculation against diphtheria and tetanus should be repeated at 14 to 16 years; re-inoculation against smallpox should occur at 6 years and again at 10 to 12 or 14 to 16 years.

In addition, they suggest tuberculosis testing at 1 year, 2 years, 4 years, and 6 years.

Recent studies show that in some groups the proportion of children not receiving recommended immunizations is substantial. A national immunization survey in 1965 found that 4 million children between one and four years of age had not had diphtheria-pertussis-tetanus or polio immunizations.[19] Even though most groups do receive the primary series of immunizations, recommended "booster" dosages are much less frequently secured.

The community health nurse should familiarize herself with the available immunization agents, with the recommendations of the local health department, and with the requirements of the board of education regarding immunization for children in school. She should work with and through school and welfare workers, school children, volunteers, and any and all channels to emphasize the importance of immunization. Her own records should contribute to knowledge of the immunization levels achieved in the community. Above all, she should locate and deal with the barriers that prevent those who need this care from actually acquiring it.

CARE OF HANDICAPPING CONDITIONS

Handicapped children may not be readily identified. Some handicaps are discovered in the course of medical evaluation very soon after birth; but other defects, such as hearing loss and mental retardation, may not be clearly demonstrated until several years have passed. The community health nurse therefore has considerable responsibility both for personal observation of the family and for sharpening and interpreting the observations of family members so they can identify any deviation from normal function that might require medical investigation.

Parents may dislike and tend to avoid the fact of a handicapping condition and, as a result, may over-represent the child's abilities or create a plausible explanation for his inabilities. This is particularly likely to happen with the mentally retarded child. Sometimes a nurse may recognize long before the parents do that the child is not developing properly. It may take persistent and careful questioning to learn all of the factors that affect the child's behavior (deafness without mental retardation, for example, may be a factor in slow development) in order to provide the physician with pertinent, complete data. Additionally, it may take skill and tact to see that the child gets care without unduly alarming the parents.

Early recognition and care of handicapping conditions is as important in treatment as it is in securing the necessary family adjustments to the condition. It is particularly important to get at hearing loss early, since deafness brings with it a degree of sensory deprivation that may seriously affect the cognitive development of the child. For that reason, screening tests for hearing loss are usually recommended between 9 and 12 months and at least once again during the preschool period. Children at special risk should be checked more frequently. These children include those whose mother had rubella or another viral disease during pregnancy, those with a family history of deafness, and those who suffered respiratory distress after a difficult delivery. (Screening tests are discussed in Chapter 24.)

The community health nursing care required for the handicapped child will vary enormously from case to case and will depend largely on the availability of nursing, social work, or educational help. In any event, the community health nurse will be one member of a group concerned with meeting the needs of the child and his family, and she will be required to plan with others to provide the care required to meet the family's total needs. The nurse will need to consider these phases of care:

1. Teaching the family how to provide required care, such as feeding, exercises, protection from injury, substitute social experiences for the child barred from usual contacts, the handling of equipment, and where to obtain special equipment (*e.g.,* cups with big handles or easily handled spoons).

2. Reassuring the family of their adequacy in the situation, constantly pointing out their successes and special contributions, putting into perspective their lapses into irritability or despondency, and pointing out the facilities available to provide help for situations the family is unable to handle.

3. Reassuring the parent of the humanness and the likability of the extremely disabled child, that he can appeal to others as well as to his family. This reassurance is sometimes made most apparent by the nurse's own attitude in dealing with the child; she should treat him not as a sick child but as one with known limitations.

4. Providing an anchor—that is, being someone who will listen, who will understand, who can be asked questions when new problems arise, who will stand by as a family makes difficult decisions and learns new attitudes and skills.

Most communities have special programs for handicapped children. Diagnostic and evaluation and treatment centers are usually available in urban communities. They may be located in the health department, in a special clinic system administered by a crippled children's authority, in a teaching hospital associated with a medical school, or in a voluntary agency. These centers are characterized by the availability of a multidiscipline staff that is able to make a comprehensive assessment of the child's potential for development and to institute wide-spectrum treatment.

Day care centers for the handicapped child may be available within a "normal" day care group; or, if the handicapping condition is very severe, there may be day care services especially for the handicapped. Such services provide an opportunity for socialization and also serve to relieve the mother from the sometimes exhausting and frustrating task of care. Voluntary groups, such as the National Association for Retarded Children, may sponsor mutual support or educational programs. The community health nurse should familiarize herself with the available facilities and help parents and teaching staff interpret the special problems and needs of each child.

The Malnourished Child.   Some problems of children are rooted in the failure of parents or other care personnel to meet the developmental and protective needs of their charges. The malnourished child may range from minimal to extreme levels of distress. Severe protein and calorie malnutrition, found too frequently in developing countries, is fortunately rare in the United States. However, it does occur, and hospital treatment is usually required to rehydrate the child and to protect him from any possible infection or illness while nutritional balance is being re-established. More often the "quieter" forms of malnutrition are found: the grossly obese child, whose gluttony may suggest either insecurity and emotional deprivation or merely the influence of parents who feel a fat child is a well child, and the child with moderate protein deficit or anemia. These less obvious kinds of malnutrition can cause considerable developmental damage, and they should not be treated lightly.

Sometimes where there is no overt evidence of malnutrition and tests for nutritional adequacy are not readily available, malnutrition can be assumed on the basis of knowledge of food intake. The community health nurse may help locate these poorly fed children. If the situation warrants it and facilities are available, the child may be referred for complete nutritional study or for counseling by a nutritionist. Alternatively, the nurse may move directly to efforts to influence parents and to institute a better diet, using the help of the nutritionist if necessary. Sometimes malnutrition is due to inadequate income, and parents who are well aware of what is needed may be unable to supply the food they would like to provide for their children. In this case, conferences with welfare agencies may locate some additional funds or food supplements. The current food stamp plan enables families to purchase more per dollar of their own expenditure. This plan is financed by federal funds and is operated by welfare agencies. However, because it requires that the family be able to put out a large share of their food expenditure in one block, the food stamp plan is often dubiously successful.

In developed countries, the problem of malnutrition is most often one of poor allocation of available money, poor habits of shopping, or food preferences rooted in tradition or culture. The child with too little protein may be plentifully supplied with candy. Changing food habits is not easy, since they tend to be socially linked and rooted in cultural habits; but trying to change the food intake of the children may motivate a change in the whole family pattern.

The Battered Child. The battered child has recently been the focus of aroused social concern. These children are abused by their parents or by other care agents, often to the point of serious injury or death. Children under three seem to be the most frequent victims. The children are usually brought by parents to the doctor or to the clinic with some plausible explanation to account for the fractures, bruises, or other evidences of injury. In most instances the child shows other signs of neglect: poor nutrition, fear at the approach of adults, or surface bruises.

There is no doubt that many cases of child abuse are not discovered. The physician or nurse may find it hard to believe what they see or to dispute the explanation of apparently sincere parents. In some cases there is a reluctance to "get involved." Recent legislation enacted in many states requires reporting child abuse and provides legal protection for the reporting agent.

Diagnosis of child abuse may not be easy; it may take a sustained medical inquiry to find evidence of repeated fractures, to make comparisons of several hospital records (remorseful or frightened parents may visit a different accident room on each occasion, hoping to avoid discovery), or to carry out careful and unhurried interviewing to uncover discrepancies between parents' reports and medical findings.

Although child abuse often comes as a surprise when it occurs in what appears to be a "good" family, in some cases it may be possible to identify a higher than usual risk of child abuse. Parents whose own upbringing was characterized by brutal treatment; who show persistent immaturity and grossly impulsive behavior; and who have a history of alcoholism, severe marital conflict, and previous child abuse are likely candidates for child abuse. Also, poorly fed or poorly diapered children, a lack of cuddling, reference to the child as "it," or sustained resentment of pregnancy and the demands of the parental role may be evidences of rejection that indicate child neglect.

Such families should be frequently visited in order for the nurse to detect evidence of abuse or neglect while at the same time trying to lessen the parental problems that are the bases of their behavior. If child abuse is suspected, careful non-accusatory interviewing may bring out an acknowledgment of the situation; and often there may be genuine concern on the part of the parent who simply reacted impulsively and who may not in fact have wanted to harm the child.

If the neglect is relatively minor, the relief of the parent through the use of day care services or a friend or relative may help. When flagrant child abuse has been verified, however, the chances of family reclamation are not great. There is a 50–50 chance of recurrence if the child is returned to his home.

Problems of child abuse are by nature multidisciplinary, and the nurse's contribution will vary with the composition of the treatment team; however, her expertise in observation, her intimate knowledge of the home situation, and her accepted role in initiating treatment will always be needed. In some instances, the nurse may be called upon to testify in court, in which case her agency will provide appropriate legal assistance.

Failure to Thrive.   Children that appear listless, show no anger when left by their parents, fail to gain weight, eat and sleep poorly, cry very little, or show excessive irritability or vomit without any discernible physical reason are initially lumped together as babies who are "failing to thrive." This condition is almost always associated with psychosocial, as well as physical, problems and requires the services of several disciplines to assess the situation and to deal with the multiple causes.

Failure to thrive is often associated with a disturbed mother-child relationship, which may result in infrequent tactile contact with the child and consequent sensory deprivation. The cause for the disturbance may be difficult to locate. The mother may have felt that this baby threatened her life or her marriage; she may not have wanted the baby; or perhaps she has been unable to respond as she felt she should to her child. As the baby shows the result of this deprivation, the mother may become more anxious and consequently even less able to establish a warm and reciprocal relationship.

Sometimes the baby's welfare assumes minor importance when other conditions are extremely threatening. The father of the family may be absent, ineffectual, or even threatening to the baby. The mother may feel socially alienated, depressed, and frustrated by conditions that she feels impotent to change and that offer no hope in the future. The baby may be in the charge of a care agent who is indifferent or insensitive to the child's needs or who has no interest in the child except as a source of income.

Because of her traditionally warm relationship with a family, the community health nurse is in a good position to look for early signs of a failure to develop a suitable mother-child relationship and of characteristic responses of the infant who is not thriving. Using available help from other disciplines, she may be able to support the mother before the situation becomes serious. The mother may be encouraged to voice her dislike or fear of the baby, to investigate the possibility of help in preventing future unwanted pregnancies, and to express her frustrations at her living conditions, even though little can be done to improve them. As the mother's acceptance of the baby grows, her fear of him and her guilt may be reduced by specific instruction in care and by reiterated statement of confidence in her ability to be a mother.

When the family is under the care of a multidiscipline group or clinic, the community health nurse can provide information about the home and the family, help explain behavior in terms of the competing emotional demands and the stresses the mother faces, or assess the mother's strength and the capacity of her husband or other family members to support her efforts. By mobilizing the help of relatives and neighbors, the nurse may alleviate some of the sources of the mother's frustration. The provision of a homemaker or the institution of day care or early school experience for older children are other examples of the kind of help needed.

Of all problems the community health nurse faces, a child's failure to thrive is probably the one that demands the broadest spectrum of interest and action, requires the most intensive work with others, and offers the highest stakes in terms of the baby's and the mother's future.

Case Load Management Is Based on a Priority System

The almost limitless opportunities offered the community health nurse to improve the health of the growing family make it immediately clear that it will not be possible for her to give all of the services she knows would be useful. For this reason, it is necessary to establish a priority system based on the likely impact of nursing service in a given situation and the realities of the nurse supply and demand. (Priority setting is discussed in more detail in Chapter 18.)

In prenatal care, lifesaving and the reduction of morbidity may have highest priority, and the risk rate becomes the criterion for selection of care. The identification of high-risk mothers has been discussed previously. In some settings it is as effective to select high-risk populations as it is to identify high-risk individuals. In very low-income areas or migrant groups, for example, women at special risk will include the majority of those involved in the reproductive process. In other situations, as in a mixed income county, the selection may be on a family by family basis.

Patients at special risk require additional care, but the intensity and urgency of the care provided by the community health nurse is dependent not only upon the risk but also upon the help provided from other sources. Thus, a mother at high risk who is seen frequently in a clinic where there is a strong surveillance and teaching program and who has great inner strength and a supportive family may need less community health nursing than does the wife whose physical risk is less but whose husband is abroad on military duty. For this reason, it is helpful to categorize families in terms of the urgency and intensity of their need for community health nursing care in order to assure differential care.

The highest priority for community nursing support may go to unwilling or obviously inadequate parents and their children, whether they are classified as high risk or not. Here, the possibility of longterm damage due to parental deprivation may be lessened by the nurse in the community. In many cases the major effect of community health nursing will not be shown by a reduction of deaths or even by a great reduction of morbidity but rather in the improvement of the quality of childbearing and child rearing.

The community health nurse is an important member of the group concerned with well-child care and parent education. As a member of this group, she not only takes responsibility for the nursing phases of the work, but she also participates in the overall planning and evaluation of the care provided. She is as responsible as is every other professional member for assuring that the total operation efficiently and effectively meets the needs of a given population.

REFERENCES

1. Bowlby, J.: Maternal Care and Mental Health. World Health Organization, Geneva, 1951.
2. Deprivation of Maternal Care: A Reassessment of its Effects. World Health Organization, Public Health Papers No. 14, Geneva, 1962.
3. Solomon P., *et al.* (eds.): Sensory Deprivation. Harvard University Press, Cambridge, 1961.
4. Gentry, Elizabeth, and Paris, Lula M.: Tools to evaluate child health development. Amer. J. Nurs., *67*:2544, December, 1967.
5. Leavitt, S. R., *et al.*: A guide to normal development in the child. Nurs. Outlook, *13*:56, September, 1965.
6. Harper, Paul: Preventive Pediatrics. Appleton-Century-Crofts, New York, 1962, p. 1.
7. Birchfield, Marilyn: A mother's views on breast feeding. Amer. J. Nurs., *63*:88, March, 1963.
8. Peters, Ann deHuff, and Chase, Charles: Patterns of health care in infancy in a rural southern county. Amer. J. Public Health, *57*:409, March, 1967.
9. Newson, John, and Newson, Elizabeth: Patterns of Infant Care. Penguin Books, Harmondsworth, Middlesex England, 1966, p. 163.
9a. Hanlon, John: Principles of Public Health Administration. 5th ed., The C. V. Mosby Co., St. Louis, 1969, pp. 373, 383.
10. Schiffer, Clara G., and Hunt, Eleanor P.: Illness Among Children. Children's Bureau Publication 405-1963. U.S. Government Printing Office, Washington, D.C., 1966, p. 3.
11. *Ibid.*, p. 46.
12. *Loc. cit.*
13. Recent Demographic Trends and Their Effect on Maternal and Child Health Needs and Services. U.S. Department of Health, Education and Welfare, U.S. Government Printing Office, Washington, D.C., 1966, p. 9.
14. Harper, *op. cit.* p. 150.
15. *Ibid.* p. 607.

16. Frazier, T. M., Davis, G. H., Goldstein, H., and Goldberg, I. D.: Cigarette smoking and prematurity: a prospective study. Amer. J. Obstet. Gynec., *81:*988, 1961.
17. The Control of Communicable Disease in Man. 11th ed., American Public Health Association, New York, 1970.
18. Report of the Committee on the Control of Infectious Diseases, 1964. American Academy of Pediatrics, New York, 1965, p. 3. (Reader: Check to see if there is a later edition.)
19. Anderson, E. H.: Commitment to child health. Amer. J. *67:*2076, October, 1968.

SUGGESTED READINGS FOR CHAPTERS 12 AND 13

Barckley, Virginia, and Campbell, Everett I.: Helping the handicapped child achieve emotional security. *In* Stewart, Dorothy, and Vincent, Pauline (eds.): Public Health Nursing. William C. Brown Company, Publishers, Dubuque, 1968, Chapter 22.
Birchfield, Marilyn: A mother's views on breast feeding. Amer. J. Nurs., *63:*88, March, 1963.
Braun, J. J.: The well baby clinic: its prospects for building ego strength. Amer. J. Public Health, *55:*1889, December, 1965.
Brim, O. G. Jr.: Education for Child Rearing. Russell Sage Foundation, New York, 1965.
Brodie, Sylvia: Patterns of Mothering. International Universities Press, New York, 1965.
Bruce, J. J.: What mothers of 6-10 year olds want to know. Nurs. Outlook, *12:*40, September, 1964.
Cahill, Imogene: Facts and fallacies about illegitimacy. Nurs. Forum, *4:*39, 1965; also in Nurs. Res., vol. 17, July-August, 1968.
Clark, Ann L., Hakerem, Helen M., Bashara, Stephanie, and Waland, Diane: Patient Studies in Maternal and Child Health Nursing: a Family-Centered Guide. J. B. Lippincott Company, Philadelphia, 1966.
Corkey, Elizabeth: A Family Planning Program for Low Income Groups. Journal of Marriage and the Family, *26:*78, November, 1964.
Expanded Nursing Role in Prenatal and Infant Care. Pediatric Nursing Currents, Ross Laboratories, Columbus, Ohio, vol. 15, no. 4, July, 1968.
Expert Committee on Midwifery: The Midwife in Maternity Care, Technical Report Series 331. World Health Organization, Geneva, 1966.
Ford, L., and Silver, H. K.: The expanded role of the nurse in child care. Nurs. Outlook, *15:*43, September, 1967.
Ford, Patricia, *et al.*: The relative roles of the public health nurse and the physician in prenatal and infant supervision. Amer. J. Public Health, *56:*1097, July, 1966.
Forfar, John: Trends and developments in child health. International Journal of Nursing Studies. Pergamon Press, Inc., New York, *3:*9, May, 1966.
Fox, Ruth, Goldman, Jack, and Brumfield, William: Determining the target population for prenatal and postnatal care. Public Health Rep., *83:*249, March, 1968.
Gentry, Elizabeth, and Paris, Lula: Tools to evaluate child development. Amer. J. Nurs., *67:*2544, December, 1967.
Goercke, Lenor S., and Stebbins, Ernest L. (eds.): Introduction to Public Health. 4th ed., The Macmillan Company, New York, 1968, Chapter 11.
Hanlon, John: Principles of Public Health Administration. 4th ed., The C. V. Mosby Co., St. Louis, 1964, Chapter 20.
Harper, Paul: Preventive Pediatrics. Appleton-Century-Crofts, New York, 1962, Chapter 1.
Illingworth, R. S.: The Development of the Infant and Young Child: Normal and Abnormal. 2nd ed., The Williams and Wilkins Co., Baltimore, 1963.
Ives, Elizabeth: Genetics and genetic counselling. Canad. J. Public Health, *57:*513, November, 1966.
Jacobziner, H.: How well are well children? Amer. J. Public Health, *53:*1937, December, 1963.
James, G., and Jacobziner, H. A.: Pediatric health service—an extension of the Child Health Conference. Amer. J. Public Health, *55:*982, July, 1965.
Knight, E.: Conferences for pregnant, unwed teenagers. Amer. J. Nurs., *65:*123, July, 1965.

Leavitt, Samuel R., Gofman, Helen, and Harris, Donya: A guide to normal development in the child. Nurs. Outlook, *13:*56, September, 1965.

Legeay, C. A.: Failure to thrive—a nursing problem. Nurs. Forum, *4:*57, 1965.

Lytle, Nancy A.: Maternal Health Nursing: a Book of Readings. William C. Brown Company, Publishers, Dubque, 1967.

Mann, D., Woodward, L. E., and Joseph, N.: Educating Expectant Parents—Some Observations and Recommendations Based on a Research Study. Visiting Nurse Association, New York, 1961.

Morris, Naomi, *et al.*: Deterrents to well child supervision. Amer. J. Public Health, *56:*1232, 1966.

Normal Adolescence. Groups for the Advancement of Psychiatry, Report no. 68, vol. 6, February, 1968.

Pamphlets for Parents. United States Department of Health, Education and Welfare, Children's Bureau, U.S. Government Printing Office, Washington, D.C.:
When Your Baby Is on the Way. Children's Bureau Publication No. 391, 1967.
Your Child Is Under One Year. Children's Bureau Publications, 1967.
Your Child from One to Three. Children's Bureau Publication No. 413, 1964 (Reprint: 1966)
Dialogue on Adolescence. Children's Bureau Publication No. 422, 1967.
When Teenagers Take Care of Children: A Guide for Babysitters, 1964.
How Title V of the Social Security Act Benefits Children, 1967.

The public health nurse in support of mothering. Pediatric Nursing Currents, Ross Laboratories, Columbus, Ohio, Part I: vol. 7, no. 8, September, 1967; Part II: vol. 7, no. 9, October, 1967.

Ribble, Margaret A.: The Rights of Infants: Early Psychological Needs and Their Satisfaction, 2nd ed., Columbia University Press, New York, 1965.

Rogers, K. D.: Preventable accidents in preschool children. *In* Stewart, Dorothy, and Vincent, Pauline (eds.): Public Health Nursing. William C. Brown Company, Publishers, Dubuque, 1968, Chapter 26.

Rose, Patricia: The high risk mother infant dyad—a challenge for nursing? Nurs. Forum, *6:*94, 1967.

Rubin, Reva: Basic maternal behavior. Nurs. Outlook, *9:*683, November, 1961.

Rubin, Reva: The family-child relationship and nursing care. Nurs. Outlook, *12:*36, September, 1964.

Schaeffer, George: The expectant father. Nurs. Outlook, *14:*46, September, 1966.

Scheffer, C. G.: Illness Among Children: Data from the U.S. National Health Survey. U.S. Department of Health, Education and Welfare, Children's Bureau, U.S. Government Printing Office, Washington, D.C., 1963.

Sears, R. R., *et al.*: Patterns of Child Rearing. Harper and Row, Publishers, New York, 1967.

Semmers, J. P.: Fourteen thousand teenage pregnancies. Amer. J. Nurs., *66:*308, February, 1966.

Spock, Benjamin: Problems of Parents. Houghton Mifflin Company, Boston, 1962.

Sundberg, Alice: Influencing prenatal behavior. Amer. J. Public Health, *56:*1218, August, 1966.

Wallace, Helen M.: Health Services for Mothers and Children. W. B. Saunders Company, Philadelphia, 1962.

White, Ruth, Tayback, Matthew, and Hetherington, Susan: Family planning as part of maternity health services in a metropolitan health department. Amer. J. Public Health, *56:*1226, August, 1966.

When Poverty Is
a Problem

Poverty is a relative term. What would be considered poverty in New York might be classified as relative affluence in Calcutta, and a level of income that would be considered poverty by a blue collar worker might well be thought quite adequate by a student or a missionary. In the United States in 1964, those households that earned $3100 or less (adjusted to the current buying power of the dollar) for a family of four were regarded as living in poverty. In that year approximately 14 percent of the population, a total of 6.8 million families, in the United States fell into this category. Poverty affects a significant minority of this nation's populace. It is important, then, that the community health nurse appreciate the nature of poverty as an aspect of the environment and as an influence upon health and the patterns of health care.

Public concern with respect to poverty has sharply increased in recent years. There is a sense of outrage at witnessing deprivation in the midst of affluence and an increasing awareness of that vicious cycle of dependence, impotence, frustration, failure, and low esteem, which tends to make poverty self-perpetuating. Public concern has prompted a concerted and vigorous effort on the part of government, voluntary agencies, professional groups, and business to alleviate the inequities. These efforts are directed against the causes as well as the symptoms of poverty; and even though many feel such efforts are not sufficiently extensive or disagree with the methods employed, few would deny the validity of the claim of the poor on society or the importance of the remedial effort. There is a conviction that the combination of American know-how backed with American affluence can conquer this age-old malady, just as it has conquered problems of health and industrial development.

The impact of poverty on the individual, neighborhood, and society extends into all aspects of life. The degree to which poverty deprives its victims of needed services and opportunities, increases their vulnerability to physical and emotional illness, and keeps individuals from the realization of their innate potential as human beings is the measure of its importance as a public health and social problem.

POVERTY WEARS MANY FACES

Poverty strikes both the white and the nonwhite, city dwellers and farm dwellers, the old and the young.

There were more white than nonwhite families living at the poverty level in the United States in 1964: in 73 percent of the families classified as poor, the head of the household was white; whereas in 27 percent he was nonwhite.[1] Yet even though the number of nonwhites living in poverty is lower than the number of whites, the significant figure is the *proportion* of each population classified as poor: 12 percent for the white population and 41 percent for the nonwhite.

A similar situation plagues the country's rural dwellers. Table 5 shows that this group has a greater proportion of families falling into the poverty classification than do the nonfarm dwellers. Whereas only 6 percent of all families in the United States have remained on farms, 13 percent of all the poor families have done so.[2] For the great majority of that 13 percent, the problem is underemployment; they are stuck in a job with low productivity and earnings as farming moves more and more to large-scale corporate operation.

Another variable the community health nurse will find will be the effect on her patients of the duration of their poverty. There are three loosely defined poverty groups. For social planning purposes the nurse may disregard the first of these, the volitional poverty group. Examples include those who elect missionary work at or below a reasonable subsistence level and those who decide to accept a training opportunity, or even those unemployed for a short period of time. The second group is composed of those who, for a generation or less, have fallen on evil

Table 5.   All Families and Poor Families: 1964*

Poor families defined as those falling below "economy level of Social Security Administration poverty index," based on income of roughly $3,100 in 1964 for a family of 4.

Characteristic	All families	Poor families	Characteristic	All families	Poor families
Number___millions__	47.8	6.8	Regional location of family:		
Percent_____	100.0	100.0	Northeast_____	25	16
Sex of head:			North Central_____	28	23
Male_____	90	74	South_____	30	48
Female_____	10	26	West_____	17	13
Color of head:			Residence of family:		
White_____	90	73	Nonfarm_____	94	87
Nonwhite_____	10	27	Farm_____	6	13
Age of head:			Earners in family:		
14 to 24 years_____	6	8	0_____	8	27
25 to 64 years_____	80	70	1_____	43	47
65 years and over__	14	22	2 or more_____	49	26
Children under 18 years:			Employment status of head:		
			Employed_____	79	53
0_____	41	33	Unemployed_____	3	5
1 or more_____	59	67	Not in labor force [1]_	18	42

[1] Includes members of the Armed Forces.

*From *Pocket Data Book, U.S.A.* U.S. Department of Commerce, Bureau of the Census, 1967, p. 193.

days. A man proud of a now obsolete skill is too old to be retrained; a man loses his job when a West Virginian mine closes down; a corner grocery or four-unit motel makes way for something more efficient, and former members of the "haves" suddenly find themselves part of the "have-nots." Theirs is a new despair. They have not yet joined the ranks of the third group, those for whom poverty has become a way of life. The impact on community health of this kind of poverty, which is both chronic and generational, is the greatest of the three. The children grow up and continue to live under the same conditions of deprivation and dependency as did their parents. Under such circumstances, members of this group tend to develop common behavioral patterns and life styles — *a culture of poverty* — that help them to survive in this hostile environment. Because of their social impact, these characteristic behaviors, values, and attitudes have been described quite fully in recent years.[3] Although not all of the poor share this culture of poverty (Lewis estimates that only about 20 percent of those living at or below the poverty line in the United States have characteristics that would so classify their way of life), many of the individual adaptive patterns that develop under such stress occur with sufficient frequency to warrant the nurse's special awareness of them when dealing with the family or community that is poor.[4] This information is valuable for planning, as it tells what is likely to be found and what approaches may be indicated for the group as a whole.

No matter how statistically significant, however, documented adaptive patterns may be unreliable guides in dealing with a particular family or a particular neighborhood. For example, self-denigration and hopelessness may characterize an urban Black ghetto, but this pattern may not occur in an Appalachian hamlet or even in another urban Negro neighborhood at the same economic level. The Appalachian resident may have a deeply rooted fatalism that is not shared by his urban counterpart in a Puerto Rican neighborhood. Poor families living in different settings may react quite differently to poverty and, therefore, also to programs for "improving" their lot.

LIFE PATTERNS OF THE POOR AFFECT HEALTH BEHAVIOR

In most respects the poor in America share the general culture of the whole American society.[5] The emphasis on achievement as desirable is held even by many whose despondency has led to apathy. The low-income parent generally wants for his children what the middle income parent wants: a good education, a professional career, and a good life; most low-income parents want the same sized family, the same material possessions, and the same status within the community as the middle income parent; and the low-income family shares the religious beliefs of other groups.

However, there are some conditions common to the poor that provoke a particular kind of adaptive behavior. The life of the poor tends to be harsh and circumscribed, and the day to day struggle for existence

leaves little time or energy for tangential interests. The uncertainty of
the future, as well as the lack of personal control over it, may engender
in this group an orientation to the present, a desire for immediate
gratification of desires. For example, the low-income family may have
learned from bitter experience that savings will be eaten up during a
strike or layoff; they consequently spend their money quickly, buying
those things that are most needed when the paycheck comes and trusting
the future to take care of itself.

Substandard and crowded housing, an environment of violence,
apathy, and distrust, poor home maintenance, and lack of home owner-
ship all too often characterize the poor neighborhood. Indeed, the term
ghetto has recently been applied (perhaps inaccurately) to low-income
neighborhoods, suggesting the confinement and sense of alienation often
felt by residents of these neighborhoods. There is little opportunity to be
alone to read or study, so school effort may become less important to
the teen-ager than his street interests The level of education among the
parents is lower than that in the general population, and adults react in
one of two ways: some belittle the school, the teacher, the texts, and the
lessons, whereas others overvalue education as a road to escape.

To compound the problem, the low-income family is likely not to be
verbally oriented. Verbal communication within the family tends to be
brief and largely confined to immediate material matters.[6] Family life
may be unstable, and in some groups consensual and transitory marital
unions are common. Affectional interchange between marital partners
and between parents and children is limited.

In many low-income families, child rearing is characterized by harsh
and immediate discipline. Frequently adults provide poor role models
for children, especially in the urban situation. The feeling of helplessness
that may attend generations of unemployment and dependency on welfare also contributes to the unfavorable climate. The role of the father in
particular is often a weak one in urban areas where it may be easier for
the wife to find work than it is for her husband. There, the mother of
young children works away from the home far more often than is true in
other socioeconomic groups.

In other poverty areas, however, the father's role may be that of a
despot. Toughness and aggressiveness are generally respected traits.
The parent-child relationship may display more parental control,
although full responsibility and often marriage come at a very early age
to children of most of the low-income families. In the farm situation the
child may be faced with excessive demands for work so that his actual
laboring hours are often as long as those of the adults. This may mean
considerable hardship for the growing child, and it almost always presents a real handicap with respect to education and social contacts with
individuals not economically disadvantaged.

Both parents and children of the urban and rural poor all too often
relinquish very early any sense of mutual responsibility. Parents lose
control of children at an early point. Thus the child, who might in other
settings be encouraged to move toward constructive outlets for his
physical or emotional energies, is in a sense deserted by those from
whom he would expect such encouragement; and he is frequently left

without the alternatives to parental love and attention that are available to children in other groups.

Because of inadequacies in the home and the frequent lack of supervised community recreational opportunities, children adopt the street as their base of operations and their peer group as models. Even very young children seek peer support rather than parental support in establishing their ideas and values. Thus the community health nurse working in a poverty area must expect to have a preponderance of multiproblem families that are apt to require more intensive and more frequent care than families in other population groups.

AWAKENED SOCIAL CONCERN

Under the leadership of President Johnson, the American people voiced their conviction that poverty should not exist in an affluent country. Public Law 88-452, the Economic Opportunity Act of 1964, is described as an act "to mobilize the human and financial resources of the Nation to combat poverty in the United States." This act, administered by the Director of the Office of Economic Opportunity, which is in the Executive Office of the President, provides for a broad attack aimed at cure rather than solely the alleviation of the condition of the poor. The act provides for:
1. Youth programs. Among them are the following:
   a. A job corps program that, through operation of conservation camps and learning centers, combines efforts at conservation of natural resources with education and vocational training and furnishes work experience and health services for young people 16 to 22 years of age.
   b. Work training programs that provide useful work experience for the unemployed in order to increase their work skills or to permit them to continue schooling.
   c. Work-study programs that provide for part-time employment in institutions of higher learning for students from low-income families.
2. Community action programs that provide incentive for both urban and rural communities to mobilize resources to combat poverty. Provision is made specifically for:
   a. Basic education programs for adults whose job potential is decreased because they are unable to read or write.
   b. Involvement of volunteers (Volunteers in Service to America) to aid community action agency centers and tutorial projects.
3. Special programs to combat poverty in rural areas through grants and loans and special assistance to migrant or seasonal workers.
4. Employment and investment incentives, including loans and guaranties to strengthen small business concerns.
5. Experimental pilot and demonstration projects designed to help unemployed heads of families and other needy persons get and hold those jobs that would enable them to support their dependents.
   The impact of the law was reinforced by the fact that it came in the

midst of a struggle to implement the civil rights legislation passed some years previously.

The 1967 Report of the Commission on Human Rights reiterated the belief that the alleviation of the causes of unequal opportunity must be the focal effort in the achievement of social justice.[7] Government-sponsored activities of many kinds sprang up (for example, Head Start, designed to help disadvantaged preschool children compete with other school entrants). Business developed scattered but individually impressive efforts to remotivate, retrain, and employ those who had "lost their knack" for work or who were unable to meet the simplest requirements for employment, such as reading directions or asking for help when they did not understand. One company, in describing its efforts, pointed out that it required great changes in their usual personnel procedures; they employed social workers or educators to help induct the new employee, and they adopted a slower pace in the training programs.[8]

It is understandable that these efforts involve the development of both hope and hostility among the victims of poverty: hope, because they see in their own education and job training the means of determining the quality of their own lives; hostility, because they are more fully aware of the irrationality of their poverty and the limited opportunity in a society notorious for its wealth. In the case of the Black American, the belief that his condition has its roots in previous injustice makes his plight seem even more intolerable and his claim on society even greater. As hope replaces fatalism and as the possibility of reversing the old adage that "the poor are always with us" becomes not a dream but a social problem, the victims and their champions turn from apathy to action. Impatience for the promised correction of long entrenched inequity rises; and anger, protest, and violence may be the reaction, especially at the point when social reform is most impressive.

POVERTY CREATES SPECIAL CONDITIONS OF WORK FOR THE COMMUNITY NURSE

By demanding special adaptations in the kinds of approaches and programs that will be suitable for low-income communities, poverty affects the worth of the community health nurse because:

1. Poverty increases the health risk of the population to a marked degree, both in general and with respect to specific disease conditions such as tuberculosis.

2. Poverty may generate attitudes and habits of response to crises that decrease acceptance and utilization of traditional health services.

3. For the nurse, poverty may create obstacles that arise from her sense of inadequacy in understanding and dealing with the problems inherent in low-income groups.

4. Poverty in itself sets constraints and potentials for nursing action that may demand particular adaptations in the nursing care of low-income communities and families.

5. Poverty creates barriers for the usual organizational approaches to the health care of populations.

Poverty Increases Health Risk

There is considerable evidence that poverty is accompanied by an unusually high rate of illness. The National Health Survey indicates that persons in families with incomes below $2000 have 2 times as many disability days, 1.6 times as many work days lost and 1.5 times as many hospital days as those with incomes of $10,000 or more.[9] A recent statement from the American Public Health Association Committee on Public Policy states "Poor families have three times more disabling heart disease, seven times more visual impairment and five times more mental disorder than the general population. Fifty percent of poor children have still not had adequate immunization. Sixty-four percent of poor children in this country have never seen a dentist."[10] Infant mortality rates average 17 percent higher among low-income groups.[11] Lepper *et al.* reported that in 24 defined poverty areas, the infant mortality rate was 60 percent higher than in other nonpoverty areas and that there were 200 percent more new cases of tuberculosis, a 100 percent higher rate for cancer of the cervix, and 450 percent more illegitimacy.[12]

Because poverty is so much more prevalent among nonwhite groups, white-nonwhite comparision is often used in discussing problems of poverty. With respect to general death rates, life expectancy, and maternal and infant deaths, there has been a consistent and persistent difference between the white and nonwhite population, which indicates that there is a substantially higher risk for nonwhite groups than for the white population.[13] However, a recent study by Ochstein and associates indicates that in at least one geographic area, low-income Negroes are more like low-income whites than they are like middle income Negroes. They also found that families living in poverty areas reported poorer health than some of those with equivalent incomes living elsewhere. In other words, the poverty environment in itself appeared to have a deleterious effect.[14] Thirty-four percent of those in the poverty areas considered their health only fair or poor, but only 18 percent of those living elsewhere reported fair or poor health.

Though estimates of the degree of health disadvantage that poverty brings may vary depending on the criteria used, the difference in health risk between low-income groups and the rest of the population is clearly substantial.

Poverty Decreases Acceptance of Health Care

One of the most bedeviling aspects of social reform is the evident unwillingness of many — whose need is obvious — to be helped at all. Although their poor health is research-documented and medical personnel stand ready, the would-be patients are delinquent for appointments and are suspicious or frankly antagonistic to the staff. Barriers to care may be organizational in nature and due to economic, geographic, or time accessibility factors; or they may stem from interpersonal or behavioral conflicts. These barriers must be understood and overcome if the nurse is to be effective in her own work and in encouraging the use of other health facilities.

Economic barriers to care may exist when there are no facilities available to the low-income family except upon payment, which they cannot provide. For example, orthodontic services may be exceedingly important to a teenage girl, yet it may not be available in a particular community except for those who can afford to pay. This condition is being somewhat bettered by recent legislation designed to improve and extend health care to those who are indigent or medically indigent. The medically indigent are those who can manage with their usual subsistence costs but cannot afford the extra expense involved when there is illness or disability.

The location of a health center may be another barrier, for transportation to a distant clinic can present a tremendous hurdle. In the city, car fare to the clinic for a mother and three children may upset a marginal budget. The rural resident may lack any transportation or must depend upon farm vehicles that are not always available. Furthermore, cost in terms of lost pay may be a very important factor when the health services are proffered only during working hours. In rural areas, a clinic visit for the whole family may be possible only at the cost of the loss of a whole day's labor.

Such organizational problems, which are the responsibility of those who administer health care, can be overcome with relative ease. Those behavioral attitudes engendered by general social deprivation present more serious barriers to the full use of available health facilities.

LOW LEVELS OF MOTIVATION

General apathy, the overwhelming force of the many other problems they face, and the minor or major difficulties encountered in securing health action combined with previous unhappy experiences in health care and a distrust of "do-gooders," frequently leave the poor family with little motivation to acquire health care. Health may have a low priority among the many conditions that lead to anxiety or discomfort. Furthermore, long-established patterns of behavior—such as resorting to use of medical care facilities only in case of critical illness—are difficult to change when, to the family, these habits do not represent a problem.

There is some indication that the level of education affects the decision to seek and to use health services, particularly preventive services. Suchman points out that lower-income group members, in addition to being less well-educated than the norm, tend to be more socially isolated, or ethnocentric, and that this ethnocentricity is related both to a lower level of knowledge about disease and to their negative health orientation.[15] Thus apathy, frustration, and ignorance discourage the use of preventive services even when they are available free of charge. In one prepaid health service, for example, it was found that low-income groups used preventive facilities less than the rest of the covered group, even though there were no financial barriers to care.[16.] However, there is at present no clear indication that educational level is associated with following prescribed regimens once the condition has been diagnosed and treatment instituted.

Coincident with his distrust of health care facilities is the poverty-dweller's impression that communication with "The Establishment" is impossible to achieve. It may, indeed, be very difficult. Differences in

background, experience, and values may get in the way of understanding; difficulties with words and their meanings may impede the
interchange of ideas; a general reliance on nonverbal behavior on the
part of the family may make it hard for them to talk freely and honestly
about their problems. Usually there are socioeconomic differences between the nurse and the family. Nurses are most likely to come from a
middle class environment and be part of the middle class culture. Since
there are relatively few nonwhite nurses, the factor of difference in color
may intrude when patients are predominantly nonwhite. Unfortunately,
communication is not necessarily guaranteed by "matching" the
provider and the recipient of service: that is, the middle class Negro
nurse may identify fully with middle class values and have had primarily
middle class life exposures, and she will find difficulty in entering into
the thinking and feelings of her low-income clients; moreover, the pov-
erty-reared health worker may expect others to match his own drive
toward upward mobility and be unable to accept a lack of aggressive
action on the part of his clients, whom he may label "irresponsible."

Working with Poverty May Create Personal Problems for the Nurse

The community nurse working in a poverty area faces personal problems and adjustments of no small magnitude. For some, there will be a
degree of cultural shock at the first acquaintance with severe impover-
ishment. The community nurse may feel even more desperation than
does the family. The insecurities that arise when the welfare check is
delayed, the father's humiliation in not being able to provide for his
family, and the desperation of the mother who cannot control her street-
oriented children may seem unsupportable to the nurse. She may suffer
from, or be revolted by, what seems to be cruel punishment of children,
even though the children themselves take it as fair and expected treatment. Unless it can be mediated, the nurse's hopelessness may interfere
with her ability to help.

Alternatively, the nurse may find it hard to accept values and behavior
foreign to her own middle class values. Concentration on the present
may seem to her an evidence of lack of responsibility rather than a
sensible accommodation to a bleak future. The unemployed head of a
family may appear shiftless, since "workers are needed so many
places"; it may be hard for the nurse to accept the problem of work
orientation and retraining even though, intellectually, she has learned
about it. The limitations on success that can be expected in many
situations may be frustrating, particularly when it appears that conditions inhibiting improvement are likely to persist.

At times of tension the nurse may encounter outright abuse and
hostility, especially in the concentrated poverty pockets of urban areas
where tensions tend to be close to the surface. She may be blamed for
racial injustices of many years ago, accused of being a "stooge" for the
police or welfare officials, or taunted as a purveyor of unwanted services.

The nurse who is confronted with hostility may find it hard to bear and difficult to deal with objectively. A sense of unfairness because her honest efforts are not appreciated may rankle, although her rational analysis of the situation indicates that she is only the symbol and not the object of the hostile reaction. She may be actually fearful of her own safety, even to the point of becoming partially immobilized. Such hostility comes less often to the nurse than to many others; her uniform is one that usually suggests help more than regulation. However, no one can expect to be immune, and the professional worker in particular must try to concentrate on the causes, rather than the expressions, of such behavior, especially when she herself is the target. The nurse's background in behavioral sciences will help develop a clearer understanding of the relation between the behavior and the reasons that cause it. Handling hostility calmly, without blame and without subsequent withdrawal of care or support, is often the first step to trust.

In dealing with consumer decisional groups, she may feel her professional expertise is not merely unused but actually belittled and that the decisions made by those receiving aid are "not good enough" and "waste good money." She sometimes finds it difficult to view the importance of the decision from the perspective of one who must value decision making and its attendant responsibility as a tool for developing self-confidence and a sense of human worth. Often the community nurse feels insecure and unable to cope with the situations she meets. She may feel she is doing things as she has been taught and that the approaches she has learned are proving inadequate to the task.

It takes a little persistence and maturity to learn to work effectively with low-income groups. Often the support of a supervisor, social worker, or psychiatrist may help the community nurse to sort things out and to achieve some perspective. Learning to set realistic goals and to seek out those problems that are amenable to present action, rather than worrying unduly about the ones that cannot be dealt with immediately; developing confidence in her patients; and, above all, seeking to increase the quality of empathy she can bring to each situation, will help offset some of the negative forces in the environment.

Poverty Sets Constraints and Creates Potentials for Nursing Intervention

When poverty is one of the factors in a situation, goal setting, developing a productive family-community nurse interchange, teaching and counseling, relating the family to the community, and evaluating their care must all be adapted to the special conditions that pertain.

It is crucial that goals for nursing care be understood and be considered relevant and achievable by the family or community involved and that the approach to a problem be broken down into steps, each of which provides an opportunity for success. In dealing with families that are for the most part beset by multiple and often reinforcing personal, social, and health problems, acceptable and achievable goals may be modest indeed. When nonhealth problems are overwhelming, it may be wise to postpone health action that would otherwise be recommended or to accept a lower level of self-determination in health matters than might be expected at a later time. A recent article on patient care in hospitals suggests focusing on a single problem that has relevance for the individual patient rather than swimming about in a sea of problems.[17] It is a good working thesis.

The establishment and maintenance of communication is crucial in adapting nursing intervention to the setting of poverty. The achievement of free communication in these circumstances is not easy. The community health nurse may represent the "other world" — the comfortable, secure, or white world — to the low-income family; and the community members may have little expectation that she can understand their problems. The nurse may also represent "the authorities" to the family and be automatically distrusted and feared. Moreover, the nurse may see the clients as "cooperative" or self-revealing to a degree that is not consistent with the norm. Sometimes professionals have an almost mystical confidence in the efficacy of their "trade skills." More than ever it is important for the nurse to listen and to try to understand the meanings, as well as the words, she hears. Sometimes it is necessary to use an "interpreter," such as an indigenous worker (paid or volunteer), who serves as a kind of spokesman for others in the group. Because this neighborhood health worker "sees it like it is" and "tells it like it is," he may get through where the professional fails. Above all, the nurse must recognize that there may be times when she cannot, in fact, truly understand the situation in its entirety.

Helping may be communication in the truest sense. The image of the nurse as one who helps immediately and tangibly can do much to diminish the distance between nurse and family. Providing as much direct help as is possible within agency policy may be more important at some points than insisting on maximum self-help on the part of the recipient.

Nursing approaches must be based on the expectation of low motivation toward noncrisis health care. "Reaching out," rather than waiting for problems to be brought up by the family, is one way to circumvent the low motivation problem. Going to the family rather than asking them to come to the office or clinic, exploring possible areas of concern about health and nonhealth problems, recognizing clues quickly, and offering specific suggestions may convey a sense of wanting to understand and to help that encourages the family to think about health care. Making it easy to take the first steps in care may be helpful: arranging for an already enrolled expectant mother to accompany the new registrant to the prenatal clinic and asking a resident in a housing unit to keep an eye out for neighbors who may need nursing care are examples of this approach. Crisis care is much more likely to be sought by low-income families. When such care is provided, it may be used as a springboard for further health action. For this reason, every effort should be made to meet these crisis situations as promptly and as fully as possible, even at the expense of the routine.

TEACHING SHOULD BE EXPLICIT, NOT DEPENDENT ON CONCEPTUALIZATION

Both the low level of educational achievement and the great impact of day to day crises among low-income groups tend to result in preoccupation with tangible immediate problems and action rather than in a conceptual or anticipatory approach to problems. For this reason, the majority of low-income families do best with health education that is directed toward defined problems that they have recognized and toward a specific course of action that they see as reasonable and possible. For example, food selection must be realistically related to welfare budgets and to the nature of the local shopping facilities and it must be in terms of essential foods rather than food elements. Constant reality testing— "Do you think this would work?" or "Will your family drink powdered milk if you fix it?"—will help to avoid mere surface acceptance of an idea without any real intent to carry out the action.

Emphasis on the reasons behind action is not inconsistent with this explicit approach; indeed, it is one of the crucial bases of learning. As health teaching progresses on the basis of the principles underlying action, the nursing services may make their own small contribution to expanding the problem-solving abilities of the educationally and socially disadvantaged.

Involvement of the individual family and of the group in its own health care is essential both to winning active patient cooperation and to replacing apathetic dependence with the ability to make responsible decisions. The purpose of good nursing practice is to enable patients to be self-sufficient. The nurse, sometimes in the course of regular family service, recognizes achievement by giving larger doses of responsibility to the head of the household. On the community level, involvement can sometimes be fostered by the development of committees or other representative groups who, with the health professionals, plan for what should be done and how to go about it.

One currently popular way of involving recipients in the care process is the employment of neighborhood residents (who are themselves in the low-income groups) in some capacity in the health service. They may serve as nurses' aides, as representatives or interpreters, or as first-line sources of information and referral.

The alert community nurse will find many ways of involving families and neighborhoods in their own care. Some of the ways that have been tried include a mothers and grandmothers committee to advise clinic personnel (it later became a regular part of clinic planning and evaluation), an everyone-bring-one approach to immunization and diagnostic health campaigns; and the use of discussion groups to recognize and utilize members' successful handling of health problems. With respect to the use of group approaches, it must be remembered that it is difficult to organize and sustain interest in groups discussing noncrisis matters among low-income populations. An aggressive "reaching out" kind of recruitment and concentration on action-oriented rather than word-oriented programs has been suggested in developing parent education programs for low-income families.[18]

Poverty May Necessitate Organizational Changes

The organization of health services frequently requires modification if participation in health care is to extend to the community as well as to the family. Such participation is required in many instances as a condition for receiving support for projects or services and is considered highly desirable by most who have had experience in working with low-income populations. The proponents of participation feel that the involvement of the recipient group in their own care builds motivation toward better care and that it prevents costly mistakes that may arise when professional workers plan for care with insufficient appreciation of the concerns and values of the group served. Undoubtedly there is some *pro forma* participation, in which the representatives of the population served simply reflect the thinking of the professional staff. But more and more, decision making is becoming a shared responsibility.

Frequently this is accomplished by committees or councils. When such mechanisms are used, it is important to clarify the nature and extent of the participation that is expected; whether or not, for example, it involves decision making or is limited to advisement. It is also the responsibility of the health operational unit to specify methods of coordinating the efforts of staff and community advisers. The health professional may find it hard to relinquish decisions on health matters or to accept a decision different from, or clearly inferior to, the one that he would have made. Sometimes there are limits set by legal or policy requirements—in the handling of communicable disease, for example. However, in the promotion of immunization against measles in a given housing unit, decisions on methods by which information can best be disseminated and the conditions under which the immunization will be provided might be much the better for the participation of the consumer group.

When such committees are considered as representatives of the community being served, it is also important that they are, in fact, representative in the eyes of their public. Sometimes the willing and vocal volunteer may not be wholly acceptable to others of his group. Representation by election or, at least, selection after a careful "feeling out" of the situation may be necessary.

One of the most appropriate areas for such cooperation is that of overcoming the previously mentioned organizational barriers to care.

Changing the place and time as well as the content of service may be necessary to meet the special needs articulated by these members of the low-income population. An excellent example of good "fit" between community and service is the "Moms and Tots" service established in Detroit by Milio.[19] The "one stop" clinic where a variety of services are offered in a single location is another recent attempt at adaptation to meet needs of low-income groups. Availability of facilities before and after the usual work hours is a feature of many comprehensive-care units. This extension of the service day does create problems, such as finding nursing personnel willing to be available during these hours, escorting women workers in unsafe areas, and deploying staff in order to have adequate skills available where they are needed;[20] The alternative to overcoming these difficulties, however, may be an ineffective service.

The increasing acceptance of the neighborhood rather than the family as the unit of care for the population is occasioning many administrative adjustments. Lepper and others describe a system built on three echelons of care: care in the home by a community nursing staff member or health adviser, care in a neighborhood health center, and care in the hospital outpatient service.[21] This system would function within a network comprised of a series of comprehensive-care centers, supported by traditional resources but having interdigitation of all facilities. Such organization makes obsolete the nurse-districting systems based on population loads. It brings each nurse into the orbit of multidiscipline planning for a population group. It almost always implies a nursing team with a large complement of short-trained workers, and with a consequent need for professional nurses to supervise and at the same time personally provide services.

The health problems of low-income families, as of all families, are inextricably interwoven with nonhealth problems. Treatment of health and nonhealth problems are often interdependent in any group. Organization of services for low-income populations therefore requires relating to the total social effort for health, welfare, education, and religious experience to an unusual degree. For example, negative reactions to school growing out of failure or social rejection may lead to delinquency and thence to specific physical and emotional health consequences. The treatment of the health problems must take into account the role played by the school, the social worker, and the court as well as the roles of peer groups, of family, of church, and other reference groups. Often several sets of medical care personnel may be involved: a comprehensive maternal and infant care project, a voluntary hospital, a family physician, a general clinic. Thus in the case of low-income families, the importance of multidiscipline case planning cannot be minimized.

Also, it is essential to carefully consider the relative weight of the many forces that are in many way operative in the situation: for instance, the approval of sexual promiscuity of the peer group versus the precepts of family or church; the kind of role model provided by adults be they parent, teacher, nurse, or famous athlete; the relative attraction of the many available protest alternatives, from burning and looting to individual and neighborhood improvement efforts. For all of these reasons, when the nurse's case load is heavy with low-income populations, her time will need to be arranged to allow for longer periods for planning and coordinating efforts with other workers and agencies than if she were working in a more favorable economic environment.

As the nurse focuses on the strengths rather than the weaknesses of her low-income clientele, she may find much richer human resources than she dreamed possible. Their preoccupation with the present may lead to a spontaneity and open enjoyment of such pleasurable experience as is available, a trait that is often absent in the future-oriented middle class culture. Their familiarity with poverty may lead the mountain family to accept privation with a dignity greater than that a suburban housewife can command when she cannot afford a mink stole. Their personal knowledge of hardship may lead a poor rural family wholeheartedly to offer their meager resources to an abused child, and their selflessness may demonstrate a sensitivity greater than that found among those living in more fortunate circumstances.

As the nurse learns the inadequacy of many of the present methods for dealing with poverty and the constant assaults on the ego that come with dependency and lack of the usual good things of life, she must marvel at those who manage to escape, and she can fully understand the courage it takes to try again when so many previous trials have failed. With each new piece of understanding, the nurse's ability to interpret the needs and to participate in social change increases.

The problems of community nursing in a poverty area are many, and the frustrations are frequent; but the potential for professional realization and personal satisfaction is enormous.

REFERENCES

1. Pocket Data Book. U.S. Department of Commerce, Bureau of the Census, U.S. Government Printing Office, Washington, D.C., 1967, p. 197.
2. *Ibid.*
3. See, for example, Harrington's The Other America or Chilman's Growing Up Poor or Besner's Economic Deprivation and Family Patterns.
4. Lewis, Oscar: LaVida. Random House, New York, 1966, p. 11.
5. Irelan, Lola M.: Escape from the slums: a focus for research. Welfare in review, 2:19, December, 1964.
6. Chilman, Catherine: Growing Up Poor. U.S. Department of Health, Education and Welfare, Welfare Publication No. 13, U.S. Government Printing Office, Washington, D.C., 1966, p. 43.
7. A Time to Listen, A Time to Act. U.S. Commission on Human Rights, U.S. Government Printing Office, Washington, D.C., 1967, p. 1.
8. Hodgson, James D., and Brenner, Marshall: Successful experience training hard core unemployed. Harvard Business Review, 46:68 and 148, September-October, 1968.
9. Welfare Trends. U.S. Department of Health, Education and Welfare, U.S. Government Printing Office, Washington, D.C., 1965, p. 11.
10. Draft of a Policy Statement on Health and Poverty. American Public Health Association. Committee on Public Policy. *In* This Is The News, March, 1968. (The statement in final form should appear after report in the Amer. J. Public Health.)
11. Welfare Trends. U.S. Department of Health, Education and Welfare, U.S. Government Printing Office, Washington, D.C., 1965, p. 6.
12. Lepper, Mark H., Lashof, Joyce, Lerner, Monroe, German, Jeremiah, and Andelman, Samuel: Approaches to meeting health needs of large poverty populations. Amer. J. Public Health, 57:1153, July, 1967.
13. Health and Welfare Indicators, June 1963. U.S. Department of Health, Education and Welfare, U.S. Government Printing Office, Washington, D.C., 1964.
14. Ochstein, H. Jr., Thanasapoulos, D. A., and Larkins, J. H.: Poverty area under the microscope. Amer. J. Public Health, 58:1815, October, 1968.
15. Suchman, E. A.: Social factors in medical deprivation. Amer. J. Public Health, 55:1725, November, 1965.
16. Nolan, R. L., *et al.:* Social class differences in utilization of pediatric services in a prepaid direct service medical care program. Amer. J. Public Health, 57:34, January, 1967.
17. Tayrien, Dorothy, and Lipchak, Amelia: The single problem approach. Amer. J. Nurs., 67:2523, December, 1967.
18. Helping Low Income Families Through Parent Education. U.S. Department of Health, Education and Welfare, Children's Bureau, U.S. Government Printing Office, Washington, D.C., 1966, p. 35.
19. Milio, Nancy: Project in a Negro ghetto. Amer. J. Nurs., 67:1006, May, 1967.
20. Personal communication. Barbara Falco, Nurse Director, Provident Neighborhood Comprehensive Health Center, Baltimore, Maryland, 1968.
21. Lepper, Mark H., Lashof, Joyce C., Lerner, Monroe, and German, Jeremiah. Approaches to meeting health needs of large poverty populations. Amer. J. Public Health, 57:1153, July, 1967.

SUGGESTED READINGS

Aponte, Harry J.: Children of society's ills. Amer. J. Nurs., 66:1749, August, 1966.

Besner, Arthur: Economic deprivation and family patterns. Welfare in Review, 3:20, September, 1965.

Chilman, Catherine S.: Growing Up Poor. U.S. Department of Health, Education and Welfare, Welfare Publication No. 13, U.S. Government Printing Office, Washington, D.C., 1966.

Chilman, Catherine S.: Social work practice with very poor families. Welfare in Review, 4:13, January, 1966.

Chilman, Catherine S.: Some differences between people and statistics. Children, 13:99, May-June, 1966.

Chilman, Catherine S., and Kraft, Ivor: Helping low income families through parent education groups. Children, 10:127, July-August, 1963.

Clark, Kenneth: Dark Ghetto. Harper and Row, Publishers, New York, 1967.

Conway, Jack: The beneficiary—the consumer. What he needs and wants. Amer. J. Public Health, 55:1782, November, 1965.

Cornely, Paul, and Bigman, S. K.: Some considerations in changing health attitudes. Children, 10:23, January-February, 1963.

Ennes, Howard: A crisis of conscience in health care. Amer. J. Public Health, 58:1809, October, 1968.

Ford, Thomas R. (ed.): The Southern Appalachian Region—A Survey. University of Kentucky Press, Lexington, 1962.

Fusco, Gene: School-Home Partnership in Depressed Urban Neighborhoods. U.S. Department of Health, Education and Welfare, U.S. Government Printing Office, Washington, D.C., 1964.

Gilbert, Arnold, and O'Rourke, Paul F.: Effects of rural poverty on the health of California's farmworkers. Public Health Rep., 83:827, October, 1968.

Glazer, Nathan, and Moynihan, Daniel: Beyond the Melting Pot. Harvard University Press, Cambridge, Massachusetts, 1963.

Harrington, Michael: The Other America. Penguin Books, Inc., Baltimore, 1963.

Humphrey, Hubert H.: The future of health services for the poor. Public Health Rep., 83:1, January, 1968.

Irelan, L. M.: Health practices of the poor. Welfare in Review, vol. 3, no. 19, October, 1965.

Jacobs, Paul: Dialogue on Poverty. The Bobbs-Merrill Co., Inc., New York, 1967.

James, George: Poverty as an obstacle to health progress in our cities. Amer. J. Public Health, 55:1757, November, 1965.

Kelly, Cynthia H.: Fighting poverty with health care. Amer. J. Nurs., 68:282, February, 1968.

Lepper, Mark H., Lashof, Joyce C., Lerner, Monroe, German, Jeremiah, and Andelman, Samuel: Approaches to meeting health needs of large poverty populations. Amer. J. Public Health, 57:1153, July, 1967.

Meissner, Hanna H.: Poverty in the Affluent Society. Harper and Row, Publishers, New York, 1966.

Milio, Nancy: Project in a Negro ghetto. Amer. J. Nurs., 67:1006, May, 1967.

Milio, Nancy: Values, social class and community health services. Nurs. Res., 16:26, 1967.

Myrdal, Gunnar: Challenge to Affluence. Random House, Inc., New York, 1965.

Reaching hard to reach families. In Stewart, Dorothy, and Vincent, Pauline (eds.): Public Health Nursing. William C. Brown Company, Publishers, Dubuque, 1968, p. 83.

Reissman, Frank: The Culturally Deprived Child. Harper and Row, Publishers, New York, 1962.

Reissman, Frank (ed.): Mental Health of the Poor: New Treatment Approaches. The Macmillan Company (Free Press), New York, 1964.

Sexton, Patricia: Spanish Harlem: Anatomy of Poverty. Harper and Row, Publishers, New York, 1965.

Slocum, Walter L.: Aspirations and Expectations of the Rural Poor—A Guide to Research. U.S. Department of Agriculture, Agricultural Economics Report No. 128, Economic Research Service, Washington, D.C., 1967.

Strauss, Robert: Poverty as an obstacle to health progress in our rural areas. Amer. J. Public Health, 55:1772, November, 1965.

Suchman, E. A.: Social factors in medical deprivation. Amer. J. Public Health, 55:1725, November, 1965.

A Time to Listen, A Time to Act. Report of the U.S. Commission on Human Rights. U.S. Government Printing Office, Washington, D.C., 1967.

Watts, Dorothy D.: Factors related to acceptance of modern medicine. Amer. J. Public Health, 56:1205, August, 1966.

Yerby, Alonzo S.: Improving care for the disadvantaged. Amer. J. Nurs., 68:1043, May, 1968.

Young, Leontine: Wednesday's Children. McGraw-Hill Book Company, 1964.

CHAPTER
15

The Community
Health Nurse in
Family Planning

Family planning has assumed an increasingly important role in the economic and social development and the health programs of nations throughout the world. As a result, it has become an area of concern for the community health nurse.

POPULATION CONTROL IS A PUBLIC PROBLEM

The rate of growth of the world's population throughout recorded history has increased in geometric proportions, as shown in Table 6. This increase, at first considered helpful, since it provided the means of developing the world's resources, is now being regarded as a threat to human health and welfare. Advances in health care that prevent untimely deaths have resulted in a faster rate of population growth, even though the birth rate remains constant; and as more infants survive to become parents, the increase is speeded up proportionately. Programs to increase the adequacy of food supplies, to improve the conditions of life, and to offer the opportunity for self-fulfillment may be negated by the overwhelming flood of mouths to feed and children to rear.

Table 6.   Doubling Time of World Population*

Period	Number of Years
? to 1650 A.D.	1700
1650 to 1850	200
1850 to 1935	85
1935 to 1970	35

*Reproduced by permission from "The Numbers of Man" by John Maier, M.D., in Rockefeller Foundation Quarterly, No. 4, 1967, p. 5.

FAMILY PLANNING IS A PART OF PUBLIC HEALTH POLICY

The following credo, drawn up by world leaders and endorsed by representatives of 30 nations on Human Rights Day, 1967, expresses the rationale for incorporating population concerns into the fabric of public policy. The statement reads:

We believe that the population problem must be recognized as a principal element in long-range national planning if governments are to achieve their economic goals and fulfill the aspirations of their people.

We believe that the majority of parents desire to have the knowledge and the means to plan their families and that the opportunity to decide the number and spacing of children is a basic human right.

We believe that lasting and meaningful peace will depend to a considerable measure upon how the challenge of population growth is met.

We believe that the objective of family planning is the enrichment of human life, not its restriction; that family planning, by assuring greater opportunity to each person, frees man to attain his individual dignity and to reach his full potential.[1]

The signatures to this document endorsed by, among others, the United States and the United Kingdom, represented more than a third of the world's population: countries both large and small, countries highly industrialized and those still mainly agricultural, countries governed by many different political and religious beliefs.

The American Medical Association recognized family planning as a component of health care; a statement, issued in 1964, says in part: "Family planning is an elective, preventive health procedure which is regarded as an integral and routine part of good medical care."[2] This belief is reflected in the fact that virtually every state and most large urban centers have some sort of family planning program. (Georgia has had a viable program since 1939.) In New York City the conviction is even more clearly expressed in the inclusion of family planning as a requirement for the comprehensive medical care given under the provisions of Medicaid.[3] Internationally, 66 governments, representing 2.5 billion people, now support family planning programs, according to a survey by the International Planned Parenthood Federation.[4]

Almost all parents in the United States, regardless of ethnic group or socioeconomic status, express the desire for two to four children.[5] Nevertheless, family size tends to be larger in the lower socioeconomic groups, and couples in the low-income category report more frequently than those in other groups that they have more children than they would like to have. Recent surveys indicate that most couples know at least one method of birth control. However, those in the middle and upper socioeconomic groups are apt to know of the more reliable methods and to have readier access to medical advice about fertility control, a fact which may account for the closer approximation of desired and actual family size in these groups.

There are now available more reliable methods for the control of conception than have been available in the past. Although few would agree that the ideal contraceptive method has been discovered, some methods in use ("the pill" and intrauterine devices) are reported to be 90 to 95 percent effective in preventing conception. Most planners agree there is need for intensive and extensive research to find methods that are simpler to prescribe and to use, that would require less reliance on patient memory and willingness to seek care at regular intervals. However, methods currently available are fairly well standardized, relatively inexpensive, and, for the most part, acceptable to the user. The more popular ones are those measures that may be used at the discretion of the female partner and independently of coitus itself.

Because of the potential effectiveness of currently available contraceptives and the promising research to produce a safer and more convenient method, the likelihood that one can successfully govern the size of his family has greatly increased. For the present, the problem facing community health nursing is one of making currently available methods known and attractive to those who wish to limit family size.

Public Health Programs Involve Service, Education, and Research

Public health programs designed to deal with this problem center about five general approaches:

1. Providing information, counseling, and supplies to groups not otherwise reached by family planning services. This may be done by enlarging the responsibility of existing clinic or counseling resources in hospitals or voluntary health and welfare organizations or by initiating a new service program.

2. Including population and family planning material in established service programs for mothers and children, prospective parents, or special population groups.

3. Increasing professional awareness of the need for and knowledge about population control. Education of on-the-job personnel in health, education, and welfare agencies and of those yet in school involves efforts such as incorporating relevant materials into the basic professional curriculum, initiating staff educational programs, and arranging special conferences to consider and act on the possibilities of integrating family planning content into ongoing programs.

4. Increasing public understanding and acceptance of services directed toward family planning and of policies directed toward control of population growth. Such efforts may be direct, as in the explanation of the physiology and methodology of birth control, or indirect, as in the development of healthy attitudes toward sex. One approach to increasing public understanding and support is the discussion group designed to find reasons for the unacceptability either of specific methods of contraception or of the program as a whole. In some localities the public attitude has been so modified as to allow community agencies to provide contraceptive advice to unmarried, sexually active teenage girls. Although public acceptance of family planning efforts is generally high, specific groups may pose special problems. For example, in one community a low-income group protested that the family planning effort was for the purpose of reducing the power of the poor by "genocide."

5. Developing research in (a) new methods for the control of conception and the direct side effects of the methods in current use, (b) efficient dissemination of such information by the health-care facility (such research might involve such questions as whether a clinic should maintain 24-hour availability or whether using public health nurses and nurse midwives for some aspects of the program would be feasible), and (c) the emotional-behavioral consequences of the unwanted pregnancy or abortion on the mother and on the family.

In each of these five phases, the community health nurse will have a part to play, for the major change in today's public health family planning center is in its availability. The previous reluctant acquiescence to a family's desire for birth control information has been replaced by a more positive approach.

THE ROLE OF THE NURSE IN FAMILY PLANNING

The Family, Not the Nurse, Must Decide

It is the right of every family to have the alternative of using or of not using birth control; this includes both those families that are on welfare and those that are self-sustaining.

The family is likewise responsible for any ethical or religious decision relative to the use of contraceptive methods. Constraints with respect to birth control are set down in the dogmata of several religious institutions. The recent attention focused on the Roman Catholic position should not obscure the fact that religious beliefs may be a factor in the decisions of many non-Catholic families as well.

The 1968 Papal Encyclical of Pope Paul VI contained a statement entitled Humanae Vitae, which declares: "Excluded is every action which either in anticipation of the conjugal act or in its accomplishment or in the development of natural consequences proposes whether as an end of or as a means, to render procreation impossible."[6] Interpretation of the implications of this pronouncement has varied among Catholic theologians from locality to locality. It would appear, however, that at least one method of contraception, periodic abstinence (the rhythm method), is widely acceptable. Consultation with local clergy represents the channel for interpreting the Encyclical when other methods are being considered.

The family is equally autonomous in its decision regarding family size. The right to have many children, as well as to restrict their number, is in most countries considered a human right that should not be denied. That the family is "on welfare" does not in any sense abrogate this right.

BOTH HUSBAND AND WIFE ARE INVOLVED

Family planning, whether it involves seeking relief from sterility or limiting family size, is a concern of both husband and wife. It will have economic, social, and psychologic ramifications that may have a profound effect on the family. Just as the failure to use effective contraceptive measures and the consequent worry about unwanted pregnancy may create marital tensions of some magnitude, the use of contraceptive methods against one's convictions may be equally destructive to the individual and may reflect itself in family relationships. Likewise, the decision of the unmarried, sexually active teenager and her parents to seek contraceptive advice may have an effect on her attitude toward marriage and family life that will carry far over into the future.

These are not matters that the nurse—or indeed anyone but the families themselves—can resolve. However, an understanding of these forces is essential for helping families to make their own decisions. Furthermore, it is important that any nursing intervention be planned to help the family both to "see the situation whole" and to support rather than to interfere with the communication between husband and wife. After all, strengthening the family is one of the major objectives in family planning.

Most Parents Want to Plan Their Families

Virtually every study of family planning indicates that the great majority of families (approximately 4 out of 5) employs one or more methods of fertility control. Experiences in Georgia and in New York City indicate that facilities which furnish such information are generally well used even when not supported by intensive educational and organizational measures.[7] Thus the problem in the United States and in similarly "developed" countries does not appear at present to be one of motivation but rather of the accessibility and acceptability of contraceptive measures.[8]

There are, of course, many reasons for wanting to limit family size. However, the overwhelming majority of parents give "the budget" as their reason. They want to have enough money to provide for a decent life and to give their children the advantages they have come to expect in an affluent society. Maternal health may be a compelling though less frequent motivation.

However, in many instances, especially among low-income groups, the desire to practice birth control is not matched by an equivalent knowledge of how to do so. Beasley and coworkers reported that only 14 percent of a group of 142 low-income randomly selected Negro women interviewed in New Orleans knew of effective birth control techniques, although the great majority (about 75 percent) indicated a desire for a limited number of pregnancies.[9] Edmands also found a disparity between desire to limit family size and sufficient knowledge to do so among a group of low-income women in Baltimore.[10] Other studies report similar findings.

There is also some indication that even when effective measures are known, they may not be used. This failure to utilize available measures is also greater among low-income groups. The reason may be personal: impulsiveness or procrastination, for example; it may be situational, as in a lack of privacy or the inaccessibility of a convenient contraceptive;

it may also be related to the method proposed by health authorities: the individual may find their specific suggestion unacceptable or difficult to carry out.

NURSING MUST "REACH OUT"

Despite the fact that many who want contraceptive advice will need only the provision of the facility where they may seek information, there is still a large group who will need to be not only informed about available resources but also prompted to use them.

Study after study reveals that the great majority — women in particular — do not want the health worker to wait for them to ask about contraceptive measures. Some may find it embarrassing to raise the question, especially if the nurse or other health worker is young and unmarried. Others may hesitate because they do not know that this is an accepted part of the public health program and may fear rejection of their request. Still others, especially those whose contact with the nurse is infrequent or those in low-income groups, may not be in the habit of being involved in their own care and may see their role in care as a passive one. In any event, it is clear that in the overwhelming majority of situations the nurse should not wait for her patients to inquire before she indicates the availability of contraceptive advice.

Sometimes others in the community may be helpful in reaching those who need information. The social worker, the neighborhood aide, and the granny midwife may all be involved in referral for care.

The Nurse Must Be Aware of Current Birth Control Methods

Methods of control vary from sterilization of either sexual partner to periodic abstinence, and the nurse should familiarize herself with methods currently popular in her own locality as well as with other methods in general use.

By far the most common methods of birth control are oral contraceptives and intrauterine devices, both of which have a high degree of reliability. The action of oral contraceptives is to prevent ovulation while permitting regular recurrence of uterine bleeding. This method at present requires a preliminary period of regulation and the careful practice of the female, who must remember to take the pills at specified periods of time.

Intrauterine devices are usually made of plastic in various shapes and are inserted through the cervical canal into the uterus. This method may be used successfully with many (but not all) women; it protects against pregnancy over a long period of time; and once the device is implanted, there is no further effort required of the user.

The rhythm method involves abstinence during the period of the menstrual cycle when conception is most likely to occur. This method is more demanding than the others because it depends upon first determining with some accuracy the woman's true menstrual cycle; the exact period of necessary abstinence may vary from 11 to 18 days. Success with this method depends upon a patient's ability and willingness to go through a period of study and to adapt her sexual behavior to the requirements of the method. This method is less reliable than oral contraception or intrauterine devices.

Sterilization is resorted to very infrequently in countries where population expansion is not creating an overwhelming problem, which is the case in the United States, the United Kingdom, and Canada. Sterilization is more likely to be promoted in countries where sources are undeveloped, food production inadequate, and conditions of life poor. It may be the method of choice when an individual cannot take responsibility for his own conduct, as is sometimes the case with the seriously mentally retarded. Finally, it has the advantage of not requiring persistent care on the part of the married partners. The disadvantages lie in finding facilities for the necessary surgical action and, for many individuals, the stress associated with the original decision.

Other methods of contraception provide for mechanical interruption of the union of the egg and sperm or depend upon spermicidal action alone and include measures such as the vaginal diaphragm, condom, and spermicidal foam. These methods are somewhat less reliable; and since they are specifically associated with each coital process, they may be less acceptable to the user.

Whatever the method, none can be relied upon for 100 percent protection against conception, and it is important that the user recognize this fact. Furthermore, no one method is suited to every patient. For this reason it is essential that the patient seek advice from a reliable health source, preferably a physician, before instituting any method of contraception.

The use of induced abortion as a means of birth control is much more controversial than is the use of other methods. Currently there is much discussion, and in many countries this has resulted in the revision of the abortion laws. The revisions generally relax the interpretation of the indications for therapeutic abortion. Induced abortion is apparently quite prevalent, and much of it is clandestine. It is estimated that there are approximately 8000 therapeutic abortions done in hospitals annually, compared to the widely varying estimates of 200,000 to 1,000,000 annual clandestine abortions.[11] Contrary to the popular stereotype, the great majority of women seeking abortion are those who already have children.

Whether medically sanctioned or not, abortion is not a simple matter. There are apt to be profound psychologic and physiologic effects on the individual and on the family. Perhaps the most effective way a community health nurse can prevent careless abortion is to help patients prevent unwanted pregnancy; that is, she can be sure that the availability of contraceptive measures is known to those who are under her care both before the advent of pregnancy (when possible) and as a regular part of prenatal and postnatal care.

The nurse, either through her own counseling or through referral to a social worker, spiritual adviser, physician, or other skilled helper, should make sure that the family knows of the possible consequences of abortion in advance of the decision. Even if abortion is medically recommended or is essential to the preservation of the mother's life or health, the family may still need support.

The Nurse Should Know the Resources for Care

In most communities there are several resources for family planning assistance. Family planning clinics provided by voluntary associations, by hospitals, or by government agencies are multiplying rapidly. In rural areas there may be mobile centers for family planning, counseling, and services, although rural facilities have on the whole increased at a slower pace than those in urban areas. Various groups operating under the aegis of the Economic Opportunity Agency include birth control referral services. Even more important, family planning is being included in general programs in obstetric and child care, in private medical practice, and in work with juveniles who are in trouble. The nurse should familiarize herself with these resources, preferably by visiting them.

The use of a particular facility by a particular family will depend on many factors. For example, some programs seem to involve a great deal of "red tape"; some are accessible on a 24-hour basis or only during evening hours; some are characterized by a high degree of personalization and warmth with an accent on counseling; others are impersonal. The type of service that appeals to one family may be considered very unsatisfactory by another family.

The nurse should ease the institution of service by familiarizing her patients with the procedures they are apt to encounter. Chesterman suggests that the nurse may help prepare the family to communicate with the service staff by giving them a chance to "rehearse."[12] She can also be responsible for seeing that her patients receive reminders of appointments and for interpreting the importance of follow-up visits that to the patient may seem no more than a way of distributing supplies; she may even help the family find a way to get to the health clinic. With migrant families she will be concerned with resources in the next stop of the migrant route so that uninterrupted care can be provided.

The nurse herself can be a resource by incorporating family planning content into whatever family service she renders; prenatal and postnatal periods, for example, offer a natural point for such content.

The nurse may serve as a member of the family planning service team. In this instance she would be providing more explicit direct care to families, and she would be expected to have some special training for this work. Nurse midwives may be particularly useful family planning team members.

IDENTIFICATION AND CORRECTION OF BARRIERS TO UTILIZATION

As has been indicated, when facilities for family planning services are available, the majority of those eligible are likely to avail themselves of the opportunity to use them. However, for some individuals and families and for some groups there will be reluctance or failure to use initial and follow-up care. Dropout rates will vary from center to center, but if the rate exceeds 20 percent, the situation should be carefully studied.

Barriers to utilization may be due to defects in the family planning resource itself. The family physician or obstetrician may be brusque, the hours may be inconvenient, or the staff may be considered lacking in humanity or warmth or may themselves feel that contraceptive practices are undesirable or immoral. The facility may be an "embarrassing" place (as is, to some persons, the welfare center), or it may lack privacy. In the case of young unmarried clients, it may not afford the special care they need. The nurse's role is pivotal: she can help to identify and remedy the clinic problems on the one hand and arrange for more acceptable sources of care for her patients on the other.

Lack of faith in professional advice may also cause a high rate of delinquency. A patient may refuse to try an alternative contraceptive method because the one previously prescribed has failed. This is particularly likely to occur if the patient had not been told of the possibility of failure with *any* method. Also, there may have been some side effects that discouraged continuation.

Misinformation, such as that which produces fear that a method may produce cancer, interfere with sexual relationships, or prevent future wanted pregnancies. also may be involved; although in urban areas particularly, recent intensive efforts have brought information to many through the mass media. Reliance on relatively ineffective methods in common practice (such as postcoital douches) may also prevent utilization of more reliable measures.

Barriers may also occur due to impulsive action or procrastination; if this is the case, the remedy must lie in changing patterns of behavior. Reminders, encouragement, and explanation by the nurse may help.

A nurse's case book can be the health authorities' most useful clue in determining the success of the program and whether or not a clinic's difficulty stems from problems within the clinic or within its patients.

Vulnerable Groups Should Receive Priority Status

Groups vulnerable to unwanted or risky pregnancy should be identified and given preferential planning and service time. Neighborhoods characterized by high maternal and infant mortality rates and a great number of unwanted pregnancies obviously warrant priority status. Areas in which repeated illegitimacy is common and families in which there is a pattern of out-of-wedlock or unwanted pregnancies represent another vulnerable group. Recent studies indicate that families who have had (or are having) their fourth child are at a critical point and often want and can benefit from family planning services.

In general, high-risk maternity patients constitute a specially vulnerable group, as do low-income groups and those living in rural areas without organized family planning services.

Whatever her role in meeting the needs of these families, the community health nurse provides valuable "back up" services for family planning.

REFERENCES

1. World Leaders Declaration on Population Presented at the United Nations on Human Rights Day, 1967. Population Council, New York, 1968, p. 13.
2. American Medical Association Renews Anti-compulsion Stand; Revises Policy on Population Control. J.A.M.A., *190*:31, December, 1964.

3. Jaffe, F. S.: Family planning and the medical assistance program. Medical Care, 6:69, January-February, 1968.
4. Urgent need for Family Planning-International Support. Nurs. Times, 64:567, April, 1968.
5. Jaffe, F. S.: A strategy for implementing family planning services in the United States. Amer. J. Public Health, 58:713 April, 1968.
6. Quoted in Population Crisis, Issued by the Population Crisis Committee of Washington, D.C., October, 1968, p. 5.
7. Jaffe, op. cit., p. 713.
8. Hutcheson, Hazel, and Wright, N. A.: Georgia's family planning program. Amer. J. Nurs., 68:332, February, 1968.
9. Beasley, J. D., et al.: Attitudes and knowledge relevant to family planning among New Orleans Negro women. Amer. J. Public Health, 56:1847, November, 1966.
10. Edmands, Elizabeth.: A study of contraceptive practices in a selected group of low income negro mothers in Baltimore. Amer. J. Public Health, 58:267, February, 1968.
11. Fonseca, J. D.: Induced abortion: nursing attitudes and action. Amer. J. Nurs., 68:1022, May, 1968.
12. Chesterman, Helen: The public health nurse and family planning. Nurs. Outlook, 12:32, September, 1964.

SUGGESTED READINGS

Amer. J. Public Health, vol. 56, Supplement to January issue, 1966, (Entire supplement).
Arnold, Elizabeth: Individualizing nursing care in family planning. Nurs. Outlook, 15:26, December, 1967.
Beasley, Joseph D., Harter, Carl, and Fisher, Ann: Attitudes and knowledge relevant to family planning among New Orleans Negro women. Amer. J. Public Health, 56:1847, November, 1966.
Chesterman, Helen: The public health nurse in family planning. Nurs. Outlook, 12:32, September, 1964.
Chilman, Catherine S.: Population dynamics in the U.S.: implementations for family planning. Welfare in Review, 4:1, June-July, 1966.
Chilman, Catherine S.: Poverty and family planning in the United States. Welfare in Review, 5:3, April, 1967.
Counseling for family planning. Amer. J. Nurs., 66:2671, December, 1966.
Draper, Elizabeth: Birth Control in the Modern World: The Role of the Individual in Population Control. Penguin Books, Inc., Baltimore, 1965.
Edmands, Elizabeth M.: A study of contraceptive practices in a selected group of urban Negro mothers in Baltimore. Amer. J. Public Health, 58:263, February, 1968.
Eliot, John W.: The development of family planning services by state and local health departments in the U.S. Amer. J. Public Health, 56:6, Supplement to January, 1966.
Family Planning Services in Public Health (Kit). Planned Parenthood—World Population, 515 Madison Avenue, New York, New York 10022.
Fischman, Susan H.: Choosing an appropriate contraceptive. Nurs. Outlook, 15:28, December, 1967.
Fonesca, J. D.: Induced abortion: nursing attitudes and action. Amer. J. Nurs., 68:1022, May, 1968.
Goerke, L. S., and Stebbins, E. L. (eds.): Introduction to Public Health. 4th ed., The Macmillan Company, New York, 1968, Chapter 14.
Hutcheson, Hazel A., and Wright, Nicholas H.: Georgia's family planning program. Amer. J. Nurs., 68:332, February, 1968.
Jaffe, F. S.: Rural Family Planning Programs. Planned Parenthood—World Population, 515 Madison Avenue, New York, New York 10022.
Jaffe, F. S.: A strategy for implementing family planning services in the United States. Amer. J. Public Health, 58:713, April, 1968.
Kirk, Dorothy N.: A family planning clinic on wheels. Nurs. Outlook, 15:36, December, 1967.

Minkler, Donald: Public policy in family planning. Nurs. Outlook, *12:*28, September, 1964.

Policy statement on population control. Amer. J. Public Health, *54:*2102, December, 1964.

Rainwater, Lee: Family Design, Marital Sexuality, Family Size and Contraception. Aldine Publishing Company, Chicago, 1956.

Siegel, Earl, and Dillehay, Ronald C.: Some approaches to family planning counseling in local health departments: a survey of public health nurses and physicians. Amer. J. Public health, *56:*1840, November, 1966.

White, Ruth M, Tayback, Matthew, and Hetherington, Susan: Family planning as part of maternity health services in a metropolitan health department. Amer. J. Public Health, *56:*1226, August, 1966.

Mental Health
and Mental
Disorder

Mental health and mental disorder are perhaps the most tantalizing of the many problems of modern community health practice. "Mental health" (or perhaps more accurately, "behavioral health") represents not only an area of community health service but also an aspect of community health practice that permeates all programs, all disciplines, and the work of all health institutions.

There is currently much soul-searching on the part of health professionals and the public about the community action that should be taken with respect to frank mental disorder and also about the care that should be provided for behavioral disturbances that never reach the level of mental illness or disability. The boundaries of mental health are so broad, the nature of mental health problems are so varied, and the care modalities so numerous and dynamic that the selection of a prudent and feasible course of action is far from simple. At the same time the impact of mental illness is so extensive and intensive that social action seems both imperative and urgent. The expectations of the public have been whetted by scientific discovery and by the reiterated evidence of linkages between mental health and social disorganization. The paradoxical result is that the public is demanding that the health system deal immediately and definitively with a problem still characterized by many unknowns.

Mental Health: Problem of Undefined Magnitude

Mental disorder is one of the most prevalent and disabling health conditions besetting modern man. The exact dimensions of the problem remain obscure, but all estimates indicate a very high rate of occurrence.

Kramer and LaPouse have pointed out the difficulties of correctly assessing the incidence and prevalence of mental disorders; LaPouse cites prevalence estimates ranging from a low of 23 per 1000 of the population, to a high of 370 per 1000.[1, 2]

One urban study reported that 81.5 percent of a population sample had some mental health problem; 23.4 percent of the population had sufficiently severe symptoms to be considered "impaired"; and 58.1 percent of the population suffered mild to moderate symptoms.[3]

In 1961 the National Committee Against Mental Illness estimated that one person in ten in the United States suffers from some form of mental illness,[4] and in 1962, the Blue Cross Organization estimated that about 3.2 million (or 17.3 per 1000) persons in the United States received some form of psychiatric care. About 62 percent of these were treated on an outpatient basis, either in a clinic or in a physician's office.[5]

Even though this figure is disturbingly high, it does not take into account many of those individuals who are treated for physical symptoms of psychologic origin but who are not considered as having a mental disorder.

The variation in estimates of mental illness is understandable, since what is labeled as "mental disorder" depends not only upon medical judgment but also upon a cultural definition of "normal" and "abnormal" as related to emotional or behavioral problems. Furthermore, medical diagnostic styles may differ widely.

Concepts of Mental Health and Mental Disorder Vary

"Mental health" may be seen by some as the absence of diagnosed mental illness or mental disorder sufficiently serious to interfere with one's usual occupation. At the other end of the semantic scale one might place Maslow's concept of "creative selfhood," a condition described by such qualitative characteristics as "superior perception of reality," "problem centering," "freshness of perception," and "richness of emotional reaction";[6] here the concept is one of developing and functioning to the capacity of one's genetic and biologic endowment. Mustard and Stebbins suggest that concepts of good mental health might include normal behavior, absence of mental disease, adjustment to environment, a perception of reality, and personality integration.[7]

Obviously, each of these concepts of mental health leads to a different decision about what should be done to promote and preserve the mental health of population groups. Thus the goal in the first case might be to prevent mental illness, to secure early and adequate care for those who do become ill, and by rehabilitative care to minimize the damage done by the disease. The goal of maximum functioning and self-realization clearly suggests a completely different order of aspiration and demands a different kind of social intervention.

The opposite of mental health, mental disorder or mental illness, is likewise difficult to define. It encompasses many diagnostic entities and a wide range of behavioral or emotional problems that never reach the stage of diagnosed illness. The senile dementia patient who is disori-

ented and dependent upon others for the simplest aspects of personal
care, the shop supervisor who adopts an autocratic and ego-diminishing
attitude toward his workers, the underachieving school child, and the
alcoholic executive all might be considered to exhibit some degree of
mental disorder.

Mental Disorder Threatens All Segments of the Population

Mental disorder and mental health problems affect all age, socioeconomic, occupational, racial, and cultural groups. The majority of the
mentally ill who require hospitalization are adults: 75 percent of those
under hospital psychiatric care are 35 years old or older, and only about
one percent are under 15.[8] However, among those receiving outpatient
care in clinics or physician's offices, the proportion of young patients
tends to be higher. With respect to problems requiring anticipatory
or preventive care, the younger age groups are also prominent, since
many of the psychiatric ills of later life have their roots in childhood
experiences.

Although more severe psychoses appear to be much more prevalent
among the lower income families, neuroses appear more often in upper
income families.[9] This statistic may, however, be due to the fact that the
economically secure group is more apt to seek care, and therefore the
neuroses are more likely to be counted. However, alcoholism is a
disease of the executive under pressure as well as of the homeless
drifter; drug abuse is a problem in the suburban school as well as in the
city school.

THE COST OF MENTAL DISORDER IS HIGH

Direct expenditures for psychiatric care from all sources in the United
States in 1962 was almost two billion dollars and represented an increase of 63 percent from 1956.[10] The indirect costs (lost wages or work
years due to prolonged absenteeism), estimated for patients in state and
county hospitals only, was over a billion dollars in 1962.

These figures represent only the monetary cost of mental illness. The
excessive use of self-prescribed or over-the-counter drug store medications by the lonesome and melancholic widow, the promotion that didn't
come because of "poor interpersonal relations," and the child warped by
a self-concept engendered by inadequate and immature parents represented wasted human potential of no small magnitude.

THE MEANS FOR ACTION ARE EXPANDING

Increasing Knowledge of Causation

The boundaries of knowledge about the nature and the impact of
mental disorder are being stretched. New discoveries about inborn meta-

bolic errors (about 60 are now known, and the number identified is growing rapidly), the effect of radiation of uterine environment, of prenatal malnutrition, and of infectious disease of the mother on the development of the fetus are all providing a broader base for protecting children from mental disorder that develops prenatally. Knowledge of the effects of phenylketonuria and of early maternal deprivation offers additional hope for the prevention of mental disorder. New appreciation of the importance of sensory stimulation in child development has made it possible to more clearly identify the "pseudoretarded" child suffering from environmental rather than biological deficiencies. The negative influence of the slum community or of the stress-loaded competition of the work community provide further channels of understanding.

In some cases, knowledge of the nature of a specific disease may be incomplete, but knowledge of treatment effects may be expanded. For example, although the etiology of schizophrenia remains obscure, great progress has been made in its treatment: hospitalization may be avoided entirely, for many others it may be shortened considerably, and disability can be sharply reduced.

The etiology of many mental disorders is still obscure, and the number of agents that may be implicated is large and nonspecific. It is the obligation of every worker in the field of mental health to keep constant vigil for unexpected behavior or for the regularly recurring conditions that may provide a small new clue to causative factors or to the effectiveness of particular methods of care.

New Treatment Modalities

The traditional one-to-one relationship of doctor to patient that characterized psychotherapy in its early phases remains one of the powerful approaches to psychiatric care. However, a growing number of other treatment modalities have appeared that are used sometimes independently and sometimes in conjunction with the traditional individual care.

Group therapy, first developed in the hospital setting, not only made it possible for the psychiatrist to treat more patients but also turned the strengths of the group itself to the therapeutic purpose. This group approach has proven useful to nonhospitalized as well as hospitalized patients and in dealing with both minor and major behavioral disorders.

Milieu therapy is based on the creation of a physical and social environment in which patients can heal themselves. The concept has implications for the home and for the community environment, as well as for the hospital.

Group "clean up campaigns" and the "rat wars" in low-income neighborhoods, "dress up day" in the school, and the development of citizens' action committees are examples of modifications in the environment that have mental health implications for the participants and, to a lesser degree, for the beneficiaries.

Family therapy, in which the family as a whole becomes the patient involved in its own treatment, allows conflicts to be brought to the surface where they can be dealt with and promotes intra-family communication and understanding. If the functioning of the family is improved, the mental health of its members is more likely to be assured. Each member, by understanding his role in the family and the way the family as a whole functions, also learns to understand himself and his relations to others.

Community psychiatry is described by Gerald Caplan in these terms: "Community psychiatry is based upon the acceptance of psychiatrists of responsibility for dealing with all the mentally disordered within the confines of a community."[11] The goal of community psychiatry is the reduction of the number of sufferers and the amount of disability and defect in the population. Thus, this approach exactly parallels the more general approaches to community health. Adelson emphasizes a comprehensive approach in community mental health, embracing prevention, a broad spectrum of services with multiple treatment modalities, highly coordinated multidisciplinary and multi-agency planning and action, and planned change as the foci of much of the effort.[12] Such community oriented approaches would provide for closer liaison among the various agencies and workers concerned with preventive and curative services for mental disorder and, hopefully, for a minimum of hospitalization consistent with treatment objectives. Such a liaison should bring psychiatric therapy and community health services closer together and promote interchange between psychiatric and general community health personnel. The community agency can provide information about families and their environment and about the values and dynamics of the micro- and the middle-sized communities. The mental health center can bring to the agency new services for patients and educational opportunities for the staff.

The Comprehensive Mental Health Center

A new and powerful resource for mental health care is the comprehensive mental health center, many units of which were developed as a result of passage of the Mental Retardation Facilities and Comprehensive Mental Health Centers Act of 1963. To qualify for federal assistance, each center is required to plan for care in conjunction with other resources and must provide at least five basic types of service:

1. Inpatient care.
2. Outpatient care.
3. Partial hospitalization (day care, night care).
4. Emergency services 24 hours a day.
5. Consultative and educational services.

In a center of this type one might expect to find services directed toward diagnosis, evaluation, and treatment, in addition to inpatient–outpatient follow-up and rehabilitation services, consultation to schools and other agencies, mental health research, inservice training of personnel, and public education. Thus it would provide for the patient a "one door," close-to-home service that would meet most, if not all, of his needs for care.

New Kinds of Workers

Only a small proportion of those requiring some kind of mental health services actually receive care. In an effort to bridge the gap, many different types of paramedical mental health workers are now being trained. Hartog has identified seven classes of mental health workers.[14] Of these, a recent addition, is the mental health technician, who is a product of a two-year course in the junior or community college. Indigenous workers with short on-the-job training have also proven helpful in crisis centers and in other care facilities. The volunteer worker, too, has taken on increased responsibilities in recent years. Such workers serve to extend services and may also be a means of placing currently unemployed people in useful work.

THE ROLE OF THE COMMUNITY HEALTH NURSE

Mental health services have traditionally held high priority in the work of the community health nurse. The mental health consultant was a familiar member of public health nursing staffs as early as the 1920's, and the use of psychiatric consultants has been frequently reported. Early efforts were directed for the most part toward minor behavior problems or toward improving nurse-family relationships. In the fifties, when the psychiatric hospital stay was shortened for many patients due to the effectiveness of drug therapies combined with home care, the services of community health nurses in more explicit care of the mentally ill patient and his family were extended. Case finding, referral, and patient–family support were extended to include supervising home care of the ill patient. It seems logical to assume that nursing input will be still further extended as mental health services increase.

A Ubiquitous Channel for Mental Health Services

The community health nurse provides a natural and highly effective channel for case finding and for a variety of other mental health services. She is accustomed to working in many different settings, with all age groups, and with people at all income levels. Her work is focused on the family and on the population as a whole and includes all phases of health care — health promotion, prevention, diagnosis and early care, continuing care, and rehabilitation. Mental health is an established concern. Previous discussions of nursing the growing family and the longterm patient make clear that many of the measures for preventing mental distress or disorder (such as preparation for predictable stress and assuring favorable emotional environment) are already integral parts of nursing service. Care of mental illness is assuming greater importance in community health nursing. A 1962 study made by the National Opinion Research Center queried 740 key officials in state and local mental and public health agencies in 50 states; at that time, 42 of the 50 state officials reported some use of nursing personnel in relation to supportive services for mental patients and their families.[15] Evans suggests that the community health nurse, by virtue of her generic public health preparation, is able with relatively little training to take on certain aspects of care of the psychiatric patient at home; and the experience of Collard and of Scarpitti *et al.* supports this view.[16–18]

As one who is close to the neighborhood and to the families in the community, she is, furthermore, in a strategic position to assist and participate in the work of a mental health center or other facility. She can help determine whether a particular family is likely to benefit or to be harmed by the hospitalization of one of its members, how presenting symptoms relate to usual behavior, and how much support and stability the family can offer to the returning psychiatric patient. She knows families well enough to estimate the likelihood of crises at points of stress and to gauge their resistance to stress. She is also in a good position to influence public opinion regarding mental health and mental health care.

THE PSYCHIATRIC NURSE SPECIALIST

Stokes and others report the use of psychiatric nurse specialists as therapists, backed up by a psychiatrist or by cotherapists in individual, group, and family therapy, in a setting in which the entire staff functioned as generic mental health workers in service groups organized to transcend hierarchical lines.[19] The nurse specialists provided consultation to community health nurses, teachers, probation workers, and group leaders, and also provided teaching and consultant services to nurses in other agencies. Generalized community health nurses carried much of the responsibility for preventive services and for prehospital and posthospital care. It seems likely that nurse specialists (practitioners) will be increasingly used in community health work.

Intervention Is Subtle and Pervasive

Roberts, discussing the care of psychiatric patients receiving visiting nurse services, pointed out that this care differed from other types of care in degree rather than in kind. This observation is equally applicable to preventive and health promotional measures directed at the improvement of mental health.[20]

NURSE-FAMILY AND NURSE-COMMUNITY INTERACTION ARE TREATMENT TOOLS

The nursing influence helps to mold family and community perceptions of behavioral problems.

The nurse–family relationship, important in any service, becomes crucial in the prevention and care of mental disorder. When incipient or frank mental disorder is present, the development of a fruitful relationship may be a subtle and difficult process. It may be necessary to win trust over and over again. Communication may be impeded by the embarrassment of the family caused by the "queer" behavior of the sick member, by longstanding habits of withdrawal from social contact, or by inability or unwillingness to face the realities of the situation. The family may be disrupted or estranged and difficult to treat as a unit.

The development of a working relationship may require that the nurse exert almost all of the effort to secure understanding and sharing of skills. She must pace the collection of information to the family's willingness to share feelings, and she must use the utmost skill and sensitivity lest she inadvertently add to the patient or family sense of anxiety or self-doubt. Similarly she must guide a community, lest its members fail to understand their obligations in the prevention of mental disorder and in the support of those needing care and rehabilitation. Her calmness and confidence are valuable adjuncts in all phases of the family-community program.

THE PATIENT

"The patient" in community health nursing services for prevention and care of mental disorder may be classified according to the kind of nursing intervention that is required.

1. *The declared patient* is the individual, group, or population that has been diagnosed as having a mental disorder. The psychiatric patient under care of the hospital, the family member coming for emergency help to the community mental health center, and the low-income area in a turmoil of hostile and violent reactions are examples of declared "patients." For this group, prompt and explicit care must be provided. Frequently these patients and families are not among those previously known to the community nurse. In a group of hospitalized patients served by public health nurses in Georgia in 1956, only about 8 percent of those referred from the hospital were previously known to the health department.[21] No generalizations can be drawn from this isolated experience, but it is likely that the community nurse's first contact with many patients will be during a critical period.

2. *The hidden patient* is the individual, group, or community that has definite symptoms of disturbed relations or perceptions but that has not been brought under care. Sometimes such patients are being treated for somatic conditions that are symptoms of psychic distress; sometimes they are concealing their symptoms deliberately or unintentionally or are unable to communicate their distress; sometimes they are known to the family or community worker but are not under care because it is felt that adequate treatment is not available. For this group, nursing observation and the knowledge of resources, as well as skill in helping others to define and accept a health problem, are exceedingly important. Since, as has already been indicated, such families may not be in the nurse's case load, the "observation" may in many instances be indirect—that is, it may consist primarily of sensitizing others to observe and report relevant facts.

3. *The potential patient* is the individual, family , or community that is especially vulnerable: those who live under conditions that place them at a greater than usual risk of mental disorder or emotional

distress and whose symptoms are not clearly indicative of need for psychiatric care. These include:

a. Patients and families of patients who have been previously hospitalized for a mental illness.

b. People under stress: those recently bereaved (especially those living alone); those with recently diagnosed catastrophic illness in the family; women at the menopause; those undergoing a sharp change in living style (sudden increase or decrease in family income, relocation, military service, or retirement); those hospitalized, or those having a family member hospitalized, for mental illness or retardation or for any other longterm or terminal condition.

c. People or groups with poor self-concepts, who are self-denigrating, oversubmissive, alienated, or suffering from anomie.

d. People with inadequate coping ability. This may be indicated by frequent unmet crises and can be characterized by children out of control; very poor money management; deliberate exposure to unwanted pregnancy; underachievement; inability to fulfill familial, community, or job roles; inability to handle crises even when anticipated; prolonged grief; overeating; excessive drinking; job delinquency; or overreaction to minor disturbances.

e. Those living in a hostile or unsatisfying environment: those living alone, especially older men and women; those living in a single-parent home; those living in a home devoid of warmth, intra-family communication, or characterized by discord, lack of balance in family power, harsh punishment, poor mothering, distorted family roles or overprotection of children; those living in socially deteriorated areas or subjected to discriminatory social action due to race or national background. All of these groups warrant a "second look" in the course of the nurse's work.

4. *The maintenance patient* is essentially the population at large, since no one is immune to the problems of stress and everyone occasionally needs unusual reassurance or support. Thus, the nurse must be concerned for the improvement of conditions necessary for the maintenance of mental health for the entire population that comes under her care.

THE GOALS

It is impossible to divorce the goals for mental health from those guiding other community health nursing services: the development of stable, mutually supportive, and warm intra-family relationships is important in child health and in mental health; the war against unsanitary housing is important in environmental control and in mental health, the preparation for the stress of death is important in geriatric care and also in mental health. Therefore the goals of mental health nursing might be generally stated as:

1. Using nursing to support the total community mental health program, in order to assure use of all available measures to prevent mental disorder or emotional malfunction.

2. Helping to preserve an intact and functioning family.

3. Supporting and assisting families in securing and participating in

treatment and in utilizing available resources to reduce emotional disability.

4. Helping to build family ability to solve problems and to deal with crises.

5. Contributing to available knowledge of the nature and causes of mental disorder and to the evaluation of prevention and treatment measures.

THE STRATEGY

To be effective, community health nursing activity in the field of mental health must be disciplined by a strategy that focuses action where it is most likely to be productive. Five strategies might be identified.

The big-merge strategy is one of joining forces in whatever way seems likely to work with the multitude of other individuals and agencies working for mental health. The efforts of the community health nurse and those of the family physician, the sanitarian, the school teacher, the many types of workers in the hospital and community mental health center, the personnel manager in industry, and the informal resources of the community must be joined so that each strengthens the work of the other. The specific role of the nurse will be exceedingly fluid in these merged efforts; sometimes she will provide information and support and sometimes leadership in patient and family-care management. The community health nurse can do much to unify the care provided by initiating case discussions or planning and evaluation sessions, developing referral procedures, or maintaining a continuing supervision of the family when services are of short duration.

The see-it-whole strategy is one of viewing mental health care in the context of the total need and the total effort and is dictated by the nature of community health nursing, which is, by definition, concerned with populations and with the whole spectrum of health services. Thus the community health nurse cannot in good conscience concern herself only with those with frank mental disorder or those who need preventive care or those in special population groups.

The it's-nursing-if-it-helps strategy is a refusal to be boxed in by traditional or outdated concepts of the boundaries of nursing function and is dictated both by the rapid changes in the nature of nursing practice and by the nature of mental health problems. In no field is it harder to draw professional boundaries. If the nurse is more readily available or in better communication with a given family, she may logically and legally do many things for them that might otherwise be considered the function of the mental health assistant, the physician, a special teacher, or the social worker. (Similarly, many functions ordinarily considered nursing may be undertaken by others when it seems to the advantage of the patient.) In this way it is possible to capitalize on the skills that are generic to the helping professions to advance the preventive or therapeutic care plan. Descriptions of current programs in mental health would suggest that community health nurses are doing far less than they could do safely and productively in the field of mental health and mental disorder.

The self-help–other-help balance strategy is another aspect of care that is generic to nursing but that also has particular importance in mental health care. Merrill has pointed out that the families in which the mother is hospitalized for schizoprenia have amazing adaptive strengths, but she wisely notes that one must also consider the possibility that if not properly used these very strengths may work to the disadvantage of the patient and the family.[22] It must, of course, be recognized that nursing itself may do harm if, for example, it provides aid that encourages a family to delay seeking medical help or if it leads to a family's over-prolonged dependence on a nurse. On the other hand, lack of immediately available support may be equally harmful. Dependency-independency needs are likely to vary widely among people with different treatment modalities, and over time. It is important that the nurse understand the strategy planned by the care team for each specific case so that she will know when to help by stepping in and when to help by stepping out.

The positive-valence-environment strategy involves manipulating the physical and social environment to produce a setting conducive to mental health and is dictated by recent treatment modalities. The school nurse, for example, might interpret to school personnel the special needs of the failing student for support and for success and help to create a supportive rather than a threatening school environment; or the community nurse might use a rat control program as a measure for developing neighbor-to-neighbor support in health matters that might increase the sense of community.

THE ACTION

Nursing action must be directed at all phases of prevention and treatment of mental illness, including the promotion of mental health.

The best avenue of prevention is good generic nursing in all areas of care. Thorough family care throughout the maternity cycle should, for example, include searching for possible genetic hazard, improving maternal nutrition, and avoiding unnecessary exposure to radiation and viral infection. A careful family health history that alerts hospital personnel to possible difficulties and the preparation of parents to fill their familial roles as competently as possible and to control family size as they see fit are good prophylaxes. Nursing care for venereal disease will help prevent neglect of syphilis. Good school or industrial nursing will help make the school and work environment a positive value in mental health. General health education will include building responsibility and competence for decision making in matters of health. Therefore, one of the things the nurse with a commitment to the improvement of community mental health must do is to review every one of her present activities for the opportunities it affords to promote mental health through direct preventive measures or through lessening adverse conditions that create undesirable stress.

The first step in providing care is finding those who need it. It is obvious that the nurse herself cannot be the sole case finder in the direct sense. However, she can be one of the important means of locating patients by alerting and enlisting many others who are in a position to observe and influence. Every person or group with whom the nurse comes in contact is a potential emissary or disciple. Louise Zabriskie, a pioneer in maternity care and a very wise and dedicated nurse, used to speak of the educational program she carried on with streetcar conductors, alerting them to refer obviously expectant mothers to sources of care. The streetcar conductor is no longer as available, but the principle remains sound: anyone in touch with the public is a potential case finder.

For them the community health nurse must try to provide knowledge of the symptoms that suggest a need for care. Hopefully, every parent, teacher, industrial foreman, high school youth, or anyone else likely to have effective entree to people should know that threats of suicide, hallucinations, delusions, assaultive or paranoid behavior, or confusion warrant immediate help and should know how to reach someone who can tell the individual where to get such help. They should know that bizarre or irresponsible behavior, frequent vague illnesses without defined disease, inability to sleep, sharp up and down moods, or withdrawal from the social group may presage difficulty. Abrupt changes in personal behavior — carelessness in dress or deportment, changes in sexual behavior, excessive anxiety or fatigue, or unusual dependence on alcohol or on drugs (whether addictive or not) — are apt to be signs of mental distress and as such merit attention. Parents and teachers in particular should be alert to the need to observe and report unusually slow development.

By including mental health content in the educational services provided to those who are in a position to influence others and by including questions about child growth and development in family or group health counseling, the influence of the nurse in detecting those who need help can be multiplied many times.

Once a patient has been referred for treatment, it is important that the nurse be prepared to engage in therapeutic care by supporting the medical regimen and by using her own skills to counsel with the patient and his family.

The degree of nursing participation in the therapeutic care of those who are mentally ill and living at home will vary. In virtually all instances the nurse will be responsible for supervising the patient and family as they carry through the recommended treatment regimen, for interpreting the rationale of the therapeutic plan (including the role drugs are to play in therapy), and for observing and reporting the patient's condition during the course of treatment.

Increasingly, the nurse is asked to participate in a broader way. Scarpitti and others reported on an experiment in which public health nurses, given a two-week orientation, acted with satisfactory results as principal care agents for schizophrenic patients at home.[23] Many other reports indicate increasing nurse responsibility in the clinic, mental health center, and in the home. The community health nurse may assist with referral to special facilities, such as day care centers, expatient clubs, or vocational training facilities.

The nurse may also provide care in the preproblem phase. For example, the individual who has shown a tendency toward self-denigration or toward belittling others may be helped to understand the probable basis for such feelings. Parents may be helped to see how belittling each other or the children may interfere with the capacity to use one's full potential and may create a reinforcing cycle of despair and doubt that lowers energy, initiative, and performance. Although such habits are often instilled during childhood and are hard to change and although they may require intensive help, in many instances the simple support and understanding provided by the nurse can do much to improve the situation.

Another point at which the nurse may provide care at the preproblem stage is at points of stress. She can help the family to tolerate the stress by encouraging them to take some kind of action in response to the situation and by preparing them in advance for inevitable later stress. The family dealing with a problem of catastrophic illness can be helped to prepare for the death of the patient or for the point when their own fatigue level has increased and their feelings of grief for the sick person are compounded by guilt at their own inability to carry on.

Sheer visibility or availability may be a great help in such preproblem situations; knowing that there is someone to call on and that help will come may be a great security builder.

The re-entry of the previously hospitalized patient into his family, work, and social group is another stressful period. The patient may be ambivalent about wanting to merge again with his world; the order and the protection of the hospital setting may be very hard to give up, particularly if the home situation is somewhat disorganized and family and friends lack appreciation of the nature of his illness. For the family, too, this is a period of stress as they try to decide what to tell the neighbors, how to act toward the returning member who may now seem a stranger because of his physical or emotional absence from them. They, too, may long for the uncomplicated life when the patient was under other care. At this point, someone to talk to, to explain and to reassure may make the stress tolerable.

The community health nurse often encounters behavior problems that result from a lack of such early care and that are of a transitory or minor nature, and she deals with them with varying degrees of support from psychiatric personnel. The nurse may deal directly with the child who invariably becomes ill on the precise day of the math examination or with the woman having mild problems associated with the menopause, and she may provide counseling and support as each individual defines and plans to meet his problem. This has been a traditional and important responsibility in community health nursing. With the extension of facilities for care of emotionally distressed children and adults, however, the nurse has a new resource for such care and may refer to others cases that previously she would have dealt with unaided.

When the nurse provides emergency care in the home or community mental health center, she must be immediately available. For this reason most centers provide 24-hour emergency care. In this setting, there is need for skill in dealing with acute psychiatric conditions and in making quick judgments. For these reasons, generalized community health nurses undertaking emergency care are usually either specifically prepared or work in cooperation with a psychiatric nurse specialist.

The Mentally Retarded Child

Mental retardation offers a special challenge to the community health nurse. Profound retardation affects all classes, but mild retardation is heavily concentrated in low-income groups, which suggests that environmental factors may be implicated.

There may be need for referral to special classes, vocational training, foster home care, sheltered employment, or institutional care. The nurse may help the family with the problems incident to the institution of such care, including dealing with the reactions of the parents and siblings as well as of the retardate himself. She can in particular help the family to understand and to deal with the pressures for a particular course of action, whether the pressure is based on competing emotional demands such as marital difficulties, on misconceptions about retardation, or on a lack of knowledge about available resources. She can also help the parents of those children who for a variety of reasons, only appear mentally retarded. *Pseudo retardation* (slow development associated with conditions other than mental disorder, such as deafness, severe motor defect, or emotional disturbance) is difficult to detect, and the nurse's observation of the child or adult in their usual environment may provide valuable clues for the clinician and prevent much unnecessary anguish, expense, and therapy.[24]

The parents of retarded children need to understand as well as love the retarded child and to appreciate the satisfaction he can achieve from small accomplishments and living routines. Parents need training, too, for they must provide the day-in–day-out activity necessary for stimulation and socialization. It is they who can offer the most encouragement and the relaxed teaching needed to push the retardate to his full capacity, to contribute to his ego development, and to improve his self-concept.

Community Attitudes Affect Mental Health Care

The importance of the community as a social environment that affects the mental health of its members has already received comment. The community health nurse is expected to exert her influence to correct detrimental community attitudes or behavior.

The community is also a provider of service; and information, impressions, and observations of the community health nurse regarding unmet needs or responses to specific programs may provide important data to community planners. The nurse may help mold public opinion by her own attitudes and by spreading information about developments in prevention and care of mental disorder and emotional disturbance. By enlisting the help of community members in providing support to the psychiatric patient returning from the hospital, she can also make clear that the great majority of psychiatric ills are not characterized by dangerous or assaultive behavior and that simple caring and helping gestures are powerful tools for rehabilitation. As the public becomes more informed, their attitude toward mental illness is likely to change, and the climate for care will improve.

Threats to the Nurse's Mental Health

Caring for the mentally disordered is a task that may occasion some uncertainty and frustration within the nurse. She may herself be fearful of mental illness and virtually immobilized when called upon to help another in mental distress; she may feel that much of the care required is not nursing, takes too much time, and interferes with the accomplishment of "real" nursing tasks or that it demands skills and knowledge beyond that expected of a nurse. She may find it hard to muster the necessary permissiveness and warmth in the face of slow progress or overt hostility, or she may feel that she cannot accept the concept of community mental health when she sees nursing as primarily a one-to-one nurse-patient interaction.

She may find it hard to accept the ambiguity of her role, the fact that some who receive care will nevertheless continue to do poorly, and that some must do without care.

The nurse may be hampered by a lack of knowledge and skill in dealing with psychiatric or behavior problems, ignorance of recent psychiatric treatment, or insecurity in evaluating patient status or progress. This feeling of inadequacy may be strengthened when families and medical personnel are not accustomed to looking to the community health nurse as a source of help in this particular field. She may not be certain about how much she should do. There are several steps she may take to remedy such conditions. She may:

1. Read about developments in psychiatric practice, treatment of addictive behavior, and mental retardation to increase her background knowledge.

2. Locate, with the help of her supervisor, consultant resources either in the agency or in the community. For example, if there is no mental health or psychiatric nurse consultant available on a regular basis to the agency, it may be possible to visit, observe, and confer with personnel at the nearest psychiatric hospital in order to "get the feel" of the problems. A local worker might help with problems of family counseling, or the psychiatric nurse or psychiatrist teaching in a nearby school of nursing may help with treatment measures.

3. Provide herself with ready reference material in areas where she feels insecure. A growth and development chart and brief notations of the action of specific drugs in current use for schizophrenia are examples of self-developed reference aids.

4. Talk out her own feelings with the nursing supervisor or other appropriate professional person, such as a consulting psychiatrist or mental health nurse consultant.

5. Get the facts—the facts about alcoholism or drug addiction, about the prevalence and incidence of mental disorders in the community, and about the characteristics of those who suffer from mental disorder.

The mental health aspects of community health care are so interwoven with every other service activity that competence in this special area is a critical issue in general nursing effectiveness. Activities that are specifically labeled "mental health" represent both a claim on community health nursing time and, at the same time, an opportunity to gain insights and skills that will carry over to many other phases of the nurse's work. Concern for improving community mental health will lead not only to seeking out those who need psychiatric help but also to modifying the community environment to make it more conducive to mental health. Here, too, the potential benefits go far beyond the immediate situation. Dealing with the ego-damaging effects of the low-income neighborhood may contribute to improvement of the health of a designated group of patients. It may also contribute to the realignment of relationships and attitudes so essential for social action and social justice. Thus the community health nurse can wisely spend much thought and care on the development of her skills in this area of professional practice.

REFERENCES

1. Kramer, A.: A discussion of the concept of incidence and prevalence related to epidemiologic studies of mental disorder. Amer. J. Public Health, 47:826, July, 1957.
2. LaPouse, Rema: Problems in studying the prevalence of psychiatric disorder. Amer. J. Public Health, 57:947, June, 1967.
3. Srole, Leo, Langner, Thomas S., Michael, Stanley C., Opler, Marvin K., and Rennee, Thomas A. C.: Mental Health in the Metropolis. McGraw-Hill Book Company, New York, 1962, p. 150.
4. What Are the Facts About Mental Illness in the United States? National Committee Against Mental Illness, Washington, D.C., 1961.
5. Blue Cross Reports, vol. 11, no. 3, July–September, 1964.
6. Maslow, Abraham: In Teevan, Richard C., and Birney, Robert C.: Theories of Motivation in Personality and Social Psychology. D. Van Nostrand Co., Inc., Princeton, 1964, p. 118.
7. Mustard, S. and Stebbins, E. L.: Introduction to Public Health. 4th ed., The Macmillan Company, New York, 1968, p. 169.
8. Hanlon, J.: Principles of Public Health Administration. 5th ed., The C. V. Mosby Co., St. Louis, 1969, p. 426.
9. Ibid.
10. Blue Cross Reports, vol. 11, No. 3, July–September, 1964.
11. Goldsmith, Stephen: Concepts of Community Psychiatry. P.H.S. Publication No. 1319, U.S. Government Printing Office, Washington, D.C., 1964.
12. Adelson, Daniel: Community mental health: a new frontier. In Kalkman, Marion E.: Psychiatric Nursing. 3rd ed., McGraw-Hill Book Company, 1967, p. 279.
13. Mental Retardation Facilities and Comprehensive Mental Health Centers Act of 1963, Public Law 88-164.
14. Hartog, J.: A classification of mental health non-professionals. Ment. Hyg., 51:517, October, 1967.
15. Williams, Richard: Trends in community psychiatry. In Bellak, L. (ed.): Handbook of Community Psychiatry. Grune and Stratton, Inc., New York, 1964, p. 349.
16. Evans, F.M.C.: The role of the Nurse in Community Mental Health. The Macmillan Company, New York, 1968, pp. 29, 38.
17. Collard, E.: The public health nurse in aftercare programs for the mentally ill. Amer. J. Public Health, 56:210, February, 1966.
18. Scarpitti, F. R., et al.: A community program for the mentally ill. Amer. J. Nurs., 65:89, June, 1965.
19. Stokes, Gertrude, et al.: A Giant Step: The Roles of Psychiatric Nurses in Community Health Centers. Faculty Press, Community Mental Health Center, Brooklyn, New York, 1969, p. 5.
20. Roberts, D. I.: Psychiatric service policy for visiting nurses. Nurs. Outlook, 4:510, September, 1956.

21. Beasley, F.: Public health nursing for families of the mentally ill. Nurs. Outlook, 2:482, September, 1954.
22. Merrill, Georgia: How fathers manage when wives are hospitalized for schizophrenia. Social Psychiatry, 4:26, 1969.
23. Scarpitti, F. R., Albini, J., Baker, E., Dinitz, S., and Pasamanick, B.: A community program for the mentally ill. Amer. J. Nurs., 65:89, June, 1965.
24. Michal-Smith, Harold: The Mentally Retarded Patient. J. B. Lippincott Co., Philadelphia, 1956, p. 41.

SUGGESTED READINGS

Abrams, Arnold, Gagnon, John H., and Levin, Joseph L.: Psychosocial aspects of addiction. Amer. J. Public Health, 58:2142, November, 1968.
Ackerman, Nathan Ward: Treating the Troubled Family. Basic Books, Inc., Publishers, New York, 1966.
Austin, Florence C., et al.: Characteristics of psychiatric patients who utilize public health nursing services. Amer. J. Public Health, 54:226, February, 1964.
Barnard, Kathryn: Teaching the retarded child is a family affair. Amer. J. Nurs., 68:305, February, 1968.
Bellak, Leopold (ed.): Handbook of Community Psychiatry and Community Mental Health. Grune and Stratton, Inc., New York, 1964.
Boone, Dorothy, and Mannino, Fortune V.: Cooperative community efforts in mental health. Public Health Rep., 80:189, March, 1965.
Bowlby, John: Maternal Care and Mental Health. 2nd ed., World Health Organization, Geneva, 1952.
Caplan, Gerald: Approach to Community Mental Health. Grune and Stratton, Inc., New York, 1961.
Caplan, Gerald: Principles of Preventive Psychiatry. Basic Books, Inc., Publishers, New York, 1964.
Collard, Eleanor: The public health nurse in aftercare programs for the mentally ill: the present status. Amer. J. Public Health, 56:210, February, 1966.
Cotter, Sister Mary Dolora: The public health nurse and community mental health. Nurs. Outlook, 16:59, April, 1968.
DeYoung, Carol D.: Nursing's contribution in family crisis treatment. Nurs. Outlook, 16:60, February, 1968.
Dutcher, Isabel, and Hakerem, Hella: Mother-child interaction in psychosomatic illness. Nurs. Forum, 7:173, February, 1966.
Ellis, N. Ried: Handbook of Mental Deficiency. McGraw-Hill Book Company, New York, 1963.
Essential Services of the Community Mental Health Center. U.S. National Institute of Mental Health, P.H.S. Publication No. 1624, U.S. Government Printing Office, Washington, D.C., 1968.
Evans, Frances Monet Carter: The Role of the Nurse in Community Mental Health. The Macmillan Company, New York, 1968.
Fackler, Eleanor: The crisis of institutionalizing a retarded child. Amer. J. Nurs., 68:1508, July, 1968.
Farberow, Norman L., and Palmer, Ruby A.: The nurse's role in the prevention of suicide. Nurs. Forum, 3:93, January, 1964.
Felix, Robert H.: Suicide: a neglected problem. Amer. J. Public Health, 55:16, January, 1965.
Freeman, Howard Edgar, and Simmons, Ozzie G.: The Mental Patient Comes Home. John Wiley and Sons, Inc., New York, 1963.
Ginott, Haim: Between Parent and Child. The Macmillan Company, New York, 1965.
Glittenberg, J.: The role of the nurse in the outpatient psychiatric clinic. Amer. J. Orthopsychiat., 33:713, July, 1963.
Greenberg, E.: Epidemiology of mental illness. International Journal of Psychiatry, 2:78, 1966.
Halpert, Harold P.: Public acceptance of the mentally ill: an exploration of attitudes. Public Health Rep., 84:59, January, 1969.
Hollingshead, August de Belmont, and Redlich, Frederick C.: Social Class and Mental Illness: A Community Study. John Wiley and Sons, Inc., New York, 1958.

Kalkman, Marion E.: Recognizing emotional problems. Amer. J. Nurs., $68:536$, March, 1968.

Katz, Elias: The Retarded Adult in the Community. Charles C Thomas, Publisher, Springfield, Illinois, 1968.

Lee, Marilyn J., and Frazier, Dorothy M.: Recognition of family-group health problems by public health nurses. Amer. J. Public Health, $53:932$, June, 1963.

Lemkau, Paul: Mental Hygiene in Public Health. 2nd ed., McGraw-Hill Book Company, New York, 1955.

Lemkau, Paul, and Crocetti, G. M.: An urban population's opinion and knowledge about mental illness. Amer. J. Psychiat. $118:692$, 1962.

Lucas, Leon: The Detroit group social activity for convalescing mental patients. Public Health Rep., $76:475$, June, 1961.

MacMahon, Brian, Johnson, Samuel, and Pugh, Thomas F.: Relation of suicide rates to social condition. Public Health Rep., $78:285$, April, 1963.

Mental Disorders: A Guide to Control Methods. American Public Health Association, New York, 1962.

Mental Illness and Its Treatment, Past and Present. U.S. National Institute of Mental Health. P.H.S. Publication No. 1345, U.S. Government Printing Office, Washington, D.C., 1965.

Neylan, Margaret P.: Anxiety. Amer. J. Nurs., $62:110$, May, 1962.

Northcutt, Travis J., et al.: Rehabilitation of former mental patients: an evaluation of a coordinated community aftercare program. Amer. J. Public Health, $55:570$, April, 1965.

The Nurse in Mental Health Practice. World Health Conference, Technical Conference on the Role of the Nurse in Mental Health Practice, Public Health Paper No. 22, World Health Organization, Geneva, 1963.

Owens, John, Nyman, Michael, Hill, E. David, and Stead, Peter: Nursing the drug addict. Nurs. Times, $64:584$, May, 1968.

Ozarin, Lucy D.: The community mental health center — a public health facility. Amer. J. Public Health, $56:26$, January, 1966.

Ozarin, Lucy D., and Levenson, Alan I.: Community mental health centers program after four year's experience. Public Health Rep., $82:941$, November, 1967.

Padilla, Elena, Elinson, Jack, and Perkins, Mervin E.: The public image of mental health professionals and acceptance of community mental health services. Amer. J. Public Health, $56:1524$, September, 1966.

Parad, Howard J. (ed.): Crisis Intervention: Selected Readings. Family Service Association of America, New York, 1965.

The Protection and Promotion of Mental Health in Schools. U.S. National Institute of Mental Health. P.H.S. Publication No. 1226, U.S. Government Printing Office, Washington, D.C., 1965 (rev.).

Quint, Jeanne C., and Strauss, Anselm L.: Nursing students, assignments, and dying patients. Nurs. Outlook, $12:24$, January, 1964.

Rohde, Ildaura Murillo: The nurse as family therapist. Nurs. Outlook, $16:49$, May, 1968.

Scarpitti, Frank R., Albini, Joseph, Baker, Elizabeth, Dinitz, Simon, and Pasamanick, Benjamin: Public health nurses in a community care program for the mentally ill. Amer. J. Nurs., $65:89$, June, 1965.

Schachter, Stanley: Obesity and eating. Science, $16:751$, August, 1968.

Stern, Edith Mendel: Mental Illness — A Guide for the Family. 5th ed., National Association for Mental Health, New York, 1968.

Stokes, Gertrude A., Williams, Florence Stoltz, Davidites, Rose Marie, Bulbulyan, Ann, and Ullman, Montague (eds.): The Role of Psychiatric Nurses in Community Mental Health Practice: A Giant Step. Faculty Press, New York, 1969.

Susser, Mervyn W.: Community Psychiatry: Epidemiologic and Social Themes. Random House, New York, 1968, pp. 3–28.

Ujhely, Gertrude B.: Grief and depression — implications for preventive and therapeutic nursing care. Nurs. Forum, $5:23$, 1966.

Ujhely, Gertrude B.: The nurse in community psychiatry. Amer. J. Nurs., $69:1001$, May, 1969.

von Bergen, Ruth: Intensive family health work. Nurs. Outlook, $11:202$, March, 1963.

Wade, Mattie L., Gillespie, Nancy S., and Sides, Murlene: How public health nurses promote mental health. Amer. J. Nurs., $63:81$, January, 1963.

Wellin, Edward, et al.: Community aspects of mental subnormality — a local health department program for retarded children. Amer. J. Public Health, $50:36$, January, 1960.

Community Diagnosis: Keystone of Public Health Practice

The basis of community health action must be an accurate assessment of the state of health of the community as a whole. For this reason, community health diagnosis is the keystone of community health practice.

In the past, estimation of the health of a population was often equated with death rates and the prevalence, incidence, and distribution of disease and disability. However, as health goals extend to encompass the improvement of the quality of health, as well as the prevention and treatment of disease, and as the impact of ecologic and psychologic forces on health and health care are more clearly understood, the concept of community health diagnosis becomes more complex.

An Ecologic Approach Is Essential

Basic to community health diagnosis today is the acceptance of the validity of the ecologic approach. The science of ecology concerns the interaction of man and his natural or man-made environment. Payne attributes much of the failure to solve the health problems of the world's peoples to the lack of this ecologic approach. He states:

> We have tended to regard man simply as a biological animal with biological needs, which can be satisfied by the expenditure of enough dollars and the provision of a few relatively simple physical necessities. We have largely ignored the fact that he is a social animal and that it may be at least as important to his health to satisfy his social needs and behavioral urges as his purely biological ones.[1]

Thus, community health diagnosis reflects not simply the additive record of health conditions and threats in a population group, but also (1) an evaluation of the dynamic situation in which that group is experiencing, adapting to, and modifying all of the biologic, physical, and social forces that have a bearing on community health and (2) the relationship and interaction of these forces.

MULTIDISCIPLINARY SKILLS ARE REQUIRED

Community health diagnosis may take place at all levels: from the judgment bulwarked by information collected by a single neighborhood worker from neighborhood residents to a full-scale report, using highly specialized and sophisticated techniques, on health and health care for a nation.

The development of a full-scale appraisal of community health involves the collection and analysis of many kinds of data and the combined judgment of several health and health-related disciplines. It will include the whole complex of public, voluntary, and private health institutions. Some of the required expertise will come from professionals in the traditional public health disciplines—the community health physicians, nurses, engineers, social workers, and biostatisticians. Some help will come from more specialized workers such as the anthropologist, the economist, the behavioral scientist, the sociologist, and the planning specialist. Also, it is increasingly apparent that community health assessment should involve the recipients of service.

A full-scale diagnosis that commands such a variety of talent is planned at relatively infrequent intervals and is likely to be sponsored by a planning group, such as a community health council or by a committee appointed by the local or state government.

The community health nurse will be involved in assessment primarily as a reporter of conditions in the area in which she works or as one who weighs the conclusions of the investigators against her own experience in the field. When a community health assessment is available, it should be studied by each community nurse as the background against which her own responsibility can be seen in perspective.

In many situations the need is for a relatively simple assessment in which one or more health workers get an estimate of the health of the neighborhood, county, or village in which they work. There may be data available that, when combined with thoughtful judgments made on the basis of observation and inquiry, provide a satisfactory basis on which to plan health programs. It is in these situations that the community health nurse is most likely to be involved in planning and carrying out an assessment of community health.

THREE CONSIDERATIONS OF COMMUNITY HEALTH
DIAGNOSIS

The community nurse should be aware of the process by which a community health diagnosis is made, for the steps will be the same at all levels even though there will be differences in the scope and sophistication of methods. Community health diagnosis is based on three interdependent, interacting, and constantly changing conditions:

1. The health status of the community, including the population's level of vulnerability.

2. Community health capability, or the ability of the community to deal with its health problems.

3. Community action potentials, or the ways and directions in which the community is likely to work on its health problems.

Any theoretical statement of the nature of an assessment will involve both data that are readily available and precise and data that are elusive and iffy in character (*i.e.,* areas in which methodology that permits a rigorous examination of the situation has been developed and areas in which educated guesses may be the best available method of investigation). Most community health leaders would agree that there is no need more pressing than the one for research that is both intensive and extensive into the nature of, and the methodology for, the assessment of community health that will provide not only a guide for action but also a much needed base for the evaluation of health care.

The Health Status of the Community

The health status of the population involves people in their environment. Consequently, the estimate of the health status of the community includes two interrelated factors: people factors and environment factors.

PEOPLE FACTORS

People factors include the following:

1. The characteristics and the growth trends of the population as a whole, including the relationships between birth and death rates and immigration and emigration rates; changes in the age, sex, or racial characteristics of the population; educational achievement levels; residence characteristics; and mobility.[2]

2. Trends in the death experience of the community, with special attention directed to untimely death.

The quality of the death experience is not necessarily shown in the death rate alone; the medical cause of death may also be a valuable indicator. For example, a high infant mortality rate or a high tuberculosis rate is generally considered evidence of inadequate preventive health services. Deaths from diseases such as measles, poliomyelitis, or diphtheria, for which preventive measures are available, are a sharp reminder of human waste, as are deaths from accidental causes. A rate used especially in developing countries as an index of untimely death is the "proportional mortality rate," developed by Swaroop.[3] This rate compares the number of deaths occurring in individuals 50 years old or older to the total number of deaths in the community. Its validity rests on the assumption that deaths in the younger age group have a higher preventability.

The medical cause of death may, however, be inadequate as a single measure of the quality of the community's death experience. If one accepts the theory of multiple causation and that the necessary and sufficient causes of disease may include personal-behavioral and social conditions as well as biologic or pathologic conditions, it is important to know what conditions, other than disease itself, are associated with a particular category of deaths. One such association that has been studied intensively is the relationship between poverty and the occurrence of certain disease entities such as tuberculosis, mental illness, and infant mortality; the relationship between cigarette smoking and death from lung cancer is another classic example. Effects of occupation and of life style, especially as related to the amount of exposure and response to stress, and the effects of climate, culture, and social integration or alienation are other areas that may affect the incidence of untimely death in a community. For this reason, it is important to know in which subgroups of the population deaths occur and the characteristics of the health behavior that may have a bearing on the prevention of untimely death. Such an analysis provides a base for remedial action.

3. The prevalence of presymptomatic illness.

There is more and more data on the existence of presymptomatic illness in population groups. Indices such as rising blood pressure, an increase in the cholesterol volume of blood, or small increases in blood sugar levels are examples of presymptomatic illness. These estimates may be made on the basis of special surveys or as part of a screening program.

4. The number and location of vulnerable or special risk groups in the community.

These are groups that do not have a disease or other condition requiring medical care but that are nevertheless at the mercy of some personal or social condition that makes them unusually susceptible to illness or lowers their capacity to deal with disease or disability. Communities characterized by extensive poverty clearly present a higher degree of vulnerability to health impairment, as do those in which the proportion of mothers with obstetric complications is great or where the number of unmarried teenage mothers is high. Relatives of diabetic patients, those markedly overweight or underweight, or those who habitually have an inappropriate food intake also fall into the increased risk group. Multiproblem families — those who are under care for a number of health or social conditions — are also considered to be a high-risk group; Gunn points out that in the multiproblem family, two types of problems may have significance for the health of the community: the first is the condition viewed as a problem by the family itself; the second is the condition viewed as problematical only by those outside the family circle.[4]

Vulnerability is also characterized by inappropriate or risky health behavior. Thus, in judging the quality of health in the population, it is helpful to know to what degree cigarette smoking, drug addiction, or excessive use of alcohol are prevalent. Careless habits with automotive vehicles may be characteristic of communities or groups; the farm area where young children are permitted to drive tractors or operate other large equipment or the high school group that takes pride in reckless driving are examples. Patterns of utilization of the available health services also reflect vulnerability levels. The extensive use of folk medicines and treatments, "shopping about" for medical care so that continuing care is made impossible, and delay in seeking care may constitute a distinct threat to health. Habits like these increase the vulnerability of the population.

5. The number and characteristics of those functioning below their potential health level. Even though this is not always an easy determination to make, the community health nurse frequently encounters individuals or groups who are obviously functioning at a level far below that which they could achieve. The chronically fatigued worker who has poor sleep habits and is unwilling to work within his physical limits, the mildly depressed housewife who sees life as an endless battle to catch up with the ironing, and the irritable, dyspeptic executive goaded to compete beyond reasonable limits are examples of functional underachievement. It is at this point that one moves from the concept of health as an avoidance of disease, disability, and death to the concept of health as a positive force for improving the quality of life.

As one peruses this list of five people factors, he sees the difficulties of community health assessment increasing. This increase may be partly due to a past preoccupation with illness and death as the principal indicators of health status and a resultant failure to move toward more precise methods for the diagnosis of the less obvious indicators of health status. However, the promotion of preventive and maintenance health care rests largely in the recognition of these less obvious deviations from health and in the development of measures to deal with them. The young worker who is helped to see the futility of accepting his chronic fatigue as inevitable may never become the tuberculosis patient who has to be identified, diagnosed, and treated. In affluent countries where disease control measures are well developed, it seems logical that these qualitative aspects of an individual's health will receive increasing attention.

ENVIRONMENT FACTORS

Environment factors include the following:

1. The physical environment, such as the purity of the air and water, the adequacy of housing, and the quality of the work and home environment.

2. The social environment, including the "metabolism" of institutions within the community, the stability of the population, the quality of social planning that attempts to prevent alienation of subgroups in the community, the effectiveness and acceptability of communication networks that provide for group identification, and the provision made for recreation.

Some environmental problems — e.g., the industrial air pollution and the community water supply — are amenable only to large-scale action. Others are matters that can be dealt with by individuals or families: air can be polluted with excessive smoke from burning leaves or with incautiously used insecticides; the quality of housing can be seriously impaired by poor maintenance practices. Rats, stairways without handrails, unvented gas heaters, and a school environment without proper handwashing equipment are examples of the kinds of environmental control problems with which the community health nurse will be concerned.

Even though it is true that in the past the major focus has been the physical aspects of the environment, the importance of the social environment and of the interdependence of physical and social aspects is increasingly clear. For example, it has been noted that although resettled slum dwellers may be in technically improved physical surroundings, they may be less happy than they were in their old environment where the social ties were different. Conversely, some who transfer from drab city slums to areas where the individuality of their dwelling is emphasized (*e.g.*, where there are separate yards for play) have improved the quality of housekeeping to a degree not seen when the move is only to another city apartment. Many housing experts now take into account the establishment of socializing centers that will take the place of the neighborhood store or the front stoop of the tenement. They now recognize the need of elderly people to see green grass from their windows and the importance of finding ways for people to get involved with the management of their environment. Welfare officials are finding that a modicum of beauty in the surroundings, in addition to the essentials for life, may be a powerful stimulus to self-respect.

The Health Capability of the Community

Health capability of a community is represented by the degree to which it is able to cope with its health problems and needs — to what extent its economic, institutional, and human resources are able to do the things required to assure the well-being of its people.

The general economy is an obvious and powerful factor in this respect. An affluent country or community almost always has greater potential for health action than does the community in which income levels are low. For health planning, it is also important to know how the wealth of the community is distributed. If the country as a whole is wealthy but the wealth is concentrated in a small privileged group, there may be large segments of the population whose situation does not reflect the general economic condition. On the other hand, a depressed economy may be reflected in general conditions of living that have a negative influence on health capability: a low level of educational achievement associated with inadequate school resources will slow down health education efforts and reduce the available pool of secondary school graduates from which the health professions recruit; poor roads or lack of public transportation may make health facilities inaccessible even when they do exist in adequate quantity and quality; inadequate nutrition may sap the energies of the population and make them indifferent to all but the most crisis-oriented health services.

INSTITUTIONAL RESOURCES

Institutional resources, such as hospital beds, nursing homes, and other community health facilities (health departments, visiting nurse associations), are apt to vary widely in quantity and quality from community to community. In addition to the actual number of facilities (or the ratio of beds or services to the population) it is important to know to what degree these facilities are obsolescent or inadequately equipped, how geographically and financially accessible they are to the people they serve, how well or how poorly they are staffed to suit their functions. For example, a community may have what appears to be a good supply of nursing homes. However, if these are proprietary (profit making) institutions that charge more than most of the people in the community can afford to pay, if they are located at great distances from the users of care, or if they are staffed so that there is virtually no professional nursing supervision, the community is not, in fact, capable of handling its problem of nursing-home care.

The ways in which resources are organized and used may be as critical as their availability. For example, if health agencies have the equipment and the know-how to provide preventive as well as curative services but programs are administered so that care is limited to those who are already ill or if the facilities are utilized by only a few of the population, the resources are still inadequate in relation to the needs of the population. If hospital beds are available for immediate care of cancer patients but admission policies are so rigid that they cause undue delay, the end result may still be insufficient. The adequacy of facilities may also be more apparent than real when there is lack of coordination, gaps and overlapping in services, or institutional isolation. For example, if a hospital has not developed adequate measures for referral, the posthospital cardiac patient may lose much of the benefit of his hospital stay, or he may have to utilize hospital services to a higher degree than should be necessary. If every institution relies only on its own information about a patient instead of using the information available from other groups, its effectiveness, as well as that of other groups, is reduced; and the institution is able to provide less care than one might expect from the ratio of the facilities to the population. Good community-wide planning maximizes the care provided.

HUMAN RESOURCES

In health care, two kinds of human resources must be considered: the professional resources of the community itself—of institutional human resources such as nurses and physicians—and the informal human resources resident in the general population.

Formal Human Resources. The availability and quality of health manpower will vary widely. The nature of the medical supply in the large city may be such that there is a great complement of specialists and very few general practitioners, ample facilities for hospital care but virtually no home visiting by the physician, excellent care for crises but little continuing health surveillance. In the rural area there may be a general practitioner available who represents a first-line health resource, but specialization backup may be at some distance. Manpower in community agencies may also vary; there may be a good supply of professional nurses but a small group from which to draw nurses' aides or other auxiliaries, a situation that might be reversed in another community. In some communities there is a strong complement of specialized workers on the health teams in hospitals and in other community health agencies, whereas in other areas there may be essentially the old "three part team" in public health—the physician, the nurse, and the sanitarian—with specialists available intermittently or by referral to another community.

With respect to health manpower, it is important to reemphasize that the organization and coordination of manpower resources is as important as the numbers and types of personnel available. If, for example, the physical therapist is available in the hospital but does not participate in the training of nurses who must provide posthospital care, there is a lack of manpower from the standpoint of the community health agency, even though the number of physical therapists is judged to be adequate for the community as a whole. If short-trained workers are organized and used with inadequate on-the-spot guidance, they may be available in adequate quantity but not in adequate quality.

Informal Human Resources.   Informal health resources have equal, if not greater, importance than professional institutional resources for health care. For example, the self-reliance and general responsibility potential of a community provides a valuable resource for health care. In a rural community where there is little affluence but also little poverty, individuals, families, and small neighborhood groups may have developed great abilities to care for their own health: older and wiser women in the community may seem a natural resource to the young wife and mother, church groups may provide home care for families when the mother is ill or otherwise unable to care for her family, and home nursing and transportation to health facilities may be undertaken by neighbors. On the other hand, in the very low income neighborhood in a large city, where educational achievement is low, dependency is high, and instability in family structure is common, the immediately available resources for self-help are more limited, and health professionals may have to provide many of the services that in other settings would be provided by the individuals themselves.

Human resources may also vary between communities made up largely of retired persons and suburban areas populated by young families. The variance grows out of the particular abilities of different age groups with respect to their own care and to their ability to help with the care of others. Again, in communities where most mothers work outside the home, less dependence on self and neighbors for health advice can be expected than in areas where most of the married women do not work.

The Health Action Potentials of the Community

Community action patterns affect health planning. Each community will differ in its patterns of health action, depending on the value people assign to health as compared to their other life needs and their characteristic way of taking action, the political system by which they govern themselves, and the habits they have developed with respect to social action. These characteristic ways of thinking and acting apply both to individuals and institutions within the community. They are of great importance in health diagnosis, since they determine the ways in which the community as a whole will respond to its health needs and the measures for improving the health situation that are likely to prove relevant, acceptable, and effective.

To use an analogy from individual diagnosis, the doctor needs to know not only the kind and severity of his patient's infection but also how well and in what ways this individual moves to deal with assaults to his life. Does he tend to give up in despair, turn to someone else to make his decisions, or delay taking required action as long as possible; or does he deal with any impairment with aggressive determination? In many instances the medical-care treatment must be as dependent upon this knowledge of the patient's ability to deal with problems as upon the accuracy of the diagnosis and the propriety of the treatment.

The assessment of the action patterns of a community involves an estimate of the basic values and beliefs about health that provide the impetus for action, the institutional system that supports the action, and the habits the community has developed for dealing with common problems.

Characteristic Beliefs and Behaviors

Within a community, there may be identifiable subgroups that develop their own ways of life and of working on their common problems. The town and gown schism is one example of this, an example that most colleges and universities are trying to eliminate. "Little Italy" or "West of the railroad tracks" or "the hollow" may be recognized by those who dwell there to have an individual identity and to merit care and social action consistent with their special values, life ways, and problems. It is important to know not only what subgroups exist but also to what degree they share in and differ from the values of the larger community, for from community values spring the community health goals—those things the community considers "good" in health care.

In some communities, traditional ways of behavior will be strictly followed, with many of the details of daily living subject to elaborate rituals and rules. In others, individuality may be stressed; or there may even be great rigidity in the need to be different. In one neighborhood, kinship bonds may be exceedingly strong; and in times of trouble, help is usually sought from a mother, an aunt or other relative, or a wise neighbor. In other communities the rule appears to be I-don't-bother-my-neighbors-and-they-don't-bother-me, and each family deals alone with its problems.

The value assigned to health care as compared with other life needs is also frequently culturally determined. In some communities health will be high in the hierarchy of life values, and health information and care will be sought and welcomed. In others areas, competing values may take precedence: the need to "get ahead" may seem more important to the business executive than does developing a way of life that will reduce stress; the struggle for sheer survival of those in pioneer or poverty situations may put all but the most immediate and urgent health needs low on the priority scale. In some communities the decisions of a

prestigious leader, such as a village priest or mayor, may influence the
behavior of the whole group; in other areas, the sources of influence are
much more diffused, a situation that prevails in large urban areas where
people tend to affiliate with and be influenced by one set of people at
work, another at church, and another at home.

These characteristic ways of behavior are exceedingly important to
the health planner. For example, if one of the health goals is that women
in certain age groups examine their breasts periodically as a means of
early detection of abnormality, education might be planned on a one-by-
one basis, with the health worker talking with individuals in their homes
or at a clinic about the reason for the procedure, the technique, and what
ought to be done should anything unusual be found. If neighborhood ties
are strong, the instruction might be given in neighborhood groups; in this
situation the educator has the advantage of reaching larger numbers and
the opportunity of using the group members themselves for mutual aid.
If the strong-leader pattern prevails, attention should be placed on
reaching and convincing the leaders before any attempt is made to
contact the target population.

THE COMMUNITY'S POLITICAL SYSTEM

The interrelationship between the political and government structure
and the people it serves is an important factor in predicting the means by
which the population will move to meet its health needs. Although
politics is often used as a derogatory term, synonymous with lack of
integrity and commitment to the public, the political system does represent the way in which a population group has organized to facilitate
collective action and to exert some control over its collective behavior.
The stability and responsiveness of the political structure has considerable effect on the ability of the community to develop continuing
and stable health programs. The way the several groups of people in the
community see "the government" also affects their expectations concerning government health action, their willingness to support and participate in government-sponsored health activities, and, often, the way in
which they relate to the health department, the school nurse, and other
government workers (*i.e.* with confidence and trust or with suspicion
and hostility).

The relationship between the political system and government units
also has an effect on the way in which the community's health tasks will
be accomplished. The degree to which health personnel are subject to
political appointment has an effect on longterm planning, since (1) political control tends to produce less continuous staffing than does the
merit system and (2) political control may attract job applicants whose
talents run more along the line of party loyalty than of professional
expertise. In general, it is considered desirable in a democracy that those
positions that are essentially policy-making in nature be tied to the
political system, since elected officials, especially those at higher levels
of responsibility, are usually committed to some kind of change and can
accomplish this best if the policy-making staff is like-minded. On the
other hand, positions that are primarily administrative and implementing
may lose much by political appointment, since the continuity of program

implementation is determined at this level and stability in the work force is beneficial. It is important to know to what extent health personnel are subject to political appointment. Also important is the degree to which the political establishment concerns itself with health programs. Do they "leave it to the experts," giving little attention or support to the programs as they develop; or do they take an active part in representing the public's needs and in striving for effective and efficient health-care systems?

THE COMMUNITY'S HABITS OF ACTION

Both the report of the National Commission on Community Health Services and the Comprehensive Health Planning Act use the phrase *partnership for health* to describe the relationship that should exist between health efforts of government at all levels and private and voluntary health services.

In the United States and Canada, as in many industralized countries of the world where private and government health-care systems are well developed, the relationship between the two is of major significance to the health of the community. This relationship may be hostile, each feeling the other is failing to act in the true interests of the community. It may be polite, being based on a scrupulous observance of declared spheres of influence, with neither party trespassing into areas that are considered the other's province. It may be a true partnership in which government agencies and voluntary agencies, private medical and health practitioners and government health employees, and hospitals and other community agencies truly combine efforts to define and correct the health problems of the community. Obviously the last pattern is the one desired, but all too often there exists something between the first and third patterns of cooperation.

To understand the health action patterns of a community, it is important to know in what ways the different levels of government interact: to know the nature of the flow of money, advisement, and support from national to state to local agencies and from the community agency to the various smaller geographic or cultural units within the community. It is important to know how the government agency interacts with the private physician: does it move to his support, provide him with consultation and patient-care services that will strengthen his work, and share responsibility with him on a planned basis; or are both groups acting as isolated entities? It is also important to know how government agencies interact with voluntary agencies: does the local health officer welcome the help of the people from the local tuberculosis association and keep them informed of the health department's plans; or does he secretly wish they would disappear and let him get on with the job? Does the government agency work with the local nurses' association on salary problems; or does it get involved only when involvement cannot be avoided?

"Who Does What" Is an Important Question.   Within each community there is apt to be a relatively small group of individuals (or institutions) that exert considerable influence on the decisions of others in the community and so become in effect the decision makers in many matters of public concern. Such a power structure has engaged the interest of sociologists for many years and has engendered some controversy over the means by which such individuals can be recognized.[5]

Recent studies indicate that power tends to be a specialized rather than a generalized attribute; the person or group exerting the influence may vary in different subgroups or in different problem areas: the individual who is in a strong position of power with respect to health decisions may not be the same one who initiates a program for city beautification. Furthermore, the person who is most vocal and most visible as a committee member may not be the one who is exerting the pressure; a behind-the-scenes leader may, in fact, have greater control. Thus, in seeking out the leadership group in a community, it is important to distinguish the figurehead from the one who truly exerts an influence on the decisions made.

Of considerable interest in recent years is the emergence of increased power among the organized poor and among students; both groups have recently exerted considerable influence on local and national decisions, the exact antithesis of their former power stance. With respect to leadership power among the poor, the change undoubtedly represents both a shift in the nature of the problems engaging the social planners and a defined public commitment to the development of leadership in this group. The result is that in many communities there is a new type of leader whose influence derives from his sharing in and knowledge of the problems of extreme poverty and whose natural capacity for leadership has been carefully fostered as a matter of social policy.

"Who Talks to Whom" Provides Action Clues.   The network of communication that is built up within families and groups has an important part to play in the development of community health plans and therefore is logically included in the community assessment process. Informal influence, such as that found within the family or work unit, has been recognized as a powerful factor in securing health action; and the degree to which such informal influence is favorable to good health practice is a matter of concern to health officials.

The patterns and the force of influence within a family differ greatly. When kinship ties are strong and communication among family members is extensive, the opinions and judgments of even the remote relative may exert considerable influence on family health decisions and attitudes. In some families, relatives are the first-line of help in emergencies of all types, and family response to the needs of its members may be prompt and generous; in other instances family ties are weak, and the first source of help or advice may be a community agency or professional worker.

Informal influence may also be exerted through friendship and organizational affiliations. Studies have shown that most people develop friendships of a continuing type. Bell and Boat[6] and Smith and co-workers[7] found that only a small proportion of the groups they studied could not identify "best friends."

In addition to individual and family communication networks, the numbers and types of groups with which community members are affiliated may have a strong influence on the way they perceive and act in health matters: the stand taken by his church may influence the individual's attitude toward contraception; the official position taken by a labor union may influence its members' judgments about the best methods for delivery of health care services; social affiliations may affect one's perception of the value of health care. Freeman and Lam-

bert have found that in at least one situation, community groups influenced health behavior to some degree.[8] Thus it is important to know
insofar as possible the channels of communication and the network of
social relationships that exist in a group as a basis for understanding the
ways in which they might be expected to take health action.

Communities Have Their Own Styles of Response.   Communities develop their own style of responding to health problems in the
way they organize to take action as well as in the characteristic course
of action followed.

Some communities tend to organize for health care on a community-
wide basis, with plans and action designed for the city or county or state
as a whole; in other areas, action may be developed within a loose
structure of community-wide planning, with considerable diversity in the
programs of smaller groups within the community; and in still other
communities, each small action group appears to go its own way with
little relationship to the plans or actions of other groups.

Some communities tend to organize for health care under well-defined
goals; others move within a vague general commitment to health care,
"rocking along" with current programs or leaving the decision to the
health administrator. When the goal-oriented approach is used, the goals
may be set by the health professionals, by representatives of the community, by a political body, or by some combination of these groups.
These goals may be minimal—to have safe streets and to be protected
from dangerously ill people and epidemics—or the goals may be much
more inclusive and operatively stated—to give the old people the medical and nursing care they need and to give mentally retarded children
educational and health opportunities to maximize their skills. Sometimes
these goals are consciously arrived at, explicitly stated, and deliberately
pursued. More often, what the community wants and is willing to support in health care is not formalized but is nevertheless expressed in
health behavior such as their patterns of utilization of available services,
their legislative action, or their response to the care provided.

Families or subgroups within the community also organize for their
own health care in different ways. They may plan on an expedient crisis
basis, using the emergency room of the local hospital as their primary
source of care; they may take a more prudent approach through prepaid
insurance and a wider use of preventive care; they may rely entirely on
the medical center specialist group for medical care or on the general
practitioner for first-line care of illness, using the medical center only for
serious problems. A recent study of 375 women in a rural county found
54 different patterns of infant health care in this group.[9]

THE NURSE'S SOURCES OF COMMUNITY HEALTH DATA

The community health nurse will find and must investigate many
sources of information that will shed light on the health situation of a
community. Official agency records, state or local published reports of
vital statistics and services provided, formal and informal conferences
with community leaders will all yield many facts and opinions that
together produce a picture of the situation.

Official Vital Statistics Provide a Useful Base

The decennial census of the United States provides detailed health and health-related information, much of which is detailed for states for local communities, such as counties and municipalities. The infrequency of the count, however, means that there will be times when the data for the local area are incomplete or inaccurate — for instance when a recent major extension of housing increases the population within a matter of months. However, the census is a valuable source of data that shows trends over time and provides the national picture as a backdrop against which the local situation may be viewed in perspective.

Local vital records or reports, generally available through the local or state health department, may prove more immediately useful. Reports of births and deaths frequently include more information than the mere fact of birth or death. A birth certificate, for instance, may include such information as whether or not the mother received prenatal care, and it may give facts about the delivery as well.

Surveys or Survey Reports Supplement Official Records

The United States Center for Health Statistics has as its purpose the continuing assembly and interpretation of health data for the population as a whole. In addition to the usual information about births, deaths, and reportable diseases, there is provision for a continuous survey of the population based on probability sampling techniques that yield data regarding the prevalence (*i.e.*, the number of individuals suffering from a particular condition at a given point in time) and incidence (*i.e.*, the number of new cases over a specified period, usually one year) or illness or disability. One segment of the program of the center is based on data collected from household interviews, the content of which may be modified from time to time to secure data of particular current interest.[10] Special surveys may be undertaken for disease-related occurrences, such as the incidence of smoking or the blood cholesterol levels of given age groups. Some of the studies combine household survey procedures and medical examination procedures. The various reports of the center are published by the Government Printing Office and are available in most health libraries and in many public libraries. Such survey data represent one of the valuable tools for public health practice.

Some local communities provide for an ongoing small sample survey that is carried out as part of the regular service. In Baltimore, Maryland, for example, a continuing household survey is carried on in which 100 families are seen each month on a carefully determined sampling basis. This sort of survey both provides cumulative data and permits a quick check on current problems affecting the total population.[11]

Special local surveys may also be organized to provide data not otherwise available or to answer specific questions. For example, a household survey might be planned to find out what differences exist in the utilization of local health resources. Surveys may be oriented to epidemiologic, behavioral, or biologic data and will vary widely in methodology. However, their two primary characteristics are that they are based on a sample that is sufficiently representative of the population being studied in order to render the findings predictive for the whole group and that the methodology is such that it minimizes the likelihood of unreliable findings.

Central Registries on Specified Conditions

Central registries may be maintained for specified conditions, such as crippling, cancer, tuberculosis, or mental illness. The purpose of such a registry is to make available at all times a count of those reported as suffering from particular diseases or impairments and the status of each case with respect to disease state and treatment. Such accounting makes it easy to plan for shifts in program as the size of the register grows or shrinks and as the characteristics of those persons listed in the register change.

Agency Records Provide Current Data

Records of hospital admissions and discharges, health department reports or case records, and insurance group records may provide data about health in the community and the services that the people are receiving. Records of illness, physical examination reports, and records of absence in schools and industries are sources of information of illness in special age or vocational groups. However, agency records that are not directly concerned with the illness and its treatment are often considered unreliable sources. For example, nursing records are probably a poor source to use for determining to what extent patient teaching programs are being implemented.

Another source of useful information is reports of screening experience — both special screening efforts and the ongoing screening that may be done in schools, industries, or in the health center for the general public.

Systematic Observation and Inquiry

Systematic observation and inquiry are good sources of community health data. For example, systematically querying prenatal patients as to their reasons for seeking medical care at the point they did may produce information on attitudes toward prenatal care. Observing which children report to the nurse in the school and the reason for their visit, combined with the teacher's judgments about the child's behavior, may help to single out children who are overanxious or underanxious about their health and help to identify those who may be unusually vulnerable. This type of inquiry can be escalated to full-scale research when the occasion warrants; Sometimes it is possible to engage in this kind of research as part of the ongoing job or to get assistance from others in the agency or from a university that may conduct the study.

Current journals, such as the nursing and public health journals, often provide information about other communities, information that may be valid in one's own setting. More specialized journals may report on community studies, such as reports of adherence to regimen among tuberculosis patients; again, these reports might have significance for one's own community.

There is a great wealth of sources. The individual involved has the responsibility of seeking out those that provide suitable data on which to base an estimate of the health of the community.

ANALYSIS OF AND INFERENCE FROM HEALTH DATA

The assembly of available factual data, of observations, and of judgments about the health conditions and the health functioning of the community is only the first step in diagnosis. The rest of the process involves the ordering and synthesis of these bits and pieces of information (which are likely to vary greatly in their quality: that is, in their reliability and generalizability) into some kind of whole that permits drawing inferences that will serve as the basis for program planning. This means that the data must be studied and related in an orderly way.

Data Must Be Seen in Perspective

Current information about health conditions and health behavior represents just one point in a long process. First, it is important to see present conditions in the perspective of time; in other words, one must recognize trends. For example, current deaths from accidental causes need to be seen in terms of the type and the number of such deaths in the past. Is the overall rate climbing or falling? Are rates for certain types of accidents changing? If the data are seen in the perspective of time, their meaning is amplified.

Second, it is important to see statistics in the perspective of the larger environmental forces that might have significance: the greater likelihood of accidental death due to an increased number of automotive vehicles; improved housing that lessens the number of home accidents; shifts in parent-youth or youth-society relationships that are conducive to aberrant behavior on the part of young people. Is the increasing syphilis rate largely accounted for by small population clusters, or is it distributed throughout the community? Is good utilization of facilities associated with their location, with the participation of the consumers in the management of the facility, or with the kind of personnel employed in the facility? The search is for those things in the environment that could be associated with an observed change, whether that change is favorable or unfavorable.

Quantitative and Qualitative Facets of the Data Must Be Balanced

The number of cases of dental caries represents a tremendous problem in terms of size. However, in terms of impact on total health, this number may carry less import than does a rising venereal disease rate. In terms of avoidability—another quality criterion—it would perhaps add up to a lesser level of importance than, say, the number of cases of measles among children. Nutritional deficiencies carry a different qualitative value in an affluent country than they would in a country where frank underfeeding is associated with economic inability to secure adequate food supplies. Therefore, unless qualitative criteria are applied, the statistical magnitude of a problem may dangerously distort its real importance.

Inferences Provide a Base for Action

Once relationships become clear, it is possible to move toward inference: the general conclusions that may be made on the basis of the data. For example, it may be apparent that a particular community will not respond well at a particular time to a crash program for tuberculosis control. This may be because they accept the disease as inevitable and that transportation and manpower deficits make it difficult to get the required medication or to provide the necessary supportive care to direct people in taking the medication. Furthermore, folk medicine may be a powerful deterrent, and the relationship between the indigenous practitioners and the organized health unit are characterized by a lack of understanding and trust. The first thrust might thus be toward caring for individuals and postponing the mass action.

In another instance the conclusion might be that it is essential to move quickly into a measles vaccination program, even though it will be difficult to get supplies and to work out satisfactory arrangements with private physicians. The public is impatient; they are used to having new discoveries placed into the program early; the product is safe; the physicians for the most part are likely to "go along" with a crash program if it is properly presented; other urgent programs will be disarranged but not seriously impeded by the requirements of this one; and a group of volunteer workers in low-income areas are anxious to have a specific program to work on. In this situation, the forces for quick action outweigh the forces for a more deliberative approach.

In other instances, inferences may be made about the possible outcomes of the program. The combination of multiple and serious health impairment, low income, negative attitudes toward authority, and a great need for identity in a low-income urban group might lead one to infer that goals should be set at a more moderate level. At the same time, service requirements may need to be built beyond the point that the health conditions themselves warrant in order to establish a level of direct help that would obviously demonstrate an honest and sustained effort to help.

The inference stage is the transition between diagnosis and program planning. It defines and sets the limitations, the imperatives, the maximizing opportunities that appear to exist, and it indicates the kinds of approaches that might be expected to be useful. Thus armed, the health worker is in a position to move to specific program planning and implementation.

The simplicity or complexity of community health diagnosis depends on the situation and on the preparation and availability of the professional worker. Some appreciation of the community in these broad terms is an essential background for the nurse as she plans for the nursing care of population groups, however large or small these groups may be. As she studies the needs for nursing care within the population for which she is responsible, she will use to some extent the observations and the processes required for more elaborate community health diagnosis.

REFERENCES

1. Payne, Anthony M. M.: The environment in human ecology: general considerations. *In* Environmental Determinants of Community Wellbeing. Pan American Health Organization, Washington, D.C., 1965, p. 3.
2. For a definition of rates and their application see Mustard, S., and Stebbins, E. L.: Introduction to Public Health. 4th ed., The Macmillan Company, 1968, pp. 97-103.
3. Swaroop, S.: Introduction to Health Statistics. The Williams and Wilkins Co., Baltimore, 1960, p. 182.
4. Gunn, Alexander: Vulnerable groups 1: problem families. Nurs. Times, *61:*1366, October, 1965.
5. See, for example, Bock, Walter: Field techniques in delineating the structure of Community Leadership. Human Organization, *24:*358, Winter, 1965; or Dahl, Robert A.: Who Governs? Democracy and Power in an American City. Yale University Press, New Haven, 1961.
6. Bell, Wendell, and Boat, Marion: Urban Neighborhoods and informal sociological relationships. Amer. J. Sociol., *62:*391, January, 1957.
7. Smith, Joel, Form, W. H., and Stons, Gregory: Local intimacy in a middle size city. Amer. J. Sociol., *60:*276, November, 1954.
8. Freeman, H. E., and Lambert, Camille: The influence of community groups on health matters. Human Organization, *24:*353, Winter, 1965.
9. Peters, Ann de Huff, and Chase, C. L.: Patterns of health care in a rural southern county. Amer. J. Public Health, *57:*409, March, 1967.
10. Health Survey Procedure. Public Health Service, National Center for Health Statistics, P.H.S. Publication No. 1000, U.S. Government Printing Office, Washington, D.C., 1964.
11. Tayback, Matthew, and Frazier, T. M.: Continuous health surveys a necessity for health administration. Public Health Rep., *77:*763, September, 1962.

SUGGESTED READINGS

Alpert, Joel, J., Kosa, John, and Haggerty, R. J.: A month of illness and health care among low income families. Public Health Rep., *82:*705, August, 1967.
Anderson, U. M., Jenss, Rachel, and Mosher, W. E.: High risk groups—definition and identification. New Eng. J. Med., *273:*308, August, 1965.
Besson, Gerald: The health illness spectrum. Amer. J. Public Health, *57:*1901, November, 1967.
Butrico, Frank A.: Environment as a health factor. *In* Porterfield, John D. (ed.): Community Health Services. Basic Books, Inc., Publishers, New York, 1966, Chapter 2.

Cornely, Paul, and Bigman, S. K.: Acquaintance with governmental health services in a low income population. Amer. J. Public Health, *52:*1877, November, 1962.

Densen, Paul M.: Health of the population. *In* Rosenau, Milton J.: Preventive Medicine and Public Health. 9th ed. by Phillip E. Sartwell and Kenneth Maxcy. Appleton-Century-Crofts, New York, 1965, Chapter 3.

Densen, Paul: Vital statistics: the accounting of health. *In* Porterfield, John D. (ed.), *op. cit.,* Chapter 16.

Duhl, Leonard (ed.): The Urban Condition. Basic Books, Inc., Publishers, New York, 1963.

Dunn, Halbert: High level wellness for man and society. Amer. J. Public Health, *49:*786, June, 1959.

Foster, George: Traditional Cultures and the Impact of Technological Change. Harper and Row, Publishers, New York, 1962, Chapters 5 to 8.

Guide to a Community Health Study. 2nd ed., American Public Health Association, Committee on Public Health Administration. New York, 1961.

Health is a Community Affair. National Commission on Community Health Services, Harvard University Press, Cambridge, Mass., 1961.

Health Survey Procedure. U.S. Department of Health, Education and Welfare, National Center for Health Statistics, P. H. S. Publication No. 1000, U.S. Government Printing Office, Washington, D.C., 1964.

Jaco, E. Gartley: Twentieth century attitudes toward health. *In* DeGroot, Leslie: Medical Care: Social and Organizational Aspects. Charles C Thomas, Springfield, Illinois, 1966, Chapter 1.

Kariel, Patricia: The dynamics of behavior in relation to health. Nurs. Outlook, *10:*402, June, 1962.

Logan, R. F. L.: Assessment of sickness and health in the community—needs and methods. Medical Care, *2:*173, July-September, 1964.

Magalhaes, Marie, and Albold, Margaret: Teaching public health nursing by the city block. Amer. J. Nurs., *62:*82, June, 1962.

Measurement of Levels of Health, Technical Report Series No. 137. World Health Organization, Geneva, 1957.

Morris, J. N.: The Uses of Epidemiology. 2nd ed., The Williams and Wilkins Co., Baltimore, 1964, Chapter 2.

Origin, Program and Operation of the U.S. National Health Survey. U.S. Department of Health, Education and Welfare, National Center for Health Statistics, P. H. S. Publication No. 1000, U.S. Government Printing Office, Washington, D.C., 1963.

Paul, B. D.: Health Culture and Community: Case Studies of Public Reactions to Health Programs. Russell Sage Foundation, New York, 1955.

Payne, Anthony M. M.: Innovation out of unity. Milbank Mem. Fund Quart., *43:*397, October, 1965, Part I.

Peters, Ann de Huff, and Chase, C. L.: Patterns of health care in infancy in a rural southern county. Amer. J. Public Health, *57:*409, March, 1967.

Rogers, Edward S.: Human Ecology and Health: An Introduction for Administrators. The Macmillan Company, New York, 1960.

Rosen, George: Health Needs and Resources in the United States. *In* DeGroot, Leslie: *op. cit.,* Chapter 20.

Sanders, Irwin T.: The community: structure and function. Nurs. Outlook, *11:*642, September, 1963.

Smolensky, Jack, and Haar, Franklin B.: Community Health. 2nd ed., W. B. Saunders Company, Philadelphia, 1967.

Suchman, Edward A.: Community Health Diagnosis. *In* Sociology in the Field of Public Health. Russell Sage Foundation, New York, 1967.

Top, Franklin H.: The farmer's health. *In* Porterfield, John D.: *op. cit.,* Chapter 13.

CHAPTER
18

Developing the
Neighborhood
Nursing Program

Even though the unit of care in community health nursing is the family, the basic planning and responsibility unit is a designated population group. The nurse's population may be those people living in a defined geographic area, such as a cluster of city blocks, a county, or a neighborhood; or it may be the population affiliated with an institution or a service, such as a school, a comprehensive health-care center, or a health insurance program. The renaissance of interest in the neighborhood as a logical and effective unit for social action makes it likely that this unit of population will increasingly be the basis of much community health nursing. For this reason, Chapter 18 will consider the neighborhood as the prototype of the populations served by the community health nurse, and program development will be discussed in this context.

Sanders points out that a community may be seen three ways: as a place, as a collection of people, or as a social system.[1] A neighborhood usually has boundaries that are recognized by its residents. The people living in the neighborhood may vary, with respect to homogeneity, from a group that shares a common cultural background and a well defined value system to a collection of many subgroups of differing backgrounds and interests. The social system will also vary from a highly separative group of families who share common shopping and social facilities but who look elsewhere for their close affectional and socializing activities to a group that is closely knit, mutually supportive, and interlaced with habitual patterns of informal interchange.

These wide variations make it necessary to see each neighborhood as a separate, collective nursing patient with special needs and special capabilities.

A Neighborhood Focus May Require Some Professional Reorientation

Nurses, like most members of the helping professions, tend to focus on individuals and families rather than on what they may see as the less personal population-in-environment unit of care. Although well sensitized to the physical and interpersonal indices of human disorder, nurses may be less attuned to the statistical cry for help that is the community's symptom of illness. A neighborhood focus places as much emphasis on the proportion of pregnant women receiving adequate nursing support as on the quality of nursing service provided to an individual family. It implies the same sensitivity to the mood and the self-respect of a neighborhood, as reflected in the appearance of streets and alleys and in the condition of its schools, as it does to the mood and self-respect of a family. It implies responsiveness to the need for concerted neighborhood action to change the dangerous play habits of children, as well as responsiveness to individual needs.

This focus requires a different nursing approach than the one-by-one approach of family care. For example, the identification and neutralization of the hostile individual or family who is not receiving care may be necessary to avoid a building of distrust of helping agencies among other potential recipients of care. The enlistment of those who exert influence in the community may require changing social patterns that are deeply ingrained.

For most, "thinking neighborhood" takes some readjustment and conscious effort, but without this point of view it is impossible to realize fully the benefits nursing can provide to the community.

THE COMMUNITY NURSE'S SHARE IN NEIGHBORHOOD PLANNING VARIES

The pattern of assignment influences the planning procedures. If the community health nurse is the sole professional nursing representative or the nursing group leader for the neighborhood, she will obviously carry the major responsibility for adapting the general program to local needs. If she is a member of a nursing group or of a multidiscipline group planning for the health care of the neighborhood, her responsibility may be smaller in scope; but she will still be expected to contribute to program planning through suggestions for change and the evaluation of new methods.

Agency tolerance for difference and experimentation affects the scope of planning responsibility. In some agencies there is great tolerance for innovation; others tend toward greater centralization of decision and methodology. However, it is safe to say that in most instances nurses in the field underestimate rather than overestimate the degree of freedom they have; usually the attitude of the central office is far less rigid than is the nurse's perception of it.

The strength and influence of community groups concerned with nursing affect the demand for change and individualized planning. For the most part neighborhood action and planning groups are geared to change and to increasing the relevance and impact of human services. They expect to be heard, to influence decision, and above all to get more of the good things of life for the community they represent. When such groups are several and active, they will expect the community health nurse to find some way of responding to their demands for increased or improved service; this would, in turn, demand adaptations in the existing nursing program.

The pattern for the delivery of nursing services requires varying degrees of "merge" in planning the nursing program. When there are several agencies providing nursing care in a neighborhood, the planning task becomes more complex, since nursing in any one agency must be related to that in all of the others in order to assure the best possible coverage. Even when there is only one designated community health nurse in a neighborhood, other health groups, such as hospital outpatient nursing services, personnel employed by the family physician, or "good neighbors" who help out in an emergency, may participate in the work of neighborhood nursing.

THE PROCESS OF DEVELOPING THE NEIGHBORHOOD NURSING PROGRAM

Neighborhood focused planning is imperative. Even though the neighborhood nursing program will be developed within the framework of the program for the larger community, the nurse will find that many adaptations are necessary if the program is to be relevant and productive.

Careful planning at the neighborhood level helps to assure that the nursing services will be accessible, acceptable, and pertinent. Even when they are in close proximity, neighborhoods are likely to differ considerably not only in the health conditions they experience but also in the degree of family independence, in patterns of use of health services, and in the sources of influence in health matters.

Planning guides the choices that have to be made. Almost never is the nurse in a situation where the demands for nursing do not outrun the available nursing time. Pressures for more nursing care or for nursing care of a specific kind come from many sources and differ from one locality to another. Each newly developed health program is "crucial"; each newly elected government official has promises to keep; and each nurse is pushed by her professional training, her professional organizations, and her professional conscience to extend and improve the services she can offer. Recent emphasis on participation and building the decisional capacity of the neighborhood as an operating group has revealed an opportunity for a new kind of nursing care. The public, too, has increased its appetite for health care, especially among the low-income groups, and is increasingly aware of its right to decide what care is required and to what they are entitled. Thus the nurse or nursing group must constantly choose among various priorities or courses of action, basing the choice on conditions specific to the neighborhood.

Planning makes performance evaluation meaningful. What is "good" community health nursing in one neighborhood may be inadequate or inappropriate in another setting, even though on the surface the communities and the services afforded seem very similar. Neighborhood focused planning helps to clarify the specific outcomes that may be used as criteria for success.

Realistic, neighborhood-based planning is an antidote to frustration. Faced with both internal and external pressures and demands, the community health nurse serving the neighborhood may run the risk of becoming frustrated or of dissipating nursing energy in scattered or low-impact activities. Planning helps to identify the things that will not be done as well as those that will be done, to indicate limits as well as hopes for nursing achievement. Defining the necessary accommodation by means of a rational process helps to relieve the nurse of unnecessary anxiety or guilt about the things that cannot be done and provides for the collection of evidence of tangible accomplishments.

In developing the neighborhood nursing program, the community health nurse will use the general processes of planning, implementation, and evaluation that have been previously discussed. She will use many of the approaches involved in community health diagnosis and, also, those that are generic to nursing and that would apply equally well in any nursing setting. However, as she draws upon these general concepts and skills and relates them to the special neighborhood conditions and her own professional style, she will fashion a program that is highly particularized.

Get the "Feel" of the Neighborhood

Nurses newly assigned to a neighborhood may have a strong compulsion to act; because there are so many problems to be dealt with and so much that could be done, there is a tendency to wade right in with advice and change. This desire to help immediately is satisfying to both the provider and the recipient of service, but it is important that the nurse not commit herself prematurely to a course of action that will later prove untenable. Precipitate action may lead to serious errors of judgment in terms of the need for and acceptability of the proposed changes.

During the first days in a new neighborhood, the community health nurse might well act like a sponge—absorbing all the sights and sounds and smells without making any effort to systematize or even to understand them. The tone of voice used in neighbor to neighbor conversation; the effort to beautify the surroundings, the way in which workers in the hospital or welfare office refer to their clients ("those people" as contrasted to "such a good mother even though she has never learned to keep house"); the ways in which people congregate on the street or in other gathering places; or the attitudes of the landlords toward children are examples of observations that may provide valuable clues to neighborhood dynamics. The nurse visiting families of a different race or nationality or social background from her own can learn much about intergroup relationships from the way in which she herself is received into a family or from the family's casual references to school or job situations.

Such reactions as these between the people or between the people and their environment have a bearing on the choice of nursing strategies; but the meaning of any single aspect of this relationship must be seen in the context of the whole. If made too soon, a systematic assessment of these factors may bias observation and obscure these interrelationships.

First impressions provide a basis for action pending more definitive study. Obviously, the community nurse is not going to postpone all action until it is possible to construct a detailed plan. During the early period in a new neighborhood it is possible to size up what seem to be the overriding problems, to get an idea of what health matters are most urgent to the people of the neighborhood, and to make a rough estimate of the ability of the population as individuals and as a community to care for its health needs. These impressions will provide a basis for immediate action and will allow the nurse to be visible and helping while taking a systematic look at nursing-action needs and alternatives.

Develop and Use a Neighborhood Data Bank

Good program development depends upon good data, and every community health nurse must allocate some time to the collection and analysis of pertinent facts about the neighborhood in which she works. One useful way of going about this is to develop a "data bank," a place where pertinent information about the neighborhood is gathered together for ready reference.

POPULATION CHARACTERISTICS

The bank should include data about both the general and the health characteristics of the population. The general characteristics of the population are important to program planning. Trends in the size of the population, age and sex distribution, family size, occupations, educational attainment, or racial or national origins influence the demands for nursing care.

Health characteristics, including trends in mortality and morbidity, illnesses causing absence from school, or health conditions for which people have been referred for nursing service, are of obvious importance. Utilization patterns — usual sources of primary medical care or the nature of the attendance group at screening services — are also clues to problems requiring nursing intervention. Patterns of family health maintenance, such as child rearing, family management, and food habits, constitute another important area of planning data.

ENVIRONMENT CHARACTERISTICS

Data about the environment should also be considered. Significant information about the physical environment might include the nature of traffic patterns (*e.g.,* the safety of crossings or high-speed freeways, general conditions of housing, the safety and adequacy of school buildings and school grounds, natural hazards, and pesticides in common use in rural areas.

Data about the social environment may include the general level of interchange among subgroups in the community, habits of recreation (whether family focused, individual, "home grown," or commercial), or intergenerational relationships.

FORMAL AND INFORMAL
NEIGHBORHOOD RESOURCES

Information about available resources for medical or health care and the conditions of their use may be supplemented by information about nonhealth groups or individuals that are available to give help. For example, it is necessary to know just which persons are eligible to use a particular clinic, when they may go, what the charges are likely to be, and to what person inquiries should be addressed. It may also be important to know that the city or state health department has a consultant in tuberculosis care who can be asked for advice, that a local industry employs a nurse who will inform workers of special health programs, or that a retired librarian may be called upon to secure books for shut-ins.

TRENDS IN SERVICE ACTIVITIES

It is not safe to assume that what has been done through community nursing service accurately reflects the current nursing needs of the population, but past activity records do reflect the expectations that have been engendered in the public with respect to nursing service. Any contemplated substantive program change must be seen in the context of these expectations and habits of use.

Information about service inputs (that is, the nursing time spent and the activities that have been undertaken) and service outputs (such as the number of cases brought to medical treatment or that show improvement) are obviously important to planning.

Systematic collection and organization of data maximizes its usefulness. It is obvious that in planning for a small population unit such as the neighborhood, information must be gathered in bits and pieces; some of the data will be specific for the neighborhood, such as that for a census tract, and some data will be extrapolated from that relating to larger population groups.

The community health nurse must see data collection as a continuing task; she must add to the available facts such new data as are uncovered and constantly update existing community information.

Depending on the nature of the data, it may be useful to tabulate it in order to provide for quick comparison (as with trends in utilization of particular services), to establish separate files (such as a resource file), or simply to file the various compilations and reports together in a readily accessible spot. The important thing is to make it easy to see the interrelatedness of these various units of information as they affect the provision of care. For example, it is important to see the changing service input trends as they relate to changes in the nature of the population or to the introduction of new sources of health care in the neighborhood. When the method of collecting and storing these data is already established, the community health nurse may need only to learn how to maintain them and to use them in a synthesized way.

Relate Nursing Efforts to Those of Other Groups

Information from the data bank will need to be supplemented with further information secured through conferences with other groups who are responsible for nursing or related programs. For instance, it is important to know if the local hospital is planning any change in program or organization that would affect the community nursing support. The nurse should inquire if the medical director in the neighborhood health unit is making plans that might require a change in the nursing support program: a special immunization campaign or potential new mental health facilities must be taken into account in the development of the neighborhood nursing program.

Engage Neighborhood Residents in Nursing

Engaging neighborhood residents in nursing is a problem of philosophy and method. Hans Spiegel recently said, "Probably no other issue is as vital to the success of solving America's urban crisis than the viable participation of urban residents in planning the neighborhoods and cities in which they live and the social programs that directly affect them."[2] This belief has been reiterated by many leaders in social planning and action and has been applied to rural as well as urban settings. Although the concept of citizen participation appears to have wide acceptance, there is little agreement on the scope of such participation or on the methods by which it might be achieved.

Community health nursing—or public health nursing—has traditionally adhered to the philosophy that the individuals and communities served should share in the decisions made about care. There is a long history of the involvement of the public in boards, committees, and other community action groups and of individuals, groups of patients, and families in their own nursing care. However, many nurses feel that this philosophy has not been implemented as fully as possible and that low-income groups in particular have not been adequately represented in community planning and action for nursing care. Recent trends in social planning suggest that much more frequent and forceful citizen involvement is likely to develop. This development offers both a challenge and an opportunity for community health nursing.

CITIZEN PARTICIPATION SERVES
PRACTICAL PURPOSES

Participation Clarifies the Needs that Nursing Should Meet. The perception of need will obviously vary between the health professional and the general neighborhood representative, since these perceptions are based in different experiences, training, and values. The professional must avoid falling into the trap of feeling that what the professional wants to do represents the "true need" and what the public wants the professional to do is the "demand." What hurts is the problem, and what hurts—whether it be the real or fancied condescension of the nurse, the absence of a night consultation service, the failure of the nurse to intercede with another agency for the family, or frank illness—is best known by these who feel the hurt. In the give and take between neighborhood representatives and the nurse or nursing group, each can put forth their facts, ideas, and feelings and, hopefully, arrive at a decision as to the nursing action that should be taken.

Participation Validates the Goals that Are Established for the Nursing Service.   Neighborhood residents are apt to make a pretty good guess as to whether or not nursing might help a situation and as to how far the residents of the neighborhood can go in coping with a problem on their own.

Participation Brings New Skills and Knowledge into Service.   In the course of dealing with the day-in-day-out problems of living in a low-income neighborhood, in an isolated rural area, or on a military post, residents learn ways of coping with the special problems they face. They know the problems of managing food stamps, of finding ways for the overworked farm boy to help at home and still join the school band, and of managing an alcoholic member of the family. Those with experience as welfare recipients know the pros and cons of the young mother's difficult decision whether to remain on welfare or to leave her child to other care and become self-supporting. Only the residents of a Hutterite community appreciate fully the pressure to maintain traditional patterns of child rearing and the problems of adapting to the world outside.

Participation Has Value in Itself.   For those who are unaccustomed to having much control over the important things in their lives, participation offers an opportunity for them to take some definite action, to feel less impotent, and to exercise their right to choose. Even when the participation is limited to criticizing the shortcomings of the present program, system, or personnel, at least it is positive action on the part of the consumer. For others more accustomed to having a voice in their own affairs, participation offers an opportunity to contribute in a meaningful way to an important service and often leads to greater health knowledge and to a greater commitment to the cause of improving the health of the public.

NEIGHBORHOOD LEADERS

The community health nurse hopes that every neighborhood resident who has any contact with nursing will participate in some way in the nursing-care program. In addition, some residents may be expected to exert unusual influence over the actions of their neighbors or to engage actively in the process of social change in the neighborhood. Sanders points out that these leaders may come in many styles, including the "top leadership" group, which has general influence in many areas; those whose leadership is exerted primarily in one system of the community, such as the health system; and those who hold elective offices or jobs that provide them with channels for influence, such as committee members or physicians, or who are recognized as spokesmen for specific groups.[3]

It is important to remember that it is not easy to separate the true from the apparent sources of leadership. The most vocal and frequently elected committee member may have status; but when decisions are made, others may play the key role. Elected committees may or may not be considered by the community as truly representing them. Also, leadership capability in many cases, especially in urban populations, may be latent. For example, in a public housing unit, the community health nurse may come upon a resident who, never before active (in the organized sense) in influencing his neighbors, when asked to help in a discussion group shows great ability at analyzing problems, seeing alternative solutions, and motivating others toward a new way of thinking.

Leadership capacity rests partly on personal endowment, on the ability and the desire to understand others and to "get through" to the strength of their impulse to act rather than withdraw in the face of a problem. The quality of the leadership will also be affected by the nature of the problems, by the leaders' knowledge of the problems, and by the ways in which their actions will affect others involved in the decision.

It is important to know to what extent those representative of or speaking for the neighborhood have had experience in problem definition and independent decision and to what extent they have — either from their general background knowledge or from materials provided them — the facts upon which a decision should rest. The neighborhood council may be working with an entirely inadequate knowledge of the financial situation of the larger community or of the long-range effects of certain actions that may be proposed. If they have lived largely in a setting in which the options for action are sharply limited, they may not be experienced in weighing alternative actions. (The community health nurse may appreciate this as she herself struggles with decisions about alternative courses of nursing action!) The nurse's persistent search for indigenous leadership must be accompanied by definite planning to develop and use the leadership available.

Training in collaborative decision making is important not only for neighborhood residents but also for professional and other service personnel who are responsible for providing the required care. The neighborhood representative needs to be provided with information and explanation about the conditions that set restraints within which decisions must be made. He must learn that any suggestion made will receive full and careful consideration, and he must distinguish between those things about which his group can make the final decision and those that must be left to the professional or paid worker. For example, no one would suppose that a neighborhood committee could decide what medication should be ordered for a specific condition or whether or not certain technical nursing procedures could be entrusted to one with less than professional preparation.

On the other side of the coin, professional workers must also be trained in the art of collaborative decision making and action. It is sometimes difficult for the professional worker, who lacks many of the experiences of his clients, to realize that the expertise of the neighborhood resident may far exceed his own in matters related to the scheduling of services or to the interpersonal relationships in the service setting.

To assure some continuity in citizen participation, the community health nurse or nursing group may want to have a citizens' advisory or action committee for nursing. This may be a separate committee that is elected or appointed by the neighborhood group, or it may be a subcommittee of the neighborhood health committee. In either case, the charge to the committee should be clearly stated. There should be provision for rotation of membership in order to increase the opportunities for participation. Regular meetings should be held, and records should be kept of the committee's actions and recommendations.

Nursing Goals and Priorities Grow Out of the Neighborhood's Needs

The listening and observant nurse will soon learn that those things she sees as nursing needs do not always coincide with those things that the neighborhood residents and their organizations see as nursing needs. In establishing goals and priorities as a base for program development, the nurse must take time and broaden her thinking so that she can see needs in a very relative sense. The object is to achieve a synthesis of her own concept of what sort of nursing care should be provided to these particular families and institutional groups with the ideas of those responsible for the overall health program development, and with the consumers' concepts of nursing care (either as they are formally expressed in committee reports or as they are deduced from nursing encounters with individuals and families).

The achievement of this synthesized view of neighborhood nursing needs requires a great deal of discussion with the relevant individuals and groups: physicians, health-care facilities personnel, welfare groups, and formal and informal action groups. It requires also that the nurse have a clear image of community health nursing practice in the conceptual sense: for instance, she should react almost automatically to the word *need* as representing a relationship between the demands set by a health condition, the ability of the family to cope with that demand, and the likelihood that nursing will affect the condition in some favorable way; she should also realize that what constitutes a "here and now" need may be totally different at another time or in another neighborhood; and she should recognize the validity of the perceived need and the legitimacy of her concern with the needs of the nonserved, as well as the served, neighborhood population. Each applicative step used in defining need should be checked out against the basic concepts that underlie nursing practice.

GOALS

On the basis of the explorations and decisions made in the course of involving institutional and citizen representatives in the nursing problem and of her own assessment of the situation, the community health nurse can develop a clearly stated set of goals and also a set of specific outcomes—*indicators*—that can be used to determine whether or not these goals have been realized.

Thus, the nurse planning for the maternity phases of the neighborhood health program might set (among others) two primary goals:

Goal I: To secure comprehensive and early medical care for expectant mothers.

Goal II: To increase family skills in early child rearing.

She might then set forth the specific outcomes toward which effort might be directed and by which progress should be measured. For example:

Indicators for Goal I

1. An increase in the proportion of those registering for care within the first trimester from the present 49 percent to 75 percent (as indicated on birth certificates).
2. Specified tests and services for at least 85 percent of those under nursing supervision.

Indicators for Goal II

1. Father interviewed by nurse or physician at least once during the pregnancy. This is obviously an indirect measure based on the supposition that involving the father as a responsible child care provider promotes better child rearing practice.
2. Parents' initial and later responses to hypothetical child rearing problems as recorded on special survey forms show an increment in the proportion of positive responses in the course of care over the first year of life. That which parents say they would do is not the equivalent of what they actually do in child rearing, so this indicator is also a secondary measure. A special survey form may be useful in areas like these in which it is unlikely that there will be sufficiently uniform conditions to supply a comparative base.

PRIORITIES

Priorities represent areas that should be given emphasis either because they represent a significant health threat or because they represent a major concern of the neighborhood residents. For instance, concentration may be placed on the care of unmarried adolescent pregnant girls or on the improvement of the food intake of expectant and nursing mothers or on interceding with community care agencies for more personalized care.

These goals and priorities should be written and on file; and they should be agreed upon by the nurse, her agency administrative personnel (which may mean her supervisor or the nursing consultant standing in for the administration), and those representatives of the neighborhood who are working with the nurse on program development.

The Action Agenda Directs Effort

Once the community health nurse has established the goals and priorities of her neighborhood program, there is need for an action agenda that will give some order to the implementation phase of the program, The action agenda is usually set up for a minimum of one year (sometimes two, if the agency is on a biennial plan and budget) with supplementary planning within shorter time units, such as a month or week or, when necessary, at even more frequent intervals. Specific schedules and plans may be drawn up on a quarterly, monthly, or weekly basis, depending on the nature of the nursing work to be done.

If the nurse is working in a large agency, there may be action agenda plans already developed within which her planning will occur; or she may find that there are general priorities or commitments and that her plan is essentially an adaptation of the larger one. The action agenda should show:

1. The general distribution of nursing time and effort as related to program and supportive responsibilities.
2. The implementation modalities that are to be used.
3. The timetable, including progress checkpoints.

THE DISTRIBUTION OF NURSING TIME

The distribution of nursing time and effort involves both fixed commitments and choices. *Fixed commitments* may be formally or informally derived. The nurse working in a neighborhood is almost always either one of a group of workers serving the neighborhood or part of an organization serving the larger community. The obligations or commitments made by the larger group will be binding upon her. Some nursing activities may be required by law—certain school examination procedures, for example. Other commitments may grow from contracts or less formal agreements: there may be a contract with an industry to provide certain home-care services to their beneficiaries, an agreement with a hospital to provide nursing support to a satellite clinic operating in the neighborhood, or an informal understanding with a neighborhood action group that specified services will be available in the evening as well as during the day.

The community health nurse should familiarize herself with the terms of these fixed commitments, know what nursing obligations are implied, and to what degree the programs may be altered within the agreements made. Time can then be allocated for these activities.

The nurse has a greater opportunity to make *choices* in the optional or flexible portion of the program. For example, the selection of expectant parents for community health nursing supervision, the intensity of care provided these families, the scheduling of services, and the choice of methods for reaching these families may be subject to the choice of the neighborhood community health nurse.

Within these optional service areas there will be some programs or aspects of programs that have a higher value than others, either intrinsically or for the present time or for the particular place. There will be population groups or mini neighborhoods whose need seems higher than that of those living elsewhere. Programing is easier if there is a classification system for identifying high priority families and populations. For example, each family or neighborhood cluster may be rated A, B, or C, depending on the intensity of their nursing need. Some agencies have established classification schemes, but for the most part these are not fully developed. Again, the community health nurse has a great opportunity to influence community health nursing practice by her own efforts in this direction. In determining the value level of a particular element of service, consideration should be given to:

1. *The urgency of the situation.* For example, the urgency of providing nutritional advisement or supplementation to the low-income expectant mother is exceedingly high—the effects of neglect are probably great—and timing is of prime importance. Suspected but still undiagnosed tuberculosis or venereal disease would fall into the same category of urgency.

2. *The likely impact of nursing intervention.* For example, the likelihood that nursing intervention will change the situation in the case of the chronic alcoholic is much less than the likelihood that nursing intervention will affect the use of available preventive health measures.

3. *The social or medical importance of the changes* that might be secured through nursing intervention. For example, the nurse may be able to persuade an elderly tuberculosis patient who is being cared for reasonably well by an equally elderly spouse to seek hospital care and more definitive treatment. When compared to the importance of the improvement of family functioning in a three-generation family faced with catastrophic illness, the former would obviously have the lesser value in terms of social benefit.

It must be reiterated that the judgment of those receiving service as well as that of health professionals is important in making these determinations.

A realistic estimate of available time is the first step in time allocation. The general time and effort distribution must take account of supportive as well as direct, service activities: time must be allowed for educational or supervisory work with auxiliaries or students, for program review and evaluation, and for writing reports. Nonservice time—travel time, sick time, and holiday time—must also be reckoned.

Thus, a nurse working in a relatively settled suburb and responsible for a population of approximately 3000 might find her time divided something like this:

Total working hours .... 1920 (240 days)
Off-the-job hours
    Holidays: 40 hours (5 days)
    Sick leave average: 48 hours (6 days)
    Total   *88 (11 days)*
Total on-the-job hours .... 1832 (229 days)
Nonservice hours
    Travel, estimated on experience: 420 hours
    Total   *420*
Total "available" on-the-job hours 1412
    Time required for supportive activities—program planning, reports, giving or receiving supervision—based on past experience.
    Average of 1.5 hours per working day: 344 hours.
    Total   *344*
Time available for direct care activities .... 1068 hours

IMPLEMENTATION MODALITIES

Implementation modalities will vary in time cost and impact value from one neighborhood to another. For example, there may be a choice between the use of a group approach and the use of an individual approach to counseling families in home care of the chronically ill. Some of the questions that might be raised include:

1. Is group contact the method of choice because it offers an opportunity to promote participation of neighborhood residents in their own care?
2. Are the people in this community likely to attend such group activities; will this program reach those who need it most?
3. Are there ready-made groups—organized church groups, for instance—in the community that might be used?
4. Does the group approach lend itself to the use of supplementary volunteer or paid services that might conserve nursing time? For example, does the adult education department of the public school system or the local chapter of the American Red Cross have facilities for offering these courses, thus conserving the time of the community health nurse?
5. Are the problems of the groups sufficiently similar so that group work will have a general appeal?
6. If the community health nurse is to undertake this program herself, will it save or cost time? If the group approach is more expensive than the individual approach, is the likely impact sufficiently greater to compensate for the difference in cost? On the basis of these two factors is the group approach a "good buy"?

These kinds of questions will help each nurse to evaluate the relative merit of a number of possible channels for service. Some general considerations about various implementation modalities are listed in Table 7.

TIMETABLE AND CHECKPOINTS

The community health nurse's calendar is usually a two-part affair: a tentative effort schedule that extends over the year and a current schedule that may be compiled for a period of a month or so. The timetable or calendar helps to keep the nursing effort on course.

All fixed commitments, such as visits to schools, clinics, and staff meetings, should be scheduled first. Plans for group instruction or group problem solving that require a longterm commitment should also be blocked out early in the planning period. More flexibly timed events, such as home visiting and other types of family-nurse conference, may then be planned around this base.

The calendar should specifically indicate "checkpoints" when time is allowed for a review of progress and for documenting and evaluating the services afforded. The frequency of such checkpoints will depend on the nature of the case load. In generalized programs in which there is considerable group work and numerous fixed commitments, a quarterly review may be adequate; in other settings, such as home-care agencies, a more frequent review may be required. The important thing is to provide for reviews in advance.

The nurse's schedule should be duplicated so that it can be made available to recipient groups, such as the neighborhood nursing committee or the school, and also to the administrative or supervisory personnel with whom the nurse is working.

Coordination—Answer to Fragmentation?

As the number of agencies and the types of service personnel continue to expand, it becomes increasingly important to assure that the various programs and services mesh in such a way that all of the resources are used efficiently to the benefit of the public. The community health nurse working in a neighborhood has a particular responsibility for the promotion of measures that will help coordinate and rationalize these many services.

Coordination of nursing effort takes place in the context of agreements and policies that are developed at broader responsibility levels: the general policy of the *whole community* with respect to the development of resources and programs and commitments to program elements, the policies and contracts of the *community agency* of which the neighborhood represents one jurisdiction, and at the *neighborhood level* where those directly responsible for providing care plan together for a mutual effort. It is at this last level that the community health nurse is most frequently directly involved, although she may suggest or help evaluate the operation of the larger system.

The barriers to interagency coordination must be identified. These barriers may include lack of any systematic means of communication, conflicting interests and goals of the various autonomous agencies providing care, or pressures upon local units from national or regional units of their organization. For example, a psychiatric hospital, under great pressure, is convinced of the need for minimizing hospital stay and looks to home-care programs to accomplish this; whereas a community health nursing service may want to protect and preserve family functioning, which may be threatened by the hospital's referral for home care.

The importance of maximal coordination cannot be overemphasized. *Maximal coordination* of nursing services directed toward the neighborhood means much more than providing for an adequate referral system. Lack of coordination wastes scarce nursing resources, decreases the likelihood that nursing services will reach all who need them, neutralizes benefits by poor follow-through, and subjects the public to the frustration and the time costs of making their way through a labyrinth of service institutions or of waiting many hours only to find they are at the wrong facility.

CRITERIA FOR EVALUATING COORDINATION

1. Wherever possible, one agency should take primary responsibility for the nursing care of a particular family or population group and for knowing the nature and extent of the nursing services given.

Table 7.   General Considerations of Various Implementation Modalities

Implementation Modality	Advantages	Disadvantages	Constraints or Problems
1. Home visits by nurse or nursing group member.	Highly individualized care. Direct observation of family functioning. Immediate adaptation to home facilities. Access to family members other than patient.	Costly in time, especially if distance is great. Indigenous non-nurse resources may not be used fully in solution of problems.	Securing adequate coverage of the population.
2. Nursing or nursing group contact in clinic, office, place of work, center, etc.	Conserves nursing time, since patient does the traveling. Easy use of other service personnel such as social worker or dentist. Use of special demonstration or teaching materials not readily transported to the home. Helps to establish family-agency ties.	Does not provide first-hand observation of family functioning. Seems less personal to the recipient of care. Works a hardship on family if carfare, baby tending, etc. are required. Does not "reach out" to those reluctant to secure care.	"Institutional flavor"; proper setting for care may be hard to achieve.
3. "Do it yourself" visits to homes by neighborhood volunteers or paid workers.	Expresses a neighborhood commitment. Easy communication, since visitor and visitee have similar backgrounds and problems. Ego-building value by providing a "giving" rather than "receiving" experience for the volunteer and a job for the paid worker. Inexpensive way to reach previously unreached groups.	Input is hard to control; the indigenous worker may communicate very well, but what is communicated may be inaccurate or harmful. Neighborhood residents may not want their neighbors to "know too much" about them. Important problems may be missed because of lack of training of visitor.	Selecting visitors trusted by the population and responsible in carrying out tasks. Professional staff must learn to accept and work with this group of workers.

Method	Advantages	Disadvantages
4. Relay service: training others to do tasks now done by nursing, as for instance training community volunteers or civic groups to do screening measures, to teach home care of the sick, etc.	Multiplier effect: allows extremely rapid dissemination of information or simple services.	May miss health problems in families. What can be taught must usually be limited to well-defined areas because judgment in health matters may be limited. Requires nursing time for development, teaching, and supervision.
5. Group instruction.	Use of demonstration equipment. Economy in use of ready-made groups. Mutual stimulation among class members.	Interests and present knowledge may vary so widely that general content is not suitable. Availability of travel, meeting places, and teaching equipment.
6. Group problem solving.	Inculcates a problem-solving approach that should carry over to new problems. Builds self-confidence of participants in health matters. Assures relevance of content.	Problems of a few may dominate all. Costly in time and may require additional preparation of nurse. Nurse must be sufficiently competent in the content. Nurse must be willing to accept validity of problems identified by group, even if they seem tangential to her.
7. "Kitchen-party," "teach-ins," or discussions: a small number of neighbors meeting in one of the participants' homes.	Commitment of groups. Lessens travel time for participants. Saves nurse's time if common problems exist. Organization and set-up time is absorbed by recipients of care.	Social, rather than learning, aspects may predominate. May lead to too great expenditure of time or money on part of hostess. Members must be used to or able to meet comfortably under such circumstances. There must be common problems in which all share an interest.
8. Calculated lack of nursing action when community interest or potential impact seems low or when family can and should take responsibility.	Conserves time for accepted perceived needs. Builds family independence and self-confidence. Avoids negative recipient response if they see the service as unnecessary.	May produce an unbalanced program. Cannot be used if the activity is in a fixed commitment class or has a high safety value. Difficult to evaluate long-term effects on nursing impact, and misjudgment may result.

2. Each agency should be apprised of nursing services provided by other agencies to clients under their care.
3. The referral system should assure that complete and specific information is transmitted to the referral agency often enough to avoid any discontinuity in care.
4. The referred family or group should be involved in the referral process, including the initial decision to refer.
5. The referral system should be as economical as possible in the professional time that it requires.
6. The right of individuals and groups to protection of privacy should be scrupulously observed in planning and referral processes.
7. The agencies involved should clarify the philosophy upon which they provide care and the nature of each agency's commitment to the community.
8. The coordinating system should be reviewed periodically to be certain that it is functioning effectively.

Coordination Methods

One of the most commonly used methods of coordination of care facilities and one which is useful in small communities with few resources or where longstanding and satisfactory working relationships have been developed is *frequent face-to-face conversation and interchange.* Thus the nurse in a rural county may "visit with" the family physician or the hospital nursing department in her area at periodic intervals, during which they discuss mutual problems with respect to referral and to coordinating their efforts. The nurse, the welfare worker, and the teacher may get together occasionally at lunch to review situations or programs in which all three have some stake. Even when more sophisticated methods are in use, this simple verbal interchange continues to play a part in the overall coordination of the program.

In the sophisticated and resource-rich community, more systematic measures may be required. These methods may include:

1. The development of a *coordinating committee* consisting of representatives from each of the agencies providing nursing care to neighborhood residents. This committee may meet regularly to agree upon procedures, records, forms, and handling of family information and to discuss problems in the coordination process. Such a committee may also develop a community-wide referral system to which all agencies would adhere.

2. The appointment of a *liaison nurse* who functions on an interagency basis. Most often this worker is found in the hospital serving the neighborhood; she is either employed by the hospital or, in some instances, by a health department or other community agency and assigned to work with the hospital. Sometimes one liaison nurse is assigned to a community agency and visits all of the hospitals used by residents of that area, or community health nurses may be assigned in rotation to this service.

The primary function of the liaison nurse is to provide a link between the hospital and the other agencies of the community. The liaison nurse, usually prepared in public health, works with the nursing and the medical staff of the hospital as they plan patient care, makes rounds, suggests points at which the community agency might be called upon to support the family during the patient's hospitalization, and reassures the patient that someone is looking after the family in his absence. She helps the community health nurse to assess the suitability of the home for the patient's return, and she encourages the staff and patient to make full use of available community services. It is her responsibility to make certain that the referrals provide complete and specific information about the care needed. She helps develop and maintain procedures for interagency communication by contributing to the development of referral forms, initiating referral, conferring as necessary with other agencies, and helping with referral to resources other than nursing. She also interprets the programs and goals of each agency to the others.

In practice it would appear that actual referrals for posthospital care fall far short of the number of persons requiring such care. One recent study, in which an experienced public health nurse evaluated the needs of 262 patients in a voluntary general hospital, revealed that 88, or 34 percent, of those evaluated were judged to have nursing needs and could benefit from nursing care after discharge. However, only 4 to 4.6 percent of those considered to need referral were actually referred for such care.[4] Mitch and Kaczala in an experiment in the use of a liaison nurse employed by the department of health in a local general hospital found great differences in need for referral between the 65 or over age group (in which 29 percent were judged to need care) and the under 65 group (in which only 4 percent were judged to need care). They noted that the introduction of this service led to the use of the referral services by 70 percent of the approximately 225 physicians on the active staff of one voluntary hospital, a rate of use far above the usual level.[5]

3. Regularly scheduled *interagency case conferences* may also provide a channel for implementing and improving the coordination effort. Thus the experience of each agency with a particular family can be shared, and common problems or service gaps can be identified. When the "patient" is a population group, a similar mechanism may be used in which agencies meet regularly to discuss their work with respect to a particular problem. For example, one conference might be on the care of the adolescent unmarried mother or on the care of the discharged mental hospital patient.

Whatever method or methods are used to assure coordination of services, it is important to check the effectiveness of the system periodically. It is good to know whether or not the users of the system are happy with it; but it is even more important to see how well the system is guiding care. The records of representative families, population groups, or recipients of a given type of service might be reviewed to establish the degree to which practice is consistent with the established criteria. What is the time lag between the identification of need for home care and the receipt of the request for such care by the community agency? How well were the identified needs of the family or group met through the combined agency effort?

The effectiveness and efficiency of the neighborhood nursing program will be largely determined by the quality of the planning that goes into its development. It is well worth the required time investment to make this development as orderly and as thoughtful as possible.

REFERENCES

1. Sanders, Irwin: Public health in the community. *In* Freeman, H. E., *et al.*: Handbook of Medical Sociology. Prentice-Hall, Inc., New Jersey, 1963, p. 371.
2. Spiegel, Hans, (ed.): Citizen Participation in Urban Development. National Training Laboratory Institute for Applied Behavorial Science (Associated with the National Education Association), Washington, D.C., 1968, vol. I, p. iii.
3. Sanders, Irwin: *op. cit.,* p. 383.
4. Hanser, J., *et al.*: Continuity of Nursing Care from Hospital to Home. National League for Nursing, Publication No. 1228, New York, 1966.
5. Mitch, Anna D., and Kaczala, Sophie: The public health nurse coordinator in a general hospital. Nurs. Outlook, *14:*34, February, 1968.

SUGGESTED READINGS

Adams, Mary, Downs, Thomas, and Deuble, H. M.: Nursing referral outcome for post-hospitalized chronically ill patients. Amer. J. Public Health, *58:*101, January, 1968.
Archer, Sarah, Jarvis-Eckert, M. A.: Health classes on wheels. Nurs. Outlook, *16:*52, April, 1968.
Auerbach, Aline B.: Parents Learn Through Discussion: Principles and Practices of Parent Group Education. John Wiley and Sons, Inc., New York, 1968, pp. 12-28.
Baca, Josephine E.: Some health beliefs of the Spanish speaking. Amer. J. Nurs., *69:*2172, October, 1969.
Burney, L. E., Bucher, R. M., Nelson, A. D., and Willis, D. P.: Planning for comprehensive health care at Temple University Hospital. Public Health Rep., *83:*439, June, 1968.
Clark, Ann: Leadership Technique in Expectant Parent Education. Springer Publishing Co., Inc., New York, 1962.
David, Janis H.: Liaison nurse. Amer. J. Nurs., *69:*2142, October, 1969.
Donnelly, Ellen M.: A cooperative program between state hospital and public health nursing agency for psychiatric after care. Amer. J. Public Health, *52:*1084, July, 1962.
Farrissey, Ruth M.: Clinic nursing in transition. Amer. J. Nurs., *67:*305, February, 1967.
Griffiths, Elsie I.: A rational approach to patient service review. Nurs. Outlook, *17:*49, April, 1969.
Hansen, Ann C., and Levy, Judith M.: Families speak for themselves. Nurs. Outlook, *9:*344, June, 1961.
Hanser, J., *et al.*: Continuity of Nursing Care from Hospital to Home. National League for Nursing, Publication No. 1228, 1966.
Hay, Stella I., and Anderson, Helen C.: Are nurses meeting patients' needs? Amer. J. Nurs., *63:*96, December, 1963.
Hochbaum. G. M.: Consumer participation in health planning: toward conceptual clarification. Amer. J. Public Health, *59:*1698, September, 1969.
Hogan, Aileen: Launching programs for expectant parents. Amer. J. Nurs., *66:*2227, October, 1966.
How to Organize and Extend Community Nursing Services for the Care of the Sick at Home. National League for Nursing, Department of Public Health Nursing, New York, 1962.
Kelly, Cynthia: Health care in the Mississippi Delta. Amer. J. Nurs., *69:*758, April, 1969.
Levine, Sol, *et al.*: Community interorganizational problems in providing medical care and social services. Amer. J. Public Health, *53:*1183, August, 1963.
Magalhaes, Maria, and Albold, Margaret: Teaching public health nursing by the city block. Amer. J. Nurs., *62:*82, June, 1962.
Mann, David: Educating Expectant Parents. Visiting Nurse Service of New York, New York, 1961.
Mickey, Janice E.: Findings of study of extra hospital nursing needs. Amer. J. Public Health, *53:*1047, July, 1963.
Milio, Nancy: A neighborhood approach to maternal and child health in the Negro ghetto. Amer. J. Public Health, *57:*618, April, 1967.

Mitch, Anna D., and Kaczala, Sophie: The public health nurse coordinator in a general hospital. Nurs. Outlook, *16:*34, February, 1968.

Neal, Helen, (ed.): Better Communication for Better Health. Columbia University Press, New York, 1962, p. 101.

Park, Wilford E.: Patient transfer form. Amer. J. Nurs., *67:*1665, August, 1967.

Paulsen, F. Robert, and Tate, Barbara: Community Planning for Nursing. National League for Nursing, New York, 1969.

Phaneuf, Marie C.: Nursing audit for evaluation of patient care. Nurs. Outlook, *14:*51, June, 1966.

Phaneuf, Maria C.: Nursing Audit Method. Nurs. Outlook, *12:*42, May, 1964.

Piskor, Barbara K., and Palleos, Sonia: The group way to banish after-stroke blues. Amer. J. Nurs., *68:*1500, July, 1968.

Rice, Donald: The nurse's role in parent education. Int. Nurs. Rev., *11:*33, July-August, 1964.

Roberts, Doris: How effective is public health nursing? Amer. J. Public Health, *52:*1077, July, 1962.

Roberts, Doris, and Hudson, Helen H.: How to Study Patient Progress. PHS Publication No. 1169, U.S. Government Printing Office, Washington, D.C., 1964.

Roth, Mitchell E., Ehringer, Robert, and Mosher, William E.: The value of coordinated and comprehensive home care. Amer. J. Public Health, *57:*1841, October, 1967.

Sanders, Irwin T.: The community structure and function. Nurs. Outlook, *11:*642, September, 1963.

Sanders, Irwin T.: Public health in the community. *In* Freeman, H. E., *et al.* (eds.): Handbook of Medical Sociology. Prentice-Hall, Inc., New Jersey, 1963, p. 369.

Schwartz, Doris R.: Communication between hospital staff and community agencies: a study of referrals to the public health nurse. Amer. J. Public Health, *50:*1122, August, 1960.

Stitt, Pauline: Who wants to know? *In* Stewart, Dorothy, and Vincent, Pauline (eds.): Public Health Nursing. William C. Brown Company, Publishers, Dubuque, 1968, p. 146.

Tayback, Mathew, and Frazier, Todd M.: Continuous health surveys a necessity for health administration. Public Health Rep., *77:*763, September, 1962.

Wolff, Ilse S.: Referral: a process and a skill. *In* Stewart, D. M., and Vincent, P. A. (eds.): Public Health Nursing. *op. cit.,* p. 130.

Wood, Audrey: Education for parenthood through the maternity services. International Journal of Nursing Studies, *3:*199, December, 1966.

Records and Reports: Boon or Bane

The family history and progress record has been previously discussed as an essential tool for family nursing care and as one part of the total record system. In this chapter, records will be discussed as they relate to the administrative, rather than to the practice, elements of nursing services.

For administrative purposes, records are apt to be focused on group phenomena, not single family phenomena; and the central concern is usually related to the care of a population or to the nursing facets of a program as a whole.

FUNCTIONS OF THE RECORD SYSTEM

The well organized and maintained recording and reporting system serves several functions:

1. The record system provides a service accounting system that documents exactly what has been done. In most local agencies, financing comes from multiple sources, including local, federal, and state funds; voluntary agency contracts; contributions; research or special project funds; and foundation grants. The administrator must account to and sometimes bill each of these agencies separately for the services they have provided. Medicare and Medicaid programs alone have added immeasurably to the amount of accounting required. Information necessary to identify the patient and his eligibility for care must be accurate and complete. Additionally, since some types of care are reimbursable, whereas some are not, information must be available about the precise care given and the level of nursing personnel that was required. Costs for certain types of visits may have to be ascertained; and here, too, the record system must supply the data upon which the answers are built.

2. The record system provides a control system that assures that the services are provided according to plan. In the process of setting goals, certain specific outcomes have been identified, often with measurable indicators of accomplishment. When screening measures are planned, for example, certain follow-up work is essential; and some check is needed to determine just how nearly the program is achieving this. Contracts with private industries or schools are often based on the provision of a defined number of nurse hours or on a defined quantity of service, and there must be a way to assure that these commitments have in fact been fulfilled. In most instances this information must be secured at periods throughout the year, in order to correct any errors of omission or misdirection of effort. The record system must supply the basic data required for making these estimations.

3. The record system provides a rich source of information for planning and evaluating the nursing service provided. Identification of the characteristics of the population served may determine whether or not the population served is indeed the one that most needs care. If nursing care were centered almost entirely on welfare clients to the neglect of the low-income, nonwelfare population, the question might be asked if the program was in fact meeting the needs of the community. Characteristics of the population being served *over time* provide a valuable clue to anticipated nursing needs. For instance, low-income populations and older populations tend to require more intensive and time-consuming nursing care than does the rest of the population, and this trend in demand is upward. A young suburban group is obviously going to have needs related to growing families and maybe to the health consequences of affluence, such as smoking, poor driving habits, or drug abuse; but here, the trend in demand for nursing care is more stable. Changes in the nature of the population being served are of particular significance; hence, the emphasis on the phrase *over time*. Groups who have not hitherto used nursing services may suddenly become frequent users, as happens when home care for psychiatric or geriatric patients is instituted.

By reviewing her own records and reports, the community health nurse has a basis for deciding the extent to which the things she is doing are relevant to the particular needs of the population she is serving, for judging whether or not the approaches appear to be suitable, for identifying the recurring problems that confront her and for deciding if these problems recur because they are not being handled as effectively as they might be, and for determining whether or not available or potential community resources are being used as fully as possible. The administrator, by reviewing the composite records of a particular service group, provides himself with the information needed to decide whether or not the level of staffing is appropriate to the work being performed. He can find in records the documentation he needs for proposing additional staff or a different kind of staff or for requesting appropriations from the agency's budget committee or the United Fund. He has a basis for considering the degree to which nursing support is contributing to each of the agency programs and whether or not additional support may have to be directed to a particular program that is either new or understaffed.

THE RECORD SYSTEM INCLUDES A VARIETY OF FORMS

The record system in any agency includes a large variety of forms, each presumably serving a particular purpose. These forms may be standard throughout the state (or other political jurisdiction) or developed specifically for each agency. The agency may adopt a record system based on the use of records from a particular source, such as the National League for Nursing, or it may select parts of the record system from many different sources. The system may be highly structured and prescribed or subject to great individual adaptation by the nurse. When computer analysis is part of the record system, certain parts of the reporting must be in standard form so that they can be easily converted to computer language.

Service Records

Service records document the care provided. They provide a register, usually in chronological order, of the services given to any population served by the nurse. Hopefully, they provide a record of the needs and goals (another facet of the documentation process) on which these services are based. They also supply the data required to describe the characteristics of the population receiving definitive nursing care. The compilation of data from these records answers the question, "In what direction did we place our nursing efforts?"

Accounting Records

Accounting records include time and effort expenditure records and fiscal records. Time and effort records center around the nurse's daily report, which may be set up in a variety of ways. In some fashion, the agency will maintain daily reports of the time worked and the services provided. Sometimes the daily time sheet provides more detailed information about time spent in various activities (travel, for instance). However, the tendency is to minimize routine daily recording and to substitute a time study based on a representative sampling of the nurse's time.

The National League for Nursing has developed a daily report form that is in wide use. (See Figure 11.) This is designed for easy transfer to cards for machine tabulation. Many agencies are using a single service form that is precoded for machine tabulation. An example of this type of card is shown in Figure 12. The nurse completes a card for each service unit and submits the forms daily.

A detailed time study may be undertaken once or twice a year for one or two weeks that are considered typical of the yearly distribution of effort. This more detailed study is used to compute the costs of particular types of activities—for example, home visits to cancer patients,

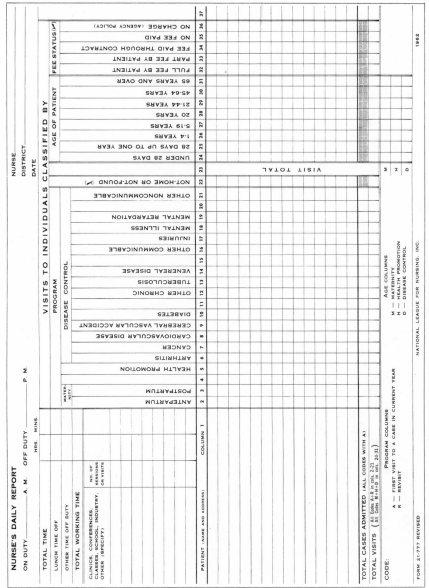

FIGURE 11. National League for Nursing daily report form.

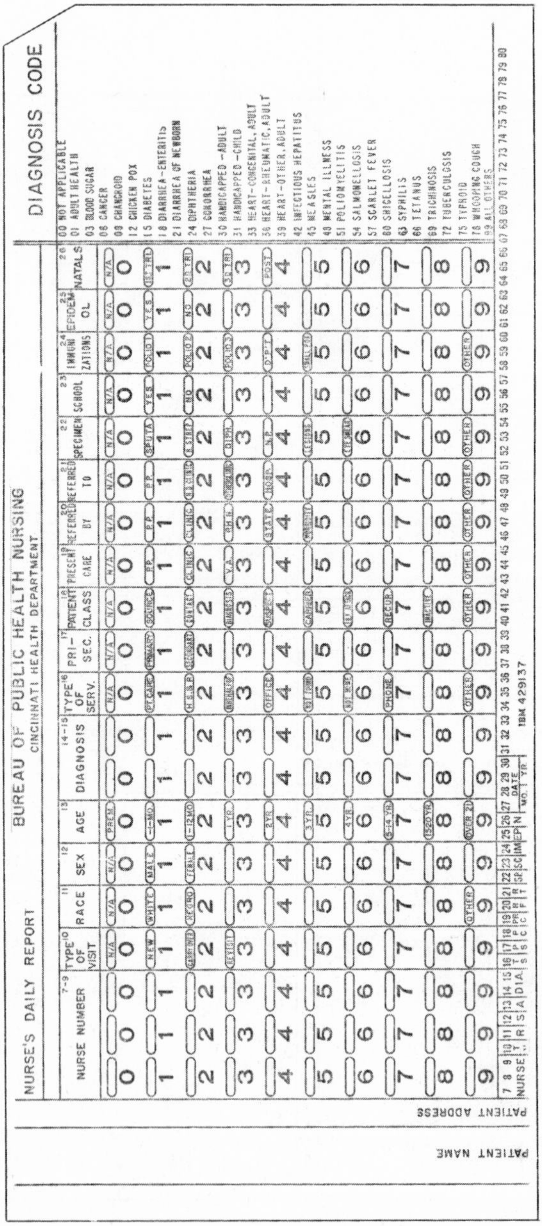

FIGURE 12. Daily report form precoded for machine tabulation. A separate card is used for each service unit.

parent education classes, or clinic sessions. It may also be used to provide information about the distribution of time in various types of activity such as preparation time, travel time, or inservice education.

The need for fiscal accounting is obvious, and the record system will provide vouchers on which to record expenditures made on behalf of the agency; purchases of equipment, car maintenance, and reimbursement for mileage when the nurse uses her own car are examples of this kind of expense. Records may also be provided for acknowledging receipt of fees when the nurse collects them directly, or provision may be made for validating bills for nursing services when the bills are submitted to the family or to a third party for payment directly to the agency.

Control Records

Control records assure that service commitments are met. *Requests for service, or referral forms requesting service,* are usually kept for a limited time and indicate the source of referral and what disposition was made of the request. A compilation of such requests may be maintained in order to estimate trends in the sources of referral, in the proportion of those referred who are already known to the service, and in the kinds of disposition made of these requests.

An index file identifies all who have been admitted for nursing service, the dates of service, and sometimes the general nature of the service provided. The case may be identified by name or by number. This makes it possible to retrieve prior records and relate the present service to past efforts. It may also yield important information about trends in the general type of service requests and persistence in the use of the agency by families or groups. This information may be stored in and retrieved from a computer, in which case the data may be more inclusive.

A case control record may be maintained in the service unit or by the individual nurse. This is usually a card containing minimal information that can be filed either by date (when localities are visited at specified times) or by the location of the case. This helps to assure that return visits will be made as planned. For cases receiving intensive nursing care, this second record may not be necessary, since it is not likely that visits planned on a daily or otherwise frequent schedule will be forgotten. However, for follow-up services or for visits that are planned at infrequent intervals, such a control file can be very useful. In some agencies a control file is kept by the supervisor or by a program director when a particular program is being given a high priority or is under special study; this kind of file may be maintained, for instance, as a control measure to assure return visits to families with tuberculosis.

Special case registers, which have been discussed previously, also serve as a control device. The register may be used to secure immediate information about the service status of any one of the cases in the register or as a means of analyzing the service status or progress of the entire group on register.

Convenience Forms

Every agency has a myriad of forms developed to facilitate the work of the staff. There may be forms for recording telephone messages or reminder lists for use in special types of visits, such as visits to a mentally retarded child and his family to estimate developmental problems or to tuberculosis contact cases. Special referral forms may be devised to ensure the inclusion of all necessary data and to provide for feedback from the agency to whom the family is referred.

These kinds of records may save considerable time and, in some cases, may lead to more systematic approaches. Their value lies in being sufficiently few in number and sufficiently easy to use so that they really do facilitate care rather than simply increase the amount of paper work.

REPORTS SYNTHESIZE AND EXPLAIN

Ongoing records are periodically synthesized into reports, which serve as a check on progress, as a guide for future action, and as a basis for reporting for the agency or program as a whole. These reports contain statistical and narrative content. They may be required on a monthly, quarterly, or annual basis. There is considerable advantage in quarterly reports, which may be incorporated into an annual report. The quarterly period is sufficiently long for some trends in, or results from, service to be apparent, and yet it is sufficiently short to permit quick rectification of misdirected activities.

Statistical Content of Reports

The quantification of nursing effort can be organized in many different ways, and the way in which it is organized will make a great difference in its usefulness. Although the agency will set certain requirements for this report, the community health nurse may have an opportunity to influence the way in which it is organized, or she may expand some aspects of the required statistical report as it relates to her own efforts in order to adapt it to her own information needs.

In most cases, statistical data are more useful if they contain an element of *comparison*. For example, the number of home visits made on behalf of school children during one year has much more meaning if it is shown in comparision with visits made during the previous year or with the number that would have been made if need were the only criterion for making the visit. The comparison might be between the proportion of visits involving care of the problems of the school child only and the proportion of visits that involved family problems as well as the difficulty that occasioned the visit, between the amount of care provided by this agency and by other agencies serving the school child, or between the average number of visits provided to the school population as compared to those made to the nonschool population. Also, the characteristics of children receiving nursing service in the school setting might be compared to the characteristics of those not receiving definitive nursing care.

Trends in the time spent on various programs, such as home care for the sick, and changes in the time and cost of particular service units, such as clinic nursing support, are most meaningful if shown over a span of several years. These figures may be important indicators of change in the clientele and their needs or of change in nursing practice.

Narrative Content of Reports

The narrative portion of the report explains and illustrates progress and problems. The narrative report should be closely related to the statistical statement. It offers, for instance, an opportunity to relate statistical findings to some of the problems incurred by the increased use of multilevel nursing personnel. The families needing higher or lower levels of care will not be neatly defined by geographic boundaries. Thus, if the same case load is served by two workers of equal preparation, the geographic area may be divided and the travel time halved. When two levels of worker are used, it is likely that each worker will have to serve throughout the entire area, with a consequent higher travel cost.

The narrative report provides an opportunity to illustrate the statistical report: the increase in personal care may be explained by describing the needs of, and the care given to, a single family; the lengthened time per home visit may be accounted for by the description of the intensity of the problems and the nature of the nursing response for families in poverty areas.

The narrative report can also describe problems or indicate changes that are not made explicit by the statistical report. For example, a description of some of the frustrations of dealing with "reluctant" families in need of preventive health care may suggest the nurse's need for further preparation or for consultative help in dealing with these problems. The narrative report also allows the identification of indigenous leaders in the community; this may be important, since they may eventually contribute to the health program even though, at first, nursing time is required to ready them for this responsibility.

This portion of the record is extremely useful to administrators, since narrative comments convey the "feel" of field problems and accomplishments and often indicate that staff education or consultative or administrative support may be needed to improve the field situation. Writing this part of the report may also clarify the nurse's own understanding of the situation.

The Annual Report

The nurse who is writing an annual report should consider it not only as the means of informing the administration and, in some cases, the public of her work but also the means of communicating to them the significance of what has been done. In addition, the annual report should identify service problems with which the nurse must deal.

The following suggestions may help to make the preparation of annual reports an exercise in problem confrontation rather than a chore.

1. Develop an outline of the content and the general method of presenting the report early in the year. The content should certainly include a report of the year's major accomplishments in both quantitative and qualitative terms, trends in service needs and activities, the relation of accomplishments to the stated goals and to the needs of the total population, and the problems and plans for the year ahead.

2. Collect information and illustrative materials throughout the year. Keep a folder handy so notes or reminders can be inserted easily.

3. Choose a style that will suit the audience. The administrator will be reviewing many such reports. He will want a succinct résumé with clear and readily located summaries of progress and problems. Reports for the general public or for citizen committees will probably be more interesting if the facts are illustrated with case materials (the identity of the cases being securely hidden) and with statistics translated to comprehensive and quickly comprehensible terms (*e.g.,* "Last year each family under care received an average of three visits; this year the average was four visits.").

4. Organize the report so that essential information is readily located. Different colored sheets may be used for the various sections of the report, a summary sheet may appear at the beginning with more detailed reports following in the same order, or the format may clearly indicate the location of special sections of the report.

5. Give recognition to other agencies, divisions, or persons who have helped with the program. If volunteers have helped, it may be useful to translate their services into professional time equivalents: the use of volunteers released X number of nurse days for other work; or, volunteers provided services that would have cost X dollars if rendered by paid staff.

RECORDS AND REPORTS PROVIDE THE BASES FOR SPECIAL STUDIES

From time to time there will be need for special studies of nursing service that require the use of recorded data. These data may include evaluative studies, cost studies, or process studies.

The Nursing Audit

The nursing audit is a prime evaluative tool. Audit methods have been used for many years in hospital and community situations. Recently this methodology has been greatly refined, particularly in its use in hospital settings. It has been used in a somewhat more limited way in community health nursing. Phaneuf has been an outstanding proponent of this method and has made many contributions to its development.[1]

The audit approach to evaluation is based upon a systematic and intensive review of a representative sample of service records; this review is performed by an expert or experts who are dissociated from the provision of the care being evaluated. The review is based upon a carefully constructed set of categories of care elements and, for each category of elements, a set of criterion measures that are considered to be indicators of the quality of the care provided. Additional criterion measures are developed for the service unit as a whole. Thus, one element of care might be "supervision of others providing nursing care," and criteria might include such measures as recorded evidence that prescribed treatments were carried out as ordered or that the supervisee was adequately checked on the treatments she was expected to provide. Some of the measures will be objective in character and clearly deducible from the record; others will be based on the judgment of the reviewer or of the review panel. The evaluations made are combined into scores for each category and for the service as a whole.

The reviewers may be professional nurses; or, when there is more than one service involved, the review board may include members of other relevant disciplines.

This methodology has several advantages. The use of "outside" reviewers helps maintain objectivity in rating, since those providing the service may have some bias arising from their closeness to the situation. The use of records rather than direct observation as the basis of the rating allows a wide range of recipients of service and types of care to be covered in a relatively short time. The scoring by category makes it possible to pinpoint areas of difficulty.

This is obviously not a method for the amateur, and arrangements for such evaluation will be made by the agency. In the multiservice agency, nursing will often be only one of the audited programs.

Self-Study

Systematic self or self-and-supervisor record review provides an overview of progress. Some of the methodology of the audit can be adapted for use by the community health nurse herself or by the nurse along with her supervisor. This approach does not have the same objectivity or the level of expertise as the audit, inasmuch as judgments of one's own work are always subject to some degree of bias. Despite these limitations, the systematic review of records can be a valuable device for estimating progress.

When such a self-study is used, efforts should be made to avoid the use of general impressions in favor of assembling from the record facts that are indicative of comprehensiveness or quality of care. One way of assuring a systematic review is to develop a schedule as a basis for the review. Figure 13 shows one approach to record analysis that was used in a well child conference.

Case No.	Date Adm.	Age Adm.	No. Appts.				Feeding		Phys. Care			Prev. Med.		Emotional Reaction			Fam. Rel.		Referral			Comments, incl. Care Other Fam. Members.
			Tot.	Kept	Canc.	Miss.	Sel.	Behav.	Bath	Sleep	Oth.	Imm.	Oth.	TCL	Relax	Sibs.	Hus-W	P-Ch	Med.	Welf.	Oth.	
1	12/5		5	4	0	1	DD (D)	D	(D)							D						
2	8/12		8	2	2	4			(D)													
3	1/18		4	4	0	0	(D)				(D)				D		(D)					Mother tries but very anxious

D = Problems discussed.
(D = Action agreed upon.
(D) = Action taken or improvements noted.

FIGURE 13.   Record analysis work sheet—well-child clinic.

CRITERIA FOR THE RECORD SYSTEM

Although the staff nurse is unlikely to be responsible for designing the record system, she may better use the system in operation if she understands the criteria the system is expected to meet. The effective and efficient record system should meet the following criteria:

1. The record system should possess sufficient uniformity to provide for easy recording, tabulation, and collation and to permit interunit and interservice comparisons. In general, records prescribe the placement and content of identifying and service data that are likely to be tabulated and compared. Thus the record may have a space for the insurance carrier, the social security number, the dates of admission and discharge from service, and the type of service provided; space for this information is often identically placed in all appropriate record forms. The purely narrative record does not lend itself to accurate and economic automatic or hand tabulation.

2. The record system should require the minimal amount of time that is consistent with the record's purpose. It is quite possible to reduce record time at the expense of reducing the effectiveness and efficiency of the service. On the other hand, unproductive record time is probably one of the greatest thieves of scarce nursing time today. Unproductive record time includes time spent hunting for records that should be readily available, making long and neat notations, the longterm storage of information that is of transitory value, time spent reading irrelevant or unimportant data, voluminous recopying of service data for transmittal to another agency when a Xerox copy or carbon copy with a gummed back would serve the purpose just as well or when the communication can be better achieved through a person-to-person contact. The format of the record affects the accuracy and time required in recording. For example, boxes providing the expected number of digits in a social security or an insurance number help prevent omission or repetition of a digit; uniform location of an item such as an address saves time because both reader and writer know where to find it. Dictation of record content may conserve scarce professional time, provided it does not encourage excessively long recording or result in significant errors in transcription.

3. The record should be quickly available to the user. Both individual service records and compiled data are useful to the degree that they are where they are needed at the time they are needed. The family history that is filed in a central location and cannot be retrieved in time to use for planning care is only half effective. The record that should be immediately available to the school teacher but that is filed in the health department several blocks away is similarly lowered in value as a tool for service planning and implementation. Compiled data, too, need to be easily available. The nurse who would like to know how her use of a home health aide is similar or different from that of other nurses finds it difficult to look at her own performance comparatively if the records are "in the computer" for months before they are available to her. Accessibility is not always easy to achieve. For instance, it seems apparent that school health records should be in school and that clinic records should be in the clinic. Yet the same information may also be needed in the general family record that is used by the nurse who is providing assistance to the family as a whole.

4. The record system should require reasonable storage space. The proliferation of records, as well as the increase in the number of people under care, may create serious problems of record storage and increased demands for clerical time. The period for which records are retained is usually a matter of agency policy; often the period of retention is as low as five years. A short retention period does save space; but it also presents problems, since community health needs and methods are changing and the period over which care is provided to a family is likely to be more prolonged. Microfilming is used in some agencies as a space saving procedure. In others, a representative sample of records that would normally be retired may be held for historic purposes or for comparisons over time. For example, it is conceivable that a full nursing record from the 1970's would be of considerable interest to nurses in the year 2000 as an indication of the general directions taken in nursing practice in an earlier period.

5. The record system should be susceptible to coordination on those parameters considered important for planning and evaluation. For example, it should be possible to pull out all of the records for a particular service (such as service to crippled children or to industrial plants) or all of the records of service to a given geographic area or population unit regardless of whether the service was provided in the school, the clinic, or the home. When automatic data processing is used, aggregations of record data are easily secured. When such processing is not available (for instance, in the small population of an individual case load), identification of special records (by color tabs or other distinguishing mark) or the assignment of a single number to all of a specific family's records, wherever they are filed, may help identify special groups quickly.

6. The record system should provide for confidentiality of record content. The assurance of privacy is one of the big problems in developing community-wide, coordinated health-care information systems, and even in a small service it is not an easy matter to deal with. For example, it may not be appropriate to open to the teaching staff in the school some of the health information held by the nurse. In some agencies, family permission must be secured before releasing information to any other person or agency. In most agencies there are regulations that limit the degree to which information may be shared; often the specific groups in the community that are eligible to have specific data are defined. In the use of data processing systems in hospitals, special keys issued only to those who are entitled to use the information, are required to activate the data-issuing mechanism. The community health nurse's individual responsibilty in this respect may be limited to careful observation of agency policies regarding release of information and, when necessary, working out special methods for storing and handling "sensitive" information.

THE COMPUTER

E.D.P. — electronic data processing — and other automated systems are assuming an increasingly important role in management, and the management of health services is no exception. Properly used, data processing promises to reduce professional and clerical paperwork, to make information available in an incredibly short time, and to provide large numbers of relationships or correlations that could not be readily secured through other methods of data handling. It is not inconceivable that at some time it will be possible to secure in minutes (if not seconds) detailed information relating to the health care provided to an individual or family from a great variety of different community health-care sources.

Although it is easy to place emphasis on the "hardware" of E.D.P. — on the incredibly rapid calculation capability, the accuracy, and storage of data — the effectiveness of any system of this kind will depend on the quality of the data that are submitted. The selectivity, the relevance, the accuracy, and the completeness of the data fed in by the various service personnel are essential to the usefulness of the compilations.

The community health nurse may find that she is required either to adapt her service records to the needs of data processing or to complete separate reporting materials for this use. She may be asked to use codes in recording to permit ready transfer of data or to make notations on cards, using a special pencil that will allow the data to be recorded directly. Because it may be easy to make errors, particularly at first, it is important that each nurse take the responsibility for careful checking to be sure there are no inaccuracies in coding or stray pencil marks that will confuse the machine.

The nursing uses of the kind of data that can be made available through electronic data processing are phenomenal. Nurses must find out what the computer can do for them: what combinations of information they may get with respect to nursing input, what material relative to the nature of the population may be useful in planning the nursing program, what within the service records offers promise of usefulness in future planning and action and so justifies computer storage. Both by suggesting what data may be fed into the processing system and by knowing about and using the data already available, the community health nurse can find the data processing system a new and powerful resource for care.

RECORDS MUST BE USED

The more records are used, the less irksome they become. Attitudes toward records and recording are probably more an outcome of the nature of the uses to which records are put than to the actual demands the record system imposes. Thus, the nurse who *uses* records — not only her own family history and progress record but also the compilations that reflect group activities and progress — is less likely to resent the time spent in recording, more apt to monitor her own recording performance, and more likely to offer useful suggestions about records and recording procedures. The habit of looking for and analyzing record data and of studying its implications for one's own work will place the individual nurse in the total picture of the health effort of which she is such an important part.

REFERENCES

1. Phaneuf, Maria: Nursing audit method. Nurs. Outlook, *12:*42, May, 1964.

SUGGESTED READINGS

Cohen, Hedwig: Records and recording. *In* Stewart, Dorothy M., and Vincent, Pauline A. (eds.): Public Health Nursing. William C. Brown Company, Publishers, Dubuque, 1968, p. 114.

Farrell, Margaret B.: Health service records at a glance. Amer. J. Nurs., *66:*312, February, 1966.

Griffith, Elsie I.: A rational approach to patient service review. Nurs. Outlook, *17:*49, April, 1969.

Hope, Penelope, and Clement, Esther M.: A records revolution in a public health nursing agency. Nurs. Outlook, *16:*52, February, 1968.

How to Organize a Record System—A Guide for Nursing Homes and Homes for the Aged. U.S. Department of Health, Education and Welfare, Division of Medical Care Administration, PHS Publication No. 1429, U.S. Government Printing Office, Washington, D.C., 1966.

Parker, Mary, Ausman, Robert K., and Ovedovitz, Irving: Automation of public health nurse reports. Public Health Rep., *80:*526, June, 1965.

Phaneuf, Maria: Analysis of a nursing audit. Nurs. Outlook, *16:*57, January, 1968.

Phaneuf, Maria: Nursing audit method. Nurs. Outlook, *12:*42, May, 1964.

Phaneuf, Maria: Nursing audit for evaluation of patient care. Nurs. Outlook, *14:*51, June, 1966.

Price, Elmina: Data processing, present and potential. Amer. J. Nurs., *67:*2558, December, 1967.

Recording the home visit. Nurs. Outlook, *15:*38, February, 1967.

Smiley, Lydia: Health records for school children. Amer. J. Nurs., *60:*918, September, 1960.

Statistical Reporting in Public Health Nursing. The National League for Nursing, New York, 1962.

Swayne, James B., Roberts, Pauline O., Edgerly, Raymond, and Yoshida, Toshiko: Development and installation of unified patient records. Public Health Rep.; *77:*201, March, 1962.

Walker, Cleopatra, and Deuble, Hazel: A schema for analysis of accident prevention activities in public health nurse's records. Nurs. Res., *17:*408, September-October, 1968.

Wolff, Ilse: Referral—a process and a method. *In* Stewart, Dorothy M., and Vincent, Pauline A. (eds.): Public Health Nursing, *op. cit.,* p. 130.

CHAPTER

20

Nursing the School Community

Nursing in the school has a long history. The first school nursing service in the United States was established in New York City in 1902 at the instigation of Lillian Wald of the Henry Street Settlement. Troubled that children with skin diseases were excluded from school for long periods of time, she offered a one-month demonstration of nursing services provided by a Henry Street nurse. This was so successful that within a few weeks 12 nurses were appointed to work in the schools.[1]

Since then, school nursing services have grown in size and scope, both as part of generalized nursing programs in communities and as a specialized service organized in departments of education. There were 15,282 nurses employed by boards of education in 1966. In addition, the 16,562 nurses employed by local special agencies carried varying degrees of responsibilities for health care of the school-age child and for nursing services to schools.[2]

Although there is much discussion as to the relative merits of having school nursing provided as a part of a generalized community nursing service or as a separate and school-based service, there is little evidence that one administrative pattern is clearly more desirable than the other. The incorporation of school nursing into the general community health programs, when a single nurse serves the school and the community at large, has the advantages of unifying in-school and out-of-school care, of some economies in nursing time, and of the allocation of nursing time in the school in accordance with a community-wide nursing priority system. The school-based program has the advantages of permitting more specialized nursing care, sometimes of readier financing (school funding may be more flexible or more assured than health agency budgets), and of allowing a closer integration of the health and educational efforts of the school on behalf of the protection and development of the school-age population. Whatever the sponsorship, both the school and the com-

munity health agencies are bound to share responsibilities for the health
of the school-age population.

The School Offers a Unique Channel for Community Nursing

A 1966 survey by the Bureau of the Census reported a school enrollment of over 55 million persons: 3 out of every 5 persons between the
ages of 5 and 34 were enrolled in school. Approximately 35.5 million
children were enrolled in elementary school, 13.4 million children were
in high schools, and 6.1 million persons were in colleges or professional
schools.[3]

Thus, the school offers a channel for human services that reaches the
great majority of children and a substantial proportion of the youth;
elementary grade schools reach virtually all of the noninstitutionalized
population in that age group.

In addition, nursing services may be made available in varying degrees
to school personnel. The school also affords a channel to other members
of the family by involving parents in the school program.

The school may become an arm of the community action, including
health action, either by serving as a center for adult education and after-
school activities or through the utilization of school children as emissaries in health educational efforts. Recent emphasis on the "community
school"—a school committed to involvement in the community it serves
as well as to the education of its pupils—has quickened this extension of
the traditional concerns of the school. Some proponents envision a
school open 12 months a year, 12 or more hours a day. Programs would
be designed for all age groups, including the aged and the very young.
The school would thus become a kind of community center. Other
agencies could participate in the programs and use the facilities of the
school and the closeness generated by the comprehensive community
approach. The potential of such access to the population staggers the
imagination!

The fact that school attendance is mandatory, added to a natural
concern for the welfare of children, produces very strong public support
for health efforts in the school. Thus is it perhaps not surprising that a
large proportion of the total available community health nursing time is
spent in the schools. In 1966, one large urban agency reported that the
school health program used more than half of the available nursing
time.[4]

The Function of the Nurse in the School Is Three Dimensional

The American Nurse's Association's official statement of functions
and qualifications for school nurses lists 20 functions that are grouped
under the general responsibility areas of assessment, planning, im-

plementation, evaluation, and study and research.[5] These are summarized in the following statement:

> In general, the functions of the school nurse are associated with the establishment and enforcement of the schools' policies and programs for the protection and promotion of health of the pupils; the maintenance of a school environment which is conducive to healthful living; the building of those components of the curriculum which have significance for health; the management of the health service including screening programs and emergency care services; the handling of special health problems; and relating the school health programs to those of the community.[6]

Thus it might be said that the functions of the nurse in the school are three dimensional: (1) to contribute to the personal health care and health education of the school population, (2) to contribute to the improvement of the physical and social environment in which the school population spends its school hours, and (3) to relate these efforts toward health improvement to those of the family and of the community at large.

The Personal Health Care and Health Education of the School Population

Ensuring a healthy school population depends on activities that are undertaken before the child is actually enrolled in school as well as on those performed at the time of the child's initial entry into the school community. Even though it is undeniably better to think of health care of children as a continuous program beginning at the point of conception, the fact is that it often takes the stimulus of impending school enrollment to get some things done. For the child entering school, it is hoped that he will have had a complete medical and dental appraisal; that he will have completed his immunization series (including recommended booster shots); and that any correctable defect, especially impairments of vision and hearing, will have been corrected.

The school nurse may confer with parents prior to the child's entry to school and help to establish special examination or immunization clinics when the services of a family physician or of other facilities are not available. Head start activities, designed to enrich the preschool years as a preparation for school, require nursing support, since health care is an integral aspect of the program.

Letters may be used to encourage parental action before school opens. When the letters are personal, warm and supportive, and provide explicit advice, they may influence a large number of parents. Parents may be asked to complete a health inventory form, or they may be supplied with forms to bring to their usual medical adviser at the time the child has his preschool medical examination.

The school health nurse contributes to the health care and health education of the school population in five ways:

1. By participating in health assessment measures, including observation, screening, medical examination, and epidemiologic investigation.

2. By providing or arranging for care of injuries and of emergency or continuing illness.
3. By counseling or arranging for counseling with students or other personnel who have health problems, including, of course, emotional health problems.
4. By involving parents, teachers, and pupils in planning and conducting health-care activities and in decision making relative to their own health.
5. By contributing to the development of health-related learning experiences for students through curriculum development; by special activities such as clubs or study groups; or through advisement with teachers or other personnel.

HEALTH ASSESSMENT OF THE SCHOOL POPULATION

Health assessment measures in the school are almost always a multiprofessional undertaking involving the child himself, his family, the teacher, school counselors, psychologists, attendance officers, school social workers, physical education instructors, and volunteer and paid assistants and technicians, as well as nurses and physicians. The school nurse, because of her awareness of the need to use all measures from the simple and incidental observation of the teacher to the multidiscipline comprehensive health examination for the detection of health aberrations, will encourage everyone in contact with the school child to be alert to any developmental or health deviation. Those in contact with the children should have available to them informational materials that will allow them to observe intelligently and that will make clear to whom they should report any observed or suspected deviation from expected health behavior.

Provisions for Observation by the Child and the Family. However effective and efficient school measures for detection of health problems may be, they cannot take the place of intelligent observation and action on the part of the pupil and his family. Even the kindergarten child can learn to recognize when he has a cold and to report this to the teacher. The nurse may reach children through the integration of this information into class content, such as personal hygiene or homemaking, or by providing opportunities for students to help with health observations or screening measures. A valuable indirect route that may be available in the secondary school is the future nurses club, the future homemakers club, or the health careers club. These social activity groups usually include students who have an interest in health and who are especially ready for health instruction. These students may also exert considerable influence on their peers in health matters.

Several methods of communication may be used to involve family members. Parents who are present at the time of school medical examinations may be advised on health symptoms or may be invited to participate more extensively in health instruction, such as classes in home nursing, or to volunteer assistance in the health program. The parent-teacher association may offer meeting time for the nurse to discuss school health problems; or the nurse may talk informally with individual parents at the time of the meetings. However, neither of these methods are likely to reach those who most need such instruction, such as those in the low-income group or those living in isolated locations, since these parents seldom attend such school activities. The nurse may have to plan to reach these parents in the home. If the nurse is carrying general, as well as school, health nursing responsibilities, she may plan to see these parents either individually or in clusters in a neighborhood; or she may enlist the aid of a nurse in the generalized program or a school health aid or a volunteer to make teaching visits to selected families.

"Notes to take home" is another measure for reaching parents with health information. This approach has the obvious advantage of reaching large numbers of parents, especially mothers. However, it is perhaps the least effective measure, since the notes may be lost or disregarded. When notes are to be used, whether sent home via the pupil or mailed, care should be taken to word them so that they convey a sense of warmth and personalization. These methods of family-nurse communication may, of course, be used for many occasions other than case finding.

Provisions for Observation by the Teacher.   The teacher, as the one in most constant contact with the child during the school day, is a key person in health observation. The community health nurse in the school may improve the quality of the teacher's observations by:

1. Arranging for the inclusion of health content in teachers' meetings. These meetings, usually held just before the start of the school year, offer an excellent opportunity for reaching teachers, especially new teachers. At this time it is possible to orient new teachers to the role and the services of the school health nurse and other health personnel, to arrange for briefing in observation techniques, and to inform teachers of the availability of nursing or other health services. Moreover, this is an opportunity for returning teachers to catch up with changes in the program or in the health personnel, and with the plans of the health-care group for the year ahead. Arrangements for such contacts are made through the school principal, school superintendent, or through the student personnel office.

2. Scheduling teacher-nurse conferences. These conferences are usually planned by the nurse and teacher with the approval of the responsible school administrator. The teacher-nurse conference is the backbone of the teacher education program. It is here that the nurse and the teacher have an opportunity to discuss the problems of individual children, especially those who appear to have health problems. It is also the occasion for a more general interchange in which each becomes informed of the problems of the other with respect to the health and education program and in which there is an opportunity to agree on courses of action that have to do with an individual child or with the class as a group.

Sometimes the problem is not so much with an individual child as it is with the group as a whole. The teacher may find a group afflicted with a contagious inattention or irritability or a class in which a few students appear to dominate the others to an undesirable degree. Sometimes culture-based group attitudes — such as attitudes toward premarital intercourse — may have health implications. Recently there have been efforts to reorganize school populations to make them more representative of the community as a whole rather than of their immediate neighborhood. In this effort, the school population becomes more diversified with respect to sociocultural backgrounds and, often, in learning interests. This may, however, create interpersonal, mental, and emotional health problems for both students and teachers.

The teacher-nurse conference should be carefully planned. The time should be set when the teacher has no scheduled class or when the children can be engaged in some activity that does not require the teacher's concentrated attention. Sometimes a teacher aide or parent volunteer can take over the class during the conference. The teacher should have had a prior opportunity to look at each child individually (usually with the guidance of a teacher observation form) for any possible health problem and to evaluate changes in those children under special observation.

Sometimes the teacher will want the nurse to meet the children as a group and may suggest that the nurse give a short talk to the class. This may serve a useful purpose, but the nurse must be careful not to divert her time to formal instruction when the real need is to explore general health matters with the teacher or to confer with individual students who have health problems.

The nurse should have reviewed her records of this particular class prior to the conference in order to bring to the conference a report on the progress made with children who are under nursing care.

The overall scheme for teacher-nurse conferences should be cleared with and understood by the school administration officer, since he is responsible for the total school effort. Anything that interrupts the usual teaching schedule or that incorporates into the school program content not under his supervision is of concern to him. His support is essential in gaining the cooperation and interest of the teaching group.

3. Alerting teachers when special observations are needed: for example, when there is an increased incidence of influenza or when teenage pregnancies are prevalent and frequently unreported. This provides an opportunity for "spot" briefing, or outlining and describing the symptoms that may be observed if, for instance, emotional problems are paramount; discussions of typical behaviors of children who are anxious, withdrawn, and depressed may help sharpen the teacher's observations.

Screening Measures.   In some states there are laws requiring that specific screening measurements be made at stated intervals. In virtually every school there are policies requiring some screening. Screening in the school setting may take many forms:

1. Informal screening of each child each day may be performed by the classroom teacher for evidence of deviance from usual health behavior.
2. Screening examinations for vision and hearing may be conducted by technicians, teachers, parents or other volunteers, or nurses.
3. Special screening measures may be instituted for a particular problem, such as tuberculosis infection, for selected children at unusual risk; for children referred by the teacher, or for specific individuals with known problems.

4. Dental screening may be conducted by the dentist, dental hygienist, or dental assistant.
5. Periodic medical examinations may be performed by the school or family physician at specified intervals.
6. Self-completed or family-completed health inventories or health histories may be required. When the family physician takes the responsibility of completing the provided form, he submits it to the school where it is then reviewed by the school nurse or school physician.

The nurse may have a major part in planning and implementing the screening program. The scheduling must be such that it interferes as little as possible with the formal educational process. Volunteers or technicians may need orientation to the programs or to the school, or they may need specific and comprehensive training by the school health personnel. The nurse must arrange to have time available not only to be present at the examination, to train or orient other workers, and to make the necessary physical arrangements but also to complete the required follow-up care for problems that are uncovered. In arranging her schedule, the nurse will want to be sure there is additional time available for this latter activity; it is of little use to discover health problems if nothing is done about them.

In general it is felt that it is beneficial for a parent to be present when the child is receiving a medical examination. This allows the health staff to clarify the health situation immediately. This parental participation is also felt to have a strong motivating force that makes correction of the problem more likely.

In carrying out screening procedures, the nurse should avoid tying herself up with the routine procedures. By delegating this kind of work to aides, volunteers, or technicians, she can be free to circulate; to talk with teachers, parents, and children; and to take the first steps in assuring follow-up care for problems.

HEALTH CARE OF THE SCHOOL POPULATION

Planning nursing care for the school population is a multifaceted task. The case load of the community health nurse in the school is the total school population, which includes both the students and the employees of the school. The extent of the responsibility of the nurse will be spelled out in policy statements; in some situations the nurse may participate in school sponsored medical examinations for teachers, whereas in other instances this is not a part of the school health program. The nurse in the school may or may not participate in preschool examination and surveillance, adult health education, or home visiting. Within these understandings, the nurse in the school will define the need for different categories of care for specified groups in the school population.

Using the measures that are available and effective in identifying health problems, it will be possible for the nurse to identify those individuals or groups who appear to have a substantive health problem or who are at unusual risk. This will include those children with multiple handicaps or health deviations, those from disorganized families who exhibit signs of social alienation, or those with chronic diseases requiring therapeutic maintenance. From this information she will develop a case load of children who are in need of intensive nursing supervision. For the remainder of the children, general surveillance will be adequate, and nursing efforts may be directed toward keeping the alertness level of teachers and parents high. Some nurses like to categorize students into three levels, thereby allowing for an intermediate service load that requires less than intensive care but more than simple surveillance.

A valuable index of need for nursing care is the absence record of individuals, groups, or specific schools. The frequency of absence in the school as a whole is, of course, important. Even more important, however, is the pattern of absence and the reasons for absence from school. The child whose absences are frequent, of short duration, and not accompanied by the need for medical care merits study with respect to general vitality level and, perhaps, attitude toward school; whereas illnesses of long duration suggest a more definitive medical problem. If the absences appear to coincide with school examinations or special programs (such as physical education), the search for causes may take a different tack. When a whole school is characterized by frequent absence — especially of girls — at points of family crisis, the need may rest in sociocultural value orientations or in the community's failure to provide adequate home help. Absence patterns that consistently affect a specific group of children might alert the nurse to the possibility of group experimentation with drugs or other unapproved activities.

   Establish a Nursing-Care Philosophy.   It is important to establish a philosophy upon which nursing care will be based and which will serve as a general guide to the nurse and to those who assist her in the provision of nursing care. This philosophy will depend somewhat upon the prevailing educational philosophy. The nursing-care philosophy might include concepts such as these:

   1. The goal of nursing care is to keep the child in school, maximize his participation in school activities, and minimize his "difference." This might lead to the decision to have handicapped children receive treatments in school rather than at home, to refer children to special classes only when these classes are necessary for the progress of the student (not to relieve the anxiety of the school staff), to deal with group attitudes toward handicapping conditions in a way that will provide sensible peer support for the handicapped child, or to make arrangements with the school cafeteria to provide special foods for children requiring them in order to avoid their having to eat apart from their classmates.

   2. Preventive and anticipatory services represent the major thrust of the school nursing program. This suggests that emergency care of children and staff be delegated where possible and that volunteer or technical assistance be maximized to reach students who are in need of more substantive health counseling. It further supposes that the nurse will have the required background of information on the conditions expected and on the preventive measures available in this group as a basis both for her own work and for the delegation of nursing work.

   3. The participation of parents and children in health decisions will be maximized. Thus, parents may serve as volunteers, older students may

teach health to younger groups, and health-care proposals will, as far as possible, be posed in terms of possible alternatives in action.

4. The family is the unit of service in the personal care aspects of nursing. This requires that the school nurse not only involve the family in the care of the child but also concern herself with the effect of the child's condition or behavior in the family and help secure required care for other members of the family.

Anticipate Required Care.   Anticipating the care likely to be required makes it possible to move smoothly into the program. The nurse should inform herself of the risks characteristic of the age groups being served, and also of any risks characteristic of this particular environment. For example, accidents are a major concern in the school-age group both as a cause of death and disability and as a cause of absence from school. This makes it obvious that provisions should be made for the nursing care and prevention of accidental injury. Emotional problems are also frequent in the school-age groups. Cancer, although of infrequent occurrence in this predominantly well group that enjoys a low death rate, is a major cause of death in the older school-age group. In certain localities there may be special problems: high incidence of drug abuse, nutritional disorders, or child neglect by affluent parents who, by substituting "things" for parental controls and concerns, produce emotional deprivation.

Careful Planning for Care.   Careful planning for care is time-consuming but pays off in the long run. The general policy relating to the nursing care provided is developed by the school medical authority; that is, either by a school medical officer or, in some cases, by a designated medical committee. However, when the school nurse provides care or treatment for a medical condition, it is important that she have, in addition to general policy, *written medical orders* for the procedure undertaken. In the case of emergency treatment, standing orders or policies may be sufficient; but for more specific or for continuing care, the orders should be explicit for the individual involved. The school nurse should report to the child's personal physician with the same regularity as would pertain were nursing service given under any other auspices. The care plan should indicate specifically what is to be done, by whom, and approximately when.

Special planning may be needed for nursing care of preschool and adult groups when they are included in the school health program. In most instances, personal health nursing care of this group will be provided from other sources or under the aegis of other programs, and the nurse in the school will limit her effort to incidental assistance or to referral.

The Health Record.   The health record is shared with discrimination. Good records contribute greatly to the effectiveness and continuity of care in the school setting. In general, a cumulative health record is combined with the general cumulative school record; and when there are special health problems that require more intensive care, there may be a special and separate health service record. For example, the child's general cumulative record might include developmental data or information on conditions that require special seating, lighting, or particular continuing observation or support by the teaching staff. This information will be immediately available to all authorized school personnel. For those students with intensive nursing needs and a separate nursing record, a notation on the cumulative record indicates that the child is in this special case load. Thus, others will be alerted to talk to the nurse if they observe any special difficulty with the child, and the nurse may still maintain this special record to ensure the confidentiality of its contents.

First-Aid Care of Emergencies and Illness.   Prompt and effective first-aid care of emergencies is essential to the safety program. Even though the nurse herself may provide emergency treatment, in most instances she must rely on others who are on the scene to give immediate care. Every school should have designated personnel who have had preparation in first-aid care and who are available to assist in emergency situations. The school may have its own policies or procedures relative to emergency care, or it may adopt the American Red Cross Textbook or other standard text as the manual for care. The American Red Cross or another organized community training facility may provide instruction, or there may be qualified first-aid instructors on the school faculty. Emergency care supplies should be available where needed and should be maintained at all times.

It is also important that there be an established procedure for notifying the family of illness or injury, for transportation of children who must go home, for procedures to follow when there is no one in the child's home during the day, and for securing necessary medical care. Sometimes there is a physician who is assigned to school health work, and who is readily available. More often there are designated physicians or institutions near the school from whom emergency care may be secured. Directions for obtaining emergency care, along with the phone number and, where relevant, the name of the person to be called, should be posted in a prominent place.

School facilities should provide a place where it is possible to isolate a child suspected of having communicable disease and a cot where children may rest if they are ill or injured. If volunteers are used for transportation, the drivers should be adequately insured.

HEALTH EDUCATION OF THE SCHOOL
POPULATION

Important to the state of health of the individual student and his family is a sufficient battery of knowledge to permit them to recognize health problems, to foresee health problems, and to take appropriate action when the need arises. Although there is no specific evidence that those who are in possession of health information act any more wisely than others in health matters, one must assume that it is important to acquaint children with the subject matter of health care as a basis for the decisions they will be required to make.

Much of the content of health education will be provided in conjunction with formal courses in family health or family living, in biology classes, in physical education classes, and in courses in the humanities and government. The nurse's function is to reinforce and supplement this general information by assisting with materials or suggested content.

The nurse's great contribution to health education will lie in educational efforts with individuals or small groups that have specific health concerns. Thus, a child coming for a bandage for a cut finger may be taught about prevention of accidents or of infection, or the young girl with frequent menstrual discomfort may be helped to a better under-standing of her own development and an increased acceptance of her feminine role.

The nurse may be asked to serve as a member of a school health committee. Such a committee is usually made up of representatives from those departments in the school that have a major concern with health and health teaching, of parents, of students, and of appropriate com-munity agencies. The committee usually reports to the administrative officer: to the school principal, if the committee is school-wide, or to the superintendent, if the committee is community-wide. The nurse whose school work represents a portion of the time spent in a generalized program should take this responsibility as seriously as does the nurse who spends her full time in the school.

EVALUATION OF NURSING PROCESS

The evaluation of nursing process and outcomes is somewhat compli-cated in the health setting because of the wide dispersion of responsi-bility. However, health progress can often be measured, even though one could not say the progress was due specifically to the nursing effort. A properly constructed record should make it easy to see at a glance whether or not the problems identified have in fact been referred for care, whether or not the care was received, and the results of care.

With nursing programs that involve a large number of students (as in follow-up care after a school medical examination), it is sometimes helpful, as an aid to measuring progress, to keep a separate "check off" index file or posting sheet in order to quickly identify the group still needing interpretation of correctional procedures.

Bryan, discussing the special problems of school nursing in culturally deprived areas, lists several indicators of parental action that were pertinent to her program.[7] Similar specific identification of desired and measurable outcomes would be most helpful in other school settings.

The nurse in the school should assure herself that care has been received when it is provided by agencies other than the school, and she should institute the requisite planning and follow-up procedures. Case conferences with nurses in the health department or the visiting nurse association or with the parents and the family medical adviser are essential. Though time-consuming, the lack of precision in care that occurs without such careful clearance is even more costly.

The effectiveness of care can be greatly improved if it is possible to identify the possible reasons or associated factors for noncompletion of recommendations for health care. Cauffman and associates, for example, found that the outcome of referral of school children for medical care was influenced by certain family characteristics and also by the way in which the referrals were made.[8] Such knowledge helps the nurse to plan more carefully in order to accommodate these impediments to care. When final outcomes are unsatisfactory due to failure of community support, the careful documentation of these conditions by the school nurse may play an important part in securing corrections.

The Improvement of the School's Physical and Social Environment

The school environment is second only to the home environment in its effect upon the health and development of children and youth. A healthful school environment should be free from hazards or barriers to health in order to be conducive to the proper physical and social development of the child and to the child's education, which is a joint commitment of the school and the home. These characteristics might describe the desirable environment in any setting, but the problems of the maintenance of a healthful environment in the school are somewhat specialized.

PHYSICAL HAZARDS

Safety in the school environment takes a prominent place in establishing a suitable environment for the child. Responsibility for maintenance of a safe environment is a responsibility which many people share: the administrative staff, who plans for new equipment and buildings; the teachers of health education, who maintain activity areas and control the behavior of children on the playground, in sports, and in other physical activities and who engage in teaching health and safety practices; the maintenance superintendent, who sees to it that good housekeeping practices reduce accident hazards; the classroom teacher, who observes and reports unsafe conditions; and the sanitarian, who inspects the premises for compliance with regulations. Often there will be a safety committee or council in the school, and the nurse's contribution may be mainly through her observation and her reporting to this committee or, sometimes, through her participation on this committee. In smaller school settings, the nurse may be required to take greater initiative in studying the safety of the environment and in securing correction of undesirable or unsafe conditions.

COMMUNICABLE DISEASES

Freedom from undue exposure to communicable disease is assured by maintaining the recommended immunization level in the school; by providing for prompt recognition (by alerted teachers and parents) of any deviation from usual health when communicable disease is prevalent; and by the exclusion from school (or temporary isolation if already at school) of those with symptoms of communicable disease.

The school nurse must be thoroughly conversant with the symptoms and treatment of communicable diseases; she must know the immunization level of the school population; and she must be aware of the state of knowledge of those responsible for the continuing screening of children. She needs also to be familiar with local regulations governing exclusion and readmission to school when communicable disease is suspected or diagnosed.

PSYCHOSOCIAL ENVIRONMENT

The psychosocial environment may have a significant impact on the health of the school child. A curriculum that is too difficult or too crowded may produce stress. A curriculum that is not sufficiently challenging or, to use the modern student phrase, "not relevant" may be equally stressful for the abler or more committed student. Schedules that do not permit interspersing of constricting and free activity or that include long class periods may also create stress. Excessive homework may also be a problem, especially when family support for such study is low.

Situations that lead to discouragement, fatigue, or loss of self-confidence or self-respect also present a health deterrent. Interpersonal stress among student groups arising from interracial or intercultural conflict, too much emphasis on formal testing, and track systems in which one group becomes known as "the dummies" or that lead to the development of sharply defined subgroups are examples of stress-producing situations that may result in emotional or social health problems.

Children's dress may also be a stress factor. Inability to secure proper clothing may cause a youngster to feel inferior; lack of cleanliness or careless dress may reflect and reemphasize a sense of defeat and lack of personal worth. Some teachers have found that "dress up days" have a very real influence on the manners and sense of self-esteem of the students, provided, of course, that the dressing up is within the capability of the children's family.

INDUCEMENTS TO GOOD HEALTH PRACTICE

The environment should offer inducements to good health practice. Adequate lighting in the school setting is crucial. Although there has been considerable disagreement as to exactly how much illumination is needed, Byrd reports American Medical Association support for the level of 10 foot candles of light in hallways and similar areas, 30 foot candles for reading, and 50 foot candles for fine work.[9] The Illuminating Engineering Society recommends 30 foot candles for reading and 100 to 150 foot candles for very fine work.[10]

Important nursing considerations are ensuring that children develop good habits in the use of available lighting, that fixtures are kept clean, that bulbs are replaced promptly, and that there is "brightness balance": that is, a balance in brightness between the seeing task area and the area immediately adjoining it (the recommended balance in reading areas is 3 to 1). Glare should be avoided.

The *seating* of school children and opportunities to move about during the classroom session are also important prerequisites to maintenance of good posture and the reduction of fatigue. Adequate facilities for handwashing, with plentiful and suitable soap and towels, are also necessary.

Provisions for in-school feeding are important. In large school systems, cafeterias may be under expert management, and the nurse's only concern may be the ways in which the facility is used: the availability of good food choices, scheduling to avoid dangerous overcrowding, and student behavior in the cafeteria as it relates to health. The sanitarian will be concerned with the preservation of good maintenance practices. The nurse, however, should be alert to the opportunity provided in the cafeteria for good food choices, the educational opportunities the food service may provide, and the quality of the socialization that occurs.

The presence of inducements to deleterious health practice may be a concern. The availability of coke and candy machines or, with college students, of cigarette vending machines may contribute negatively to the health environment.

The existence of good role models in the teaching, administrative, and student personnel staff is also a powerful factor in health behavior. The example set by the teaching and the administrative staff and the degree to which they are able to incorporate sound health teaching into the total curriculum have a profound impact on children's perceptions of health and of health care. The teacher's lesson that school children should stay at home to avoid infecting others when they have evidence of a communicable disease makes little impression if she herself comes to school coughing and sneezing with a cold. The school counselor who thinks that venereal disease and out-of-wedlock pregnancy happen only to children who are "not nice" will fail to recognize the possibility of such a condition in some socioeconomic groups or may convey her own attitude to such an extent that the child's ability to use adult help is limited. Attitudes toward health are "caught not taught," and the school group must recognize that teaching health involves this very important aspect of setting a good example.

Teachers and others coming into contact with children should be aware of health resources and of the nurse's role in using such resources. In a survey in three Oregon counties, Forbes found that many teachers didn't know the role of the nurse; there was serious lack of communication on health matters between the teacher and the nurse.[11]

The nurse should seek out all possible measures for establishing and reinforcing a joint approach to health problems. Circulating the annual report of the nurse to the teaching staff or using teacher's meetings or teacher-nurse conferences to discuss the plans for the nursing service in the school are examples of approaches that might be used. When any unusual circumstances arise, the nurse, acting in coordination with the school medical adviser, may send a reminder to teachers. For example, if a polio immunization program is being started in the community, the teachers might be informed of the importance of this preventive measure, the method that is being used, and the children or adults who should be encouraged to secure immunization. If nutritional conditions among students appear to be below par, suggestions about observation of children for symptoms of malnutrition or about the use of hot lunch supplementary feeding programs may help. The nurse might work with a nutritionist in the school or in the local or state health department to be sure the materials she is using are pertinent and up-to-date.

Students are also a valuable health resource. A valuable channel for the school nurse is the membership of the future nurses club or the health careers club. These clubs attract students who have a special interest in health and who may later enter one of the health occupations. The school nurse is often the sponsor for these groups. Help with materials and further information may be secured from the National Health Council or from the National League for Nursing.

Students may serve as volunteers in various health activities in or out of the school. When students are expected to observe or work in community agencies as part of the education program, the nurse may help the instructional staff in arranging such observations and, for some students, experience in health agencies.

The nurse may also be called upon to help teachers and students with special projects in other subject matter areas in which the content involves health. For example, a history student might be interested in health conditions at a given era, or a science student may be interested in some of the health problems of space exploration.

The Relationship of School Nursing to the Health of the Family and the Community

A supportive and participating community is an essential environmental condition. The ability of the school to contribute to the health of the child will depend upon community support in providing funds and in setting general policy regarding conditions for school health care.

A community that is interested in what the school is doing for their children, in understanding the basis for the school health program, and in participating in its development and evaluation can profoundly influence service outcomes.

The nurse may contribute to securing a supportive and participating community by using her work with children as a channel to "reach out" to the parents and to the neighborhood. Mothers and fathers may be invited to conferences where decisions are being made about school examinations and the ways in which parents will be notified and asked to participate. A group of parents may volunteer to interpret the upcoming program to other mothers in their neighborhood and may encourage them to participate by attending the examination session.

The nurse can also do much to interpret the school health program and the needs and plans of the school community to official and voluntary agencies in the community, to parents or to those whose children are not in school, and to the family physician, who may need to follow up on the problems uncovered in a school examination or who, in some instances, may be resentful of the school's interference with the care of his patients.

The nurse may also attend and become involved in the general community activities of the school apart from their health aspects, or she may engage in community teaching such as home-nursing classes. Thus, she may come to know and to appreciate the parents and neighbors and help them to recognize the very real interest of the school in them and in their welfare.

Through the health program in the school, the nurse contributes to the general health care of the school-age child. Through service planning sessions, case discussion, and referral, the nurse in the school keeps other health agencies informed as to the needs and the problems of school-age children and plans the school nursing program in such a way as to support the general community efforts on behalf of the school-age child. Data regarding nursing needs or health conditions found in the school are helpful to the generalized community health nurse in program planning, just as the activities of the school health nurse with respect to such community activities as vaccination for poliomyelitis contribute substantially to the total community effort.

In summary, the school must be seen as a powerful channel for reaching the public with important health information and guidance. It offers an opportunity not only to assure each child of the opportunity to maximize his learning experience free from unnecessary disease and accident, but also a chance to increase his ability to cope with health conditions that cannot be remedied and to prepare him for the important health decisions he must make immediately and later, when he reaches adulthood. The school also provides direct access to adults in the school environment, the home, and the community.

REFERENCES

1. Roberts, Mary: American Nursing: History and Interpretation. The Macmillan Company, New York, 1954, p. 84.
2. Facts About Nursing, (1967 ed.). American Nurses Association, New York, 1968, p. 15.
3. Statist. Bull. Metrop. Life Insur. Co., *48:*4, September, 1967.
4. School Health Personnel Utilization Project: Report on Phase 1. Medical and Health Research Association of New York City, New York, 1966, p. 3.
5. Functions and Qualifications for School Nurses. American Nurses Association, New York, 1966.
6. School Nursing. American Nurses Association, New York, 1965.
7. Bryan, Doris: Redirection of school nursing services in culturally deprived neighborhoods. Amer. J. Public Health, *57:*1164, July, 1967.
8. Cauffman, Joy, Peterson, E. L., and Emrich, J. A.: Medical care of school children: factors influencing outcome of referral from a school health program. Amer. J. Public Health, *57:*60, January, 1967.
9. Byrd, Oliver E.: School Health Administration. 4th ed., W. B. Saunders Company, Philadelphia, 1966, p. 388.
10. American Institute of Architects: Standards of School Lighting. Illuminating Engineering Society and National Council for School Nurse Construction, New York, 1962.
11. Forbes, Orcilla: The role and functions of the school nurse as perceived by 115 public school teachers from three selected counties. J. Sch. Health, *37:*101, February, 1967.

SUGGESTED READINGS

Brion, Helen H., Johnson, Margaret, and Bardin, Rhea: A day in the life of a school nurse teacher. Nurs. Outlook, *15:*58, August, 1967.
Brunswick, Ann F.: Health needs of adolescents: how the adolescent sees them. Amer. J. Public Health, *59:*1730, September, 1969.
Bryan, Doris, and Cook, Thelma: Redirection of school nursing services in a culturally deprived neighborhood. Amer. J. Public Health, *57:*1164, July, 1967.
Byrd, Oliver E.: School Health Administration. W. B. Saunders Company, Philadelphia, 1964.
Cauffman, Joy, G., Peterson, Eleanora, and Emrick, John: Medical care of school children: factors influencing outcome of referral from a school health program. Amer. J. Public Health, *57:*60, January, 1967.
Cromwell, Gertrude: The Nurse in the School Health Program. W. B. Saunders Company, Philadelphia, 1963.

DeChantal, Sister M. Jane: School nurse-teacher relationship on the elementary level. J. Sch. Health, *32:*81, March, 1962.

Dialogue on Adolescence. U.S. Department of Health, Education and Welfare. Children's Bureau Publication No. 442, U.S. Government Printing Office, Washington, D.C., 1967.

Dithridge, Eileen H.: Administration of school health services: a review. Nurs. Outlook, *14:*50, May, 1966.

Dunphy, Barbara A.: In defense of school nurses aides. Amer. J. Nurs., *66:*1338, June, 1966.

Forbes, Orcilla: The role and functions of the school nurse as perceived by 115 public school teachers from three selected counties. J. Sch. Health, *37:*101, February, 1967.

Fredlund, Delphie: The route to effective school nursing. Nurs. Outlook, *15:*24, August, 1967.

Gabrielson, Ira, Levin, Lowell, and Ellison, Margaret: Factors affecting school health follow up. Amer. J. Public Health, *57:*48, January, 1967.

Gendel, Evalyn S.: Effective interaction for school health. Amer. J. Public Health, *56:*2133, December, 1966.

Grout, Ruth: Health Teaching in Schools. 5th ed., W. B. Saunders Company, Philadelphia, 1968.

Guthrie, E. H., Schultz, C. S., and Davis, R. L.: Research needs and bottlenecks in school health. Amer. J. Public Health, *51:*1525, October, 1961.

Hammar, S. L., and Eddy, Jo Ann: Nursing Care of the Adolescent. Springer Publishing Co, Inc., New York, 1966.

Hoenig, Leah: A hearing program for school children. Amer. J. Nurs., *63:*85, May, 1963.

Llewellyn, Charles E., Persons, Elbert L., and Helmick, Caroline: The mental health program in a college health service. Ment. Hyg., *48:*93, January, 1964.

Mannerstedt, Gordon, and Spillane, Alice: Family doctor or school physician. J. Sch. Health, *32:*215, June, 1962.

McFadden, Grace M.: The part time nurse in the school, why and how. Nurs. Outlook, *12:*62, October, 1964.

Mental Health in the Schools. Association of State and Territorial Health Officers, Association of State and Territorial Mental Health Authorities, and Council of Chief State School Officers, Washington, D.C., 1966.

Miner, Jan: Wyoming school nurse. Amer. J. Nurs., *65:*95, September, 1965.

Obertuffer, Delbert, and Beyrer, Mary: School Health Education. Harper and Row, Publishers, New York, 1966.

Ojemann, Ralph H. (ed.): The School and the Treatment Facility in Preventive Psychiatry. University of Iowa Press, Iowa City, 1966.

Reading, Sadie: The blue and the gray. Nurs. Outlook, *10:*664, October, 1962.

Richie, Jeanne: School nursing: a generalized or a specialized service? Amer. J. Public Health, *51:*1251, September, 1961.

Rogers, K. D., and Reese, Grace: Health studies of presumably normal high school students, Part 2: Absence from school. Amer. J. Dis. Child., *108:*598, December, 1964.

Rosner, Lester J, Pitkin, Olive E., McFadden, Grace, Rosenbluth, Lucille, and O'Brien, Margaret: Better use of health professionals in New York City schools. Public Health Rep., *84:*729, August, 1969.

Salisbury, Arthur, and Berg, Robert B.: Health defects and need for treatment of adolescents in low income families. Public Health Rep., *84:*705, August, 1969.

School Health Program: An Outline for School and Community. U.S. Department of Health, Education and Welfare, Children's Bureau Publication No. 834, U.S. Government Printing Office, Washington, D.C., 1966.

School Home Partnership in Depressed Neighborhoods. U.S. Department of Health, Education and Welfare, Office of Education, U.S. Government Printing Office, Washington, D.C., 1964.

Smiley, Lyda M.: Health records for school children. Amer. J. Nurs., *60:*1256, September, 1960.

Stine, Oscar, Rider, Rowland V., and Sweeney, Eileen: School leaving due to pregnancy in an urban adolescent population. Amer. J. Public Health, *54:*1, January, 1964.

Stitt, Pauline, and Schultz, Carl S.: Five fold focus on child health. Nurs. Outlook, *15:*29, August, 1967.

Stobo, Elizabeth C.: Trends in the preparation and qualifications of the school nurse. Amer. J. Public Health, *59:*669, April, 1969.

Stramler, Mary: A tuberculosis detection program and the school nurse. J. Sch. Health, *34:*481, December, 1964.

Tipple, Dorothy: The school nurse as a counselor. Amer. J. Nurs., *63:*110, September, 1963.

Weber, Elmer W. (ed.): Health of the School Child. Charles C Thomas, Springfield, Illinois, 1964.

Wheatley, George, and Hallock, Grace: Health Observation of School Children. 3rd ed., McGraw-Hill Book Company, New York, 1965.

Wilcox, Elaine: Patient follow up: procedures, techniques, and devices for improvement. Amer. J. Public Health, *55:*1741, November, 1965.

Wilson, Charles C., (ed.): School Health Services, 2nd ed. A publication of the joint committee on health problems in education (National Education Association and American Medical Association). The National Education Association, Washington, D.C., 1964.

Yankauer, A. L., and Lawrence, R.: A study of the periodic school medical examination: methodology and initial findings. Amer. J. Public Health, *45:*71, January, 1955.

CHAPTER

21

The Community
Health Nurse in
the Occupational
Health Setting

The health of those who work is a vital public concern. There are over 80 million people in the work force in the United States; this figure includes all segments of the adult population — men and women, of low and high income, of urban and rural residence. Almost a third of their life is spent at work. They need — and they expect — a safe work environment that is conducive to good physical and mental health. Health insurance and health care are important fringe benefits. Furthermore, work in itself and the ability to stay at work are of deep importance to most adults: it is, for the head of the family, a symbol of his role as provider; for the professional worker, it is an outlet for his creative skills; and for the mother, it may be a chance to get more things for the children or to get away from the isolation of the home setting.

For employers, the health of the worker is inextricably linked with production; absence or inefficiency due to poor health may lead to expensive lags in production and affect many workers other than the one who is ill or injured. For the country, the achievement of full production is a necessary condition for improving the standard of living of the population. Therefore, the health of those who work is a pressing government concern as well.

Nursing has been an accepted component of industrial health services for a long time. The first industrial nurse in the United States, Miss Ada Stewart, was employed by the Vermont Marble Company in 1895. The work she did was largely visiting nursing and would probably be described today as "generalized public health nursing."

SOME CURRENT TRENDS AND PROBLEMS

Perhaps the most significant trend affecting occupational health is the broadening of the perceived mission of this service. Lavenne describes the trend in this way: "Industrial medicine . . . began with accidents in works and factories, went on to occupational diseases and their prevention, and now must concern itself more and more with questions of adaptation of work to man, and man's adaptation to his work."[1]

There has even been a new term coined to describe the process of achieving this mutual adaptation: *ergonomics,* the application of biologic and engineering sciences to achieve the best adjustment of man to his work, and to improve efficiency and well-being.[2]

As a result of this broadened concept, new approaches to worker health care are being developed and are using a variety of professional skills. The control of tractor accidents, for example, might be approached by the engineer through an analysis of the relationship of the tractor to the individual who runs it, the protection afforded by a rigid cab as compared to an open seat, the accessibility of the controls, and the stability of the equipment on rough terrain. Simultaneously, the epidemiologist might study the natural history of tractor accidents — when they happen, to whom, and in what kind of situation — in search of the causes or related factors. Such studies have shown, for example, that women and children are at greater risk when driving tractors than are adult males. The social scientist might study the human factors involved, such as the cultural or behavioral conditions that affect the occurrence of accidents. From these studies there may emerge a variety of approaches to accident control: a new design for tractors; regulations regarding manufacture and use; the development of a tractor safety education program involving schools, agricultural agencies, and manufacturers; or a method of reporting and analyzing tractor accidents in order to provide better control information.

A second trend affecting occupational health programs is the rapid extension of production technology. The picking of tomatoes is moving toward automated, rather than hand, processes. The capacity to produce tomatoes of uniform size, a necessary precursor to automated picking, is within sight. This changes the whole nature of the occupational health problem of the tomato harvester. Workers will need training in the handling and maintenance of equipment and in habits that will decrease accidents. The increased speed of harvesting will make even more difficult the problem of adequate housing and sanitation for workers present only a fraction of the year; it may even make the migrant crew obsolete. Similarly, explorations of space have created many problems of extreme noise, the need to adapt to weightless states, and the necessity for rigorous adherence to specified safety procedures. The nurse in occupational health must develop special knowledge of the science areas that are related to the work processes, and she must be constantly relearning the conditions of the work situation as they affect health.

A third trend affecting the occupational health program is the great extension of insurance coverage for the working population. Although compensation insurance, which provides benefits for work-related accident or illness, has long been common, more extensive general health (or more properly, illness) insurance is now prevalent. This provides greater coverage for nonindustrial health problems and may extend insurance coverage to the family of the worker.

Large industries are tending toward reasonably comprehensive in-plant care of employees, but the problem of providing care to the small plant is still largely unresolved. It is in this sphere that there may be the greatest potential for imaginative use of nursing personnel.

OBJECTIVES OF THE OCCUPATIONAL HEALTH PROGRAM

As a member of the occupational health-care group, the nurse shares in the implementation of the objectives of the occupational health program. These are:

1. To protect employees from health hazards arising from occupational processes or environment.
2. To assure that the job assignment of each worker is suited to his physical and mental capacity and his emotional make up.
3. To assure adequate care and rehabilitation for occupational injury and illness and for the nonoccupational conditions that are specified in the organization's policies.
4. To contribute to each worker's ability to cope with his own and his family's health needs.[3]

Brown's definition of occupational health nursing reflects this broad mandate: "Occupational health nursing is the application of nursing principles and procedures for the promotion, restoration, and maintenance of optimum health of employees at their places of employment."[4]

The primary difference between occupational health nursing and health care of the presumably well adult population who are not at work lies in the work setting and the demands it places on the worker. The ready access, which is provided by the work setting, to a large segment of the population makes occupational health care an exceedingly attractive channel for public health effort.

THE HEALTH PROBLEMS OF PEOPLE AT WORK

The health problems of people at work are of two types: those that characterize all adults of working age and those that are generated by the work environment or work processes.

Problems Brought to the Job

The mortality rates in the working population follow those of the general population; heart disease, cancer, stroke, and accidents are the leading causes of death. Upper respiratory infections play a major role in illness and cause interruption of work or decreased work efficiency. Emotional problems affect a large proportion of the working population. Other common problems of this age group include alcohol or drug abuse, venereal disease, poor living habits with respect to nutrition, and lack of rest and weight control that lead to stress, fatigue, or lowered resistance to disease.

These problems are of concern to the occupational health-care group because they result not only in hardship to the individual and his family but also in absenteeism, an inability to maintain satisfactory work performance, and a need for changes in work assignment.

From a public health point of view, this age group represents a major channel for early recognition and control of longterm illness, since it is during these years that the symptomless evidence of disease may first appear and that deleterious health practices have such a profound effect.

Within each work group there will be subgroups who bring particular problems to the job. The worker recruited from a very low income neighborhood may bring with him the problems characteristic of the poverty syndrome; women of childbearing age will bring the problems associated with pregnancy and child rearing; the executive may bring a stressful attitude deriving from the keen drive for success that so often characterizes this group.

Problems Generated by the Job

Job-induced health problems may arise from the use of toxic or irritating materials or from exposure to extremes of heat, cold, light, or noise. The work processes involved may make such exposure unavoidable, and the counteractive measures of wearing protective clothing or adopting an attitude of constant vigilance may in turn create a degree of stress.

Accident risk—varying from the major possibility of mine collapse to the minor probability of paper cuts—may also be associated with work conditions. Machines may be dangerous in themselves, and require constant care on the part of the worker.

Stress may also arise from highly competitive or monotonous work or work that does not permit the individual to make choices. Processes that make a man feel like a machine instead of a person and poor interpersonal relationships among workers also appear to have negative effects on worker morale and health.

Thus, in analyzing the work to be done, the nurse in occupational health must look both at the conditions affecting people in the age and sex group that is characteristic of a specific working population and at the culture and the social environment of the community as a whole. She must then look at the health implications of the work environment: the physical characteristics of the plant, the processes and the materials involved, and the interpersonal environment that prevails.

DEVELOPING THE NURSING PROGRAM IN AN OCCUPATIONAL HEALTH SETTING

Identification of Nursing Needs

As in any other setting, the nursing needs of the work population will represent the relationship between the health problems of the group; the degree to which they are able to cope with these problems; the services provided by other health workers; and the capacity of the occupational nursing staff in terms of time, skills, and authorization. The pattern developed will vary from plant to plant. The following construct represents typical needs in the occupational setting.

EMERGENCY CARE

Needs for emergency care will be present in some degree in all settings. However, there will be great differences in the nature of the accident risk. In a steel plant, for example, major accidents may be a primary concern; whereas in a bank, the accidents will be for the most part minor in nature. The need for emergency care of illness will also vary greatly. When the work force contains a significant complement of older workers, care for coronary attack or stroke may be required often enough to necessitate special preparation to deal with these problems expeditiously. When the work force is largely female and young, minor illnesses will more likely be the pattern. It is important to know the nature, as well as the extent, of the emergency care load in order to determine the degree to which the nurse or other professional health worker must plan to provide care and the extent to which reliance may be placed on first-aid personnel equipped with short training. It is important to know the kinds of accidents that are most common: for instance, whether most accidents are falls from high equipment, foreign objects in the eye due to failure to wear safety goggles, or dermatitis arising from the use of irritating substances. A careful review of accident and emergency records for the past year will tell the nurse much about what to expect in the way of needs for emergency care.

NON-EMERGENCY CARE

Needs for other than emergency nursing care of occupational or nonoccupational illness or injury include case finding, prevention, and care. Case finding needs are based on expected or possible incidence of specific conditions, which, in turn, are estimated on the basis of the incidence of these conditions in the general public in the age, sex, and racial groups represented in the industry and also on the basis of the conditions that might be anticipated as a result of the particular industrial processes used. Again, a review of a sampling of records of those receiving service during the previous year and an analysis of medical examination results will provide much information. The frequency and patterning of absences will also be a clue to illness patterns of the group.

It is harder to get a base for the estimation of emotional or health behavioral problems. The identification of such problems seems to be as much a factor of the interests and background of the nurse as of the particular population served. However, it is often possible to identify subgroups in the work population that might be expected to have higher than usual needs in this direction. Very young workers—messengers, wrappers, librarian aides, for example—are one such group. The nurse's own experience is probably the best index to the extent of this type of need.

HEALTH EDUCATION

Health counseling or health education needs are identified by the problems uncovered in screening or medical examination programs and by the expected health problems of analogous age and socioeconomic groups in the general population. Records of the previous year indicate the rate of positive findings in medical examinations or screening procedures and the counseling or educational services that were previously provided. However, in most instances, records will indicate a below-optimum level of recognition of such need. Direct observation, such as observation of food choices in the cafeteria, weight trends, or on-the-job behavior, may provide further clues.

The need for referral to other than nursing care, either in or out of the plant, may be estimated by reviewing a sample of records to determine whether or not referral would have been useful. Even readily available sources in the plant, such as a nutritionist or psychologist, may be inadequately used; and referral to community agencies or family physicians may be minimal. Again, past practice may or may not be a good index of the level of the need, since nurses vary widely in their sensitivity to referral needs.

PREVENTIVE CARE

The need for specific preventive measures may be estimated by comparing the actual recorded experience of the group against a list of desirable preventive measures for the age group involved. Desirable measures might include:
1. Medical examination: annually or biennially.
2. Immunization: recommended schedules may be secured from the medical director, from the local or state health department, or from a medical advisory panel.
3. Periodic screening: depending on medical advice, the age of the group, and the nature of the industry might include screening for specific occupational hazards such as toxic effects of materials used or contact dermatitis, vision and hearing tests, weight checks, cervical smears for detection of cancer, tuberculin testing or x-ray examination, tonometry for detection of glaucoma, tests for diabetes, blood pressure determination, and hemoglobin determination.

NEEDS OF THE ORGANIZATION

Support of general personnel and production measures of the firm may also require special nursing measures. If the industry is making a special effort to employ socially disadvantaged groups, for example, the nurse might be expected to develop a special intensive health counseling plan and to arrange her own program to reach these workers early and frequently. She might visit the homes in order to understand the problems this group faces in adapting to regular work or to identify and deal with family health or health-related problems that may be impeding an individual's work progress. A program of weight control and dietary reform for executives might be backed up by nursing action to secure the cooperation of the wives. She might encourage wives to use the service of the agricultural extension staff or of a gas or electric company in planning family fare consistent with the dietary plan for the head of the family. New recruits in a military setting might receive a little extra nursing attention or referral to volunteer sources of support as a tiding over measure until they accustom themselves to being away from their homes and families; some will never have had that experience before.

Interpretation of the firm's policies and of legal rights and obligations of employers and employees may sometimes be indicated to explain why certain procedures are necessary.

In the process of seeking out nursing needs, the nurse will be able to identify individuals and groups that are at special risk or who need more than the usual amount of nursing care or support. From this she will build the register of cases requiring intensive or continuing supervision.

Nursing Goals

Nursing goals should be explicit and time-related. Once the nursing needs are determined, it is possible to take a realistic look at what can reasonably be accomplished through nursing in a given time period. The nurse will then want to establish for her guidance a set of specific goals (or desired nursing outputs). These goals will, of course, be influenced by the company's philosophy of care. Thus she may want to set as a goal that 80 percent or 90 percent of pregnant workers will be under medical care within the first trimester, that the rate of eye accidents associated with failure to wear goggles will be reduced by x percent, that recommended immunizaton procedures will be offered to the entire working staff, and that 75 percent will accept these immunization procedures. Specific goals help lend direction to the nursing activities and provide a basis for evaluation and for interpretation of the service to nonhealth personnel.

Establishment of the Health-Care Relationship Network

Establishing the health-care relationship network in the industrial setting takes time and thought. Within the plant the nurse is working with new partners. The physician director upon whom she is accustomed to depend for many decisions may, in many instances, be there only on a part-time or an on-call basis. The safety engineer, the systems analyst, the personnel director, the shop steward (union representative), the foreman and various management officers, the industrial psychologist or vocational counselor, the rehabilitation worker, and the insurance company health consultant staff offer new kinds of support and in turn expect different things from the nurse than may have been expected by the usual community health working group. The nurse needs to know and to be known by each of these people; she must understand their relative contributions to employee health and establish ways of reporting to and planning with them that are both effective and efficient in the use of time.

At the same time, the health of the worker represents only one facet of the health care of the family, and the health care of the industrial community represents only one part of the total community health care. Relationships with hospitals, clinics, voluntary and official health and welfare agencies, educational facilities, and private family physicians must be established and maintained at an easy and productive level.

Person-to-person contact, careful information exchange, and case conferences will work here, as they do in the general community health program, to provide a good base for a congenial and effective working relationship.

Arrangement of Nursing Activities

It is axiomatic that nursing time is never adequate to do all that could be done. The occupational health nurse, like all others, will have to select among alternative actions in order to get the greatest results for the nursing time invested. A list of those individuals or groups with unusual need for nursing care will serve as a starting point in arranging activities.

Other basic considerations are to achieve visibility and coverage. Much of what the occupational health nurse is able to do results from a good understanding of her function by those who use nursing care or who are responsible for referring others for such care. Referral for nursing care is more likely to be pertinent if the nurse is known to workers and management groups. Getting around the plant may have a high priority, since it provides an opportunity to observe conditions that affect health and also makes the nurse a familiar figure to the work force. When there is more than one work shift or when the work force is scattered through several locations, the nurse will also want to be sure that she is available to all of the various groups that are entitled to use her services. This may affect the scheduling of conference time in order to reach those who change shifts in the early morning or the late afternoon. The arrangement and planning of nursing activities must also take account of the need to respect the integrity of the work flow. For example, pulling one member out of a production line for a conference on prenatal care may disarrange the work of several others in her unit. Arranging these activities in conjunction with the work supervisor will avoid such conflict.

Policies and Standing Orders

Policies and standing orders should be in writing and complete. Sometimes, especially in small plants, the nurse must work in the absence of an on-the-spot physician. It is important that she safeguard the patient and protect her own professional integrity by having clearly written policies and standing orders. Such statements, however, cannot be substituted, either professionally or legally, for the nurse's own professional judgment. There may be occasions when standing orders should not be followed: for example, if there is some indication of sensitivity to a common drug. However, well-written and frequently reviewed policies are an essential base for action. Written and signed standing orders are essential for the safety of the patient, and they also serve to interpret to others the limits of the nurse's authority with respect to dispensing drugs or to taking other action in the absence of an immediate medical diagnosis.

The Nurse's Role in Safety Provision

Safety is everybody's business in the occupational setting. In many instances, first-aid care is given by short-trained workers in the work unit. Much safety teaching is done on the spot by the foreman or the training officer as he introduces the new worker to the job or as he engages in a continuing reinforcement of the safety education program. One training officer stated that the habit of safety is caught as well as taught, pointing out the importance of having every one set a good example to others in safety practice.

The nurse may be responsible for the coordination of first-aid efforts and for maintaining first-aid supplies. Whether or not it is written into her job description, the nurse in occupational health must be constantly alert to breaks in the safety system and take her part in assuring as far as possible that accidents are prevented and that they are treated promptly and properly when they do occur.

The provisions of workman's compensation laws vary from state to state, but in general they provide for liability of the employer for certain medical and disability benefits to employees suffering industrial injuries. To be compensable, the injury must arise out of or in the course of employment. In general, the same benefits apply whether or not the injured person was negligent.

Some nursing time should be allowed to add to the knowledge of occupational health. Although few nurses in occupational health have had the opportunity to engage in rigorous research, virtually every one has a chance to add to knowledge of the health problems and health care of the working population. This may take the form of participating in epidemiologic investigations, such as tracing the factors associated with an outbreak of dermatitis; of evaluating different methods of providing care, such as involving the worker himself in health decisions as compared to keeping the majority of decisions in the hands of the health professionals; or of describing and analyzing absence patterns.

Health Records

Records play an especially significant role in occupational health services. They provide an official record that may protect the rights of the employee and of the employer, and they may serve as legal evidence regarding the circumstances surrounding a particular injury or illness. Since the nurse is often the first observer at the time of injury or illness, her record is particularly valuable.

The cumulative health record of the employee is important in understanding his health progress and in relating changes in his health to changes in the work situation. Since many adults do not visit a personal physician consistently, the well-kept occupational health record may provide the only reasonably comprehensive picture of an individual's health progress; as such, it could be an invaluable aid to his physician or to the hospital medical staff should he require intensive care.

The analysis of health records has already been mentioned as an excellent basis for establishing health needs, for planning health programs, for documenting the need for extra plant care facilities, and for evaluating the nursing and health services provided.

Health records should be considered to be confidential documents. When a health condition requires work adjustment, the condition and the limits it imposes may be interpreted by the physician in a written statement to management, but the record itself should be available only to qualified health personnel. Policies relating to the divulgence of health information should be clearly stated and rigorously followed. Sometimes this confidential health information takes the form of a record analysis of the reasons for the patterns of absence, the characteristics of an "absence prone" group, or of a record audit in which someone outside is requested to analyze the service provided as it relates to personnel needs.

Whatever the form, the nurse in in a good position to add to the knowledge about the needs for and processes of occupational health care. The nurse trained in community health is especially helpful in dealing with areas of health care as distinguished from care of disease or injury.

THE NURSE IN OCCUPATIONAL HEALTH MAY NEED SPECIAL PREPARATION

The nurse in the occupational setting faces practice problems somewhat different from those she would expect to find in other settings. She is much more "on her own." One recent study involving over 10,000 occupational health nurse respondents indicated that most nurses work without supervision: 40 percent of the respondents reported that they worked alone, and another 16 percent stated that they worked with other nurses but without a supervisor. Furthermore, only one fourth worked with a full-time physician, and nearly a third reported that they had no physician available on a regular basis; however, 95 percent had a physician at least on call.[5] Thus many nurses in the occupational setting will need more than the usual nursing preparation.

New and constantly changing methods of production and of manpower utilization create health and nursing needs of considerable complexity. The nurse in the occupational setting needs to be unusually aware of physiologic responses to the conditions of work, such as the effects of heat, cold, stress, and noise; she needs a sufficient grasp of biochemistry to recognize the potential or actual toxic effects of materials used in the particular occupational setting; she must be very familiar with emergency nursing; and she must understand the dynamics of production and of management in order to fit her program into the whole fabric of the productive effort.

The need for the nurse to make preliminary diagnostic decisions has already been noted. This, too, suggests the need for special preparation in relevant clinical fields. The administrative responsibilities of the occupational health nurse who works alone or without the structure of an organized occupational health program are also great; they may range from program development and budgeting to setting up first-aid stations or clinics. An analysis of the areas of knowledge or skills required in this field has recently been developed by a special committee of the American Nurses' Association and should be read by anyone contemplating employment in occupational nursing.[6] There is no doubt that formal post-baccalaureate education could make a significant contribution to the development of requisite competencies.

In her own development, as in so many other things, the occupational nurse must be on her own. Most large city and state health departments and some insurance carriers have nurse consultants who may be called upon for help. When community nursing agencies supply part-time nursing to industry, they are likely to have a nurse knowledgeable in the occupational health field to direct the work and to provide leadership to others engaged in the occupational health program. Professional associations in nursing and in public health, including the American Association of Industrial Nurses, will have publications and programs. Experts in other fields within the industry may make willing and valuable consultants. Each nurse must seek out and use these sources for professional support.

SPECIAL WORK GROUPS

Every work group has its own special problems, but there are some work groups in which the risks are sufficiently unique to warrant special discussion.

Farm Workers

In 1964 about 6.8 million people worked on farms.[7] The special conditions imposed by their work creates health needs that involve nursing. One special hazard faced by farm workers is that of accident. Because of the distance of the farm from centers of population and the shortage of skilled workers, the farmer is forced to do many things that, in the urban environment, would be undertaken by specialists. He is, at once, electrician, carpenter, mechanic, operator of large equipment, animal keeper, and manager. Although a small number of farmers have had specific training and might be classified as professional or scientific farmers, for the most part training has been a family or self-initiated process. Even those who have degrees in agriculture may have had little preparation for the many technical things they must do. Because farming is a family occupation, women and children may be temporary members of the work force. They may, for example, drive tractors or handle other large equipment at peak periods of the farm cycle. Thus the danger of accident is higher on farms than in other settings.

The farm worker is also exposed to dusts, pollens, and to a variety of chemicals that may have harmful health effects, some of which are cumulative. Insecticides, rodenticides, and pesticides are examples of such materials.

Another hazard faced by the farm worker is exposure to diseases of animals that may be transmissible to man: for instance, anthrax, rabies, or tularemia.

Perhaps as much a problem as any of these exposures to harm is the inaccessibility of health care. The number of hospitals available to farm residents has been greatly increased through federal support for construction and, to a limited degree, for operation of rural hospitals, but the distance involved often leads to sparing use of these facilities.

The number of physicians available is less than in urban centers, and the age of the physicians that are available tends to be higher. The result may be that care is delayed or that home remedies are used, especially during busy seasons. The fatalism that seems to characterize the farm group may also contribute to a failure to deal with disease until it is well advanced or severely incapacitating.

Migrant Workers

The health problems of migrant agricultural workers are sufficiently different to require special programs. More than 700 of the nation's 3,100 counties depend on farm workers from outside the local area during the peak harvest season.[8] This work is provided largely by migrant laborers who travel in defined "streams" or routes as they move from one harvest area to the next. (See Figure 14.) It is estimated that approximately three quarters of a million people move in the migrant stream each year.[9]

The migrant laborer travels with his family. He is recruited and supervised by a "crew leader," who deals with the farm owners and serves as a leader of the work group. It is the crew leader who owns much of the equipment, such as the buses and trucks in which the group travels. He is the camp manager; he provides food and the transportation from the campsite to the fields; he allocates the work; and he serves as a banker and as an intermediary with the employer and with the communities to which the migrants travel.

The agricultural migrant population is poor and, for the most part, unskilled. Many are separated from the mainstream of the communities they serve by language barriers or by cultural patterns. Most have little formal education.

The migrant's record for health is poor. In 1964, maternal deaths among the migrant population were 4.4 per 10,000 live births, compared to 3.5 in the general population; infant deaths were 30.6 per 1000 live births, compared to the national figure of 24.8; tuberculosis mortality

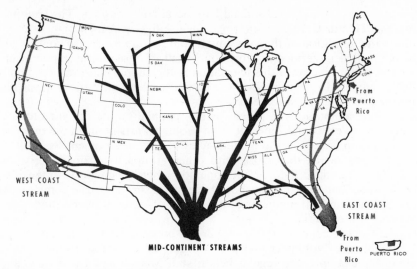

FIGURE 14.   Travel patterns of seasonal migratory agricultural workers. (From *Migrant Health Program Current Operations and Additional Needs.* U.S. Department of Health, Education and Welfare, U.S. Government Printing Office, Washington, D. C., December, 1967.)

was 26 per 100,000 population, compared to 10 per 100,000 of the general population. Mortality from accidents was also high: 156 per 100,000 population, compared with 54 per 100,000 for the general population.[10]

The problems that the migrants bring with them are aggravated by the conditions of the work itself. For the most part, work is on a piecework basis, and pay is determined by the amount each one harvests. This tends to encourage long hours; the traditional farmer's day of "can't see to can't see" often prevails. It also encourages children's participation in the labor; children over 9 years of age are generally included in the work in the fields.

Because the work requires a large number of workers for a very short period of time, housing is apt to be isolated from the general community and minimal in construction and equipment. Crowded conditions prevail, and facilities for cooking are often primitive. Local and state regulations do require specific provisions for sanitation, but these laws vary greatly.

Often migrant workers find they are not socially welcome in the communities they serve; they may be considered "wild" or "different." Residence requirements may bar them from health or welfare services. Their frequent moves make it extremely difficult to maintain continuity of care.

The federal government has long been concerned about the plight of the migrant worker, and the Migrant Health Act of 1962 and the amendments to this act greatly expanded federal activity in this area. The goal of this legislation is to raise the level of the health services provided to migrants to the level of those provided to the general population. Direct services may be sponsored by federal funds; or, more commonly, state programs are partially subsidized by federal contributions. The Comprehensive Health Care Act and many legislative actions designed to improve the condition of the very low income group have also contributed to intensified government efforts on behalf of agricultural migrant families. A potent factor in this legislation is the support afforded for family health clinics. In many areas these clinics are held after the working day in order to reach all who need help.

Nursing adaptations required for this population are designed to deal with the poverty syndrome and with problems arising from the mobility of the group and from the inadequacies of the environment.

The approaches that work with other groups living in poverty are equally pertinent to the migrant population (see Chapter 13). Intensified care, "reaching out," taking special care to assure that true communication exists, and strengthening the family's sense of worth and competence are essential.

Because the needs of this group are so great, most agencies find that a combination of volunteer and paid workers are required. In one area in Ohio, for example, the regular health staff was supplemented by volunteer groups who recorded stories and songs in Spanish for a Spanish-American group of children left in camp while their parents were in the field; besides providing entertainment, this activity helped to strengthen the migrant workers' sense of identity with a specific culture.[11] Sometimes lawyers serve as volunteers, since migrants often need help in understanding their legal rights and obligations. Literacy and homemaking classes may be organized to supplement the health services. The problems of sanitation and nutrition are unusually great for this group. Even such simple things as handwashing may be hard to arrange. Parents will need considerable help in adapting the family diet to foods that can be prepared with the limited equipment and time available. Such changes of habit are not easily accomplished. Powdered milk, for example, is inexpensive, is usable when refrigeration is limited, and can be easily transported. However, for families who are unaccustomed to its use, the taste may be unacceptable. Also, the need for milk may not even be recognized.

Child care represents another grave concern. Children are often inadequately protected against communicable disease, are fed under unsanitary conditions, and are inadequately supervised when the parents are at work in the fields. Day care centers are badly needed, but they are difficult to organize. In some communities, volunteers acting under the aegis of local social agencies or the VISTA program have provided day care services for children of migrant workers.

Family planning is another service that frequently misses the migrant group. Their isolation and transitory stay in the community make it difficult to locate sources for family planning and to secure the necessary follow-up care.

Although the diseases from which the agricultural migrant population suffers will probably parallel those of others who are poor and in farm work, communications problems may increase the difficulty of identifying problems and providing care. The short stay and often the cultural and language barriers of the migrant preclude the slow development of trust and the easy interchange that grows with familiarity and extended contact over a long period of time. Thus the nurse has to seek more diligently for possible problems. There are, for example, great differences among camps in the number of venereal disease cases reported. There is little reason to suppose that there is an actual difference in the occurrence of these diseases; rather, the difference in rate is more likely the result of failure to report symptoms that require care.

The need for emotional support and motivation toward health care is also extremely high in this group. The migrant life is so rigorous that the need for other than frankly curative health care may have a low priority. The social isolation in, and sometimes frank rejection by, the communities in which they work can only be emotionally damaging. With such pressures, health care requires an exceptional effort on the part of all of the health professional group.

With the migrant population, the need to provide for continuity of care is paramount. Since the stream transcends state lines and covers many communities in the course of the year, continuity is difficult to achieve. The nurse working with the migrant group should familiarize herself with the stations along the stream and establish communication with the health organizations and personnel who will care for the family later. Referral forms and procedures may need to be developed. The United States Public Health Service encourages the use of a wallet-sized personal history to be carried by each person as he moves along the migrant stream. This is a valuable adjunct to agency records. If, in addition, each nurse takes the responsibility for informing the health organization at the next station on the stream about those who require special care and, as far as possible, refers the family needing care to a particular person, continuity of care is more likely to be achieved.

It would be an error, however, to assume that the failure of families to seek or to secure care in the new community is due entirely to mechanical failure of the referral system. All too often the worker and his family do not truly understand the nature of their problem or are not persuaded of its importance or of the need for care. Careful teaching, demonstrated concern on the part of health personnel, and the use of interpreters to assure that the message is understood are essential to secure the motivation required for the family to seek follow-up care.

The Small Industry

The small industry may take special planning. Approximately two thirds of all employees work in industries that are too small to maintain their own preventive health services.[12] For some of these, part-time nursing service is usually provided by arrangement with a local nursing organization. Hours and conditions of the service are agreed upon by the agency and the industry, and contracts are drawn up. The hours may vary, but one typical agency assigns six hours of nursing time and one hour of physician time for each 100 employees.[13] In these industries the nurse is usually the only immediately available representative of health services and the first source of health care. She will work with a designated physician, physician panel, or clinic from whom she will secure standing orders and policies relative to referral for medical care. For many of the health education aspects of the work, she will be "on her own."

When such service is provided through an agency, there is usually one person with special preparation in occupational health nursing who serves in a supervisory and coordinating role and who either provides the service or works with the nurse that is actually visiting the plant and providing service. The nurse in this setting carries the same responsibilities that would characterize work in any other occupational health setting. She has the same responsibility for assuring that emergency care is available and safe, for promoting the general health of the workers, for protecting them against hazards in the environment, and for providing intensive care to those with special problems. Because she is the only health worker in the setting on a regular basis, and also because she may be only a part-time employee, it is especially important that the nurse in this type of industrial establishment make herself visible and take the time to familiarize herself thoroughly with the work force and with the work processes. Because of the absence of specialists in personnel, in safety, and in management, she will have more than the usual responsibility for initiating certain facets of the program or for proposing changes that will improve care. For example, a system for employee counseling and health education may need to be established from scratch, or a totally inadequate record system may have to be updated in order to underpin the day to day responsibilities of the nurse's job.

REFERENCES

1. Lavenne, F.: Down the mines: heat, dust and danger. World Health, March, 1969, p. 28.
2. Carpenter, David: Machines made to measure. World Health, March, 1969, p. 6.
3. These objectives have been adapted from the statement of objectives in the American Medical Association publication entitled Scope: Objectives and Functions of Occupational Health Programs. American Medical Association, Chicago, 1960, p. 2.
4. Brown, Mary Louise. *In* Functions, Standards and Qualifications for Occupational Health Nurses. American Nurses' Association, New York, 1960, p. 4.
5. Gray, Jean: Why define occupational health nursing? Nurs. Outlook, *15:*52, October, 1967.
6. Occupational Health Nursing Section. Selected Areas of Knowledge or Skill Basic to Effective Practice of Occupational Health Nursing. American Nurses' Association, New York, 1966.
7. Top, Franklin: The farmers health. *In* Porterfield, John (ed.): Community Health: Its Needs and Resources. Basic Books, Inc., Publishers, New York, 1966, p. 140.
8. Hospital Survey and Construction Act, Public Law 725.
9. Migrant Health Program. Current Operations and Additional Needs. U.S. Department of Health, Education and Welfare, U.S. Government Printing Office, Washington, D.C., December, 1967, p. 3.
10. Migrant Health Program. Current Operations and Additional Needs. *op. cit.,* p. 12.
11. Ohio's Health, *17:*1, May, 1967.
12. Part-Time Nursing in Industry. U.S. Department of Health, Education and Welfare, PHS Publication No. 1296, U.S. Government Printing Office, Washington, D.C., 1965.
13. Brown, M. L.: Occupational health problems in small employee groups. Arch. Environ. Health, *3:*79, 1961.

SUGGESTED READINGS

Bauer, Mary Lou, and Brown, Mary Louise: Occupational Health Nurses: An Initial Study. PHS Publication No. 1470, U.S. Government Printing Office, Washington, D.C., 1966.
Brown, Mary Louise: Nursing in occupational health. Public Health Rep., *79:*967, November, 1964.
Brown, Mary Louise: Occupational Health Nursing. Springer Publishing Co., Inc., New York, 1956.
Brown, Mary Louise: Occupational health problems in small employee groups. Arch. Environ. Health, *3:*79, July, 1961.
Cassel, John: The use of medical records: opportunity for epidemiological studies. J. Occup. Med., *5:*185, April, 1963.
Chapman, A. L.: Migrant health project in Pennsylvania, 1963. Public Health Rep., *79:*561, July, 1964.
Chladek, Marian: Nursing service for migrant workers. Amer. J. Nurs., *65:*62, June, 1965.
Delgado, G., Brumback, C. L., and Deaver, M. B.: Eating patterns among migrant families. Public Health Rep., *76:*349, April, 1961.
Farrell, Margaret: Hospital employees get sick too. Amer. J. Nurs., *60:*1622, November, 1960.
Functions and Qualifications for an Occupational Health Nurse in a One Nurse Service. American Nurses' Association, New York, 1968.
Functions, Standards and Qualifications for Occupational Health Nurses. American Nurses' Association, Occupational Health Nurses Section, New York, 1960.
Harper, George L.: A comprehensive care program for migrant farmworkers. Public Health Rep., *84:*690, August, 1969.
Health Services and the Migrant. Currents in Public Health, Ross Laboratories, Columbus, Ohio, vol. 3, no. 2, February, 1963.
Hornung, Gertrude: The nursing diagnosis—an exercise in judgment. Nurs., Outlook, *4:*29, January, 1956.
Johnston, H. L., and Lindsay, J. R.: Meeting the health needs of the migrant worker. Hospitals, *39:*78, July, 1965.
Koch, William: Dignity of Their Own. Friendship Press, New York, 1966.
The Legal Scope of Industrial Nursing Practice. American Medical Association, Chicago, 1959.
Levinson, Harry: Emotional Health In the World of Work. Harper and Row, Publishers, New York, 1964.
Lindsay, J. Robert, and Johnston, Helen L.: The health of the migrant worker. J. Occup. Med., *8:*27, January, 1966.
McKiever, Margaret: The health of women who work. PHS Publication No. 1314, U.S. Government Printing Office, Washington, D.C., 1965.
McKiever, Margaret, and Siegel, Gordon: Occupational Health Services for Employees: A Guide for State and Local Governments. PHS Publication No. 1041, U.S. Government Printing Office, Washington, D.C., 1963.
McKiever, Margaret: Trends in Employee Health Services. PHS Publication No. 1330, U.S. Government Printing Office, Washington, D.C., 1965.
Nursing Part Time in Industry. U.S. Department of Health, Education and Welfare, PHS Publication No. 1296 (prepared in cooperation with the National League for Nursing), U.S. Government Printing Office, Washington, D.C., 1965.
Piper, Doris, and Corrado, Vivien P.: Space age nursing. Int. Nurs. Rev., *15:*368, October, 1968.
Porter, E. R.: When cultures meet—mountain and urban. Nurs. Outlook, *11:*418, June, 1963.
Recommended job responsibilities: staff nurse. Amer. Ass. Industr. Nurses J., *8:*19, November, 1960.
The Role of the Nurse in Occupational Health Nursing. U.S. Department of Health, Education and Welfare, Public Health Service, National Center for Urban and Industrial Health, Cincinnati, Ohio.
Rural Migrants to Urban Centers. Currents in Public Health, Ross Laboratories, Columbus, Ohio, vol. 4 no. 3, March, 1964.
Scope, objectives and functions of occupational health programs. J.A.M.A., *174:*533,

October, 1960. (This information is also published as a pamphlet by the A.M.A., Council on Occupational Health, 1960.)

Selected Areas of Knowledge or Skill Basic to Effective Practice of Occupational Health Nursing. American Nurses' Association, Occupational Health Nursing Section, New York, 1966.

Shostack, A. B., and Gomberg, William, (eds.): Blue Collar World. Prentice-Hall, Inc., New Jersey, 1964.

Striegel, Bernadine: Correlated Activities in an Employee Health Program. A Guide for Management (Physician and the Nurse). Metropolitan Life Insurance Company, New York, 1962.

Top, Franklin: The farmer's health. *In* Porterfield, John (ed.): Community Health — Its Resources and Needs. Basic Books, Inc., Publishers, New York, 1966, p. 140.

Zintz, Miles: Education Across Cultures. William C. Brown Company, Publishers, Dubuque, 1963.

The Nursing Home: A Special Population

In the United States in 1964 there were an estimated 17,400 nursing homes serving approximately 554,000 patients.[1] The number of these institutions is growing. The increase in the aging population, the unavailability of family care due to increasing employment of women outside the home, and the public concern for the plight of the aging and the elderly sick that has resulted in greatly increased support for care have all conspired to create a sharp demand for care that is less sophisticated than that of the hospital and that is suited particularly to the needs of the patient whose problems are more social than medical.

The nursing home industry, having had few planning restraints, has grown haphazardly. For the most part these institutions have been proprietary — that is, run for profit — although there is a trend toward the incorporation of such facilities into government health systems.

Many nursing agencies carry some responsibility for service to nursing homes. In a 1962 survey of nursing agencies (including government, voluntary, and combined agencies), of 622 agencies responding, 50.7 percent reported some program for assistance to nursing homes.[2] The community health nurse should therefore expect to be concerned with this particular population group.

THE NURSING HOME IS AN INTEGRAL LINK IN THE HEALTH CARE SYSTEM

The nursing home is an institution for the provision of residential care to individuals who require medical or nursing services but who do not require the special equipment or intensive care ordinarily afforded by the hospital. Although the term is used very loosely, and studies may use different bases, the term "nursing home" does not usually include long-term care hospitals that provide intensive care or purely domiciliary institutions in which the residents are provided with board and room and in which health services are incidental to the main purpose of the institution.

Types of Nursing Homes

Nursing homes vary widely in size, in the type of patient they are prepared to receive, in the quality and sophistication of the care they provide, and in sources of support. However, they may be roughly grouped into three categories:

1. *The skilled nursing-care home,* in which residents receive a level of nursing care that requires professional nursing supervision. In this type of institution it is expected that there will be at least one registered nurse employed full time and that there will be licensed practical nurses for those times that the registered nurse is not immediately available.

2. *The personal-care-with-nursing home,* in which there may be a substantial number of residents who require minimal or intermittent nursing and personal care assistance. In such institutions there may be no registered nurse employed, and care may be provided by a combination of licensed practical nurses and aides. Of the 468 nursing homes accredited by the National Council for Accreditation of Nursing Homes in 1964, about half (237), representing 13,430 beds, fell into this category.[3]

3. *The personal care home,* in which the residents need assistance with daily living activities but do not require nursing care *per se,* except on the same basis as would be required with any population group of this age.

The provisions of the amendments to the Social Security Act provide for reimbursement of agencies defined as "extended care facilities." (Public Law 89-97, Sec. 1861j.) This term embraces the skilled nursing-care home and the rehabilitation centers. It does not include nursing homes in which skilled nursing care is not required.

Nursing-Home Care Is Incorporated into Ongoing Programs

Within a health agency, several program units will be concerned with nursing-home care. Even though each health department or visiting nurse association has its own system for program identification, the following are typical programs that have some interest or activity related to nursing homes.

1. Disease control programs. Since nursing homes are used predominantly by older members of the population, disease control activities directed toward chronic or infectious diseases (which represent a particular hazard to the elderly) would include programs for the nursing-home population as a vulnerable group.

2. Medical-care programs. The experience of some countries indicates that the use of facilities such as nursing homes can be very flexible, with constant reassessment of the desirability of nursing-home

care as an alternative to hospital care, home care, foster home care, psychiatric hospital care, or domiciliary group care. Thus all of the units in the medical-care program might be expected to have some relationship with nursing home facilities, and many units will provide some care to nursing-home residents.

3. Mental health programs. Many elderly residents of nursing homes have had psychiatric episodes, develop psychiatric problems in the course of nursing-home care, or have psychosocial problems requiring mental health approaches for their solution.

4. Geriatric health maintenance programs. Geriatric clinics for the presumably well elderly patient are growing in number and in the scope of services provided. Geriatric health maintenance programs are also very much interwoven with the work of the family physician, the visiting nurse association and other community health services.

5. Research programs concerned with growth and development (including the aging process) or with methods of delivery of health services.

CHARACTERISTICS OF THE NURSING HOME POPULATION

The nursing home population has special characteristics. The population of the nursing home with which the community health nurse will be concerned includes patients, staff, and visitors.

The Residents

The special characteristics of nursing home residents create special nursing problems. It is obviously impossible to generalize regarding the group in a particular nursing home, but recent studies and reports provide some common characteristics that are significant in planning for nursing care.

1. Nursing home residents are preponderantly elderly. In a study of 90 patients in skilled nursing homes, reported by Miller and coworkers, the average age of the residents was between 78 and 80 years; and in an earlier study by Solon and coworkers, 90 percent of those in proprietary homes were 65 years or older.[4, 5]

2. Most residents in nursing homes have one or more chronic illnesses of a nature that does not require intensive medical care. Psychiatric disorder, stroke, emphysema, cancer, heart disease, and glaucoma are often found.

3. General debility and sensory impairment are frequent. Patients complain of nervousness, weakness, dizziness, and fatigue. Hearing and sight are often impaired, and mental acuity may be reduced. Confusion, disorientation, and memory loss are common.

4. For the minority of patients whose mobility is sharply restricted or who are bedridden, there is risk of decubiti, muscle contracture, or other effects of prolonged bed rest. Often patients are admitted with these conditions, following inadequate home care.

5. Virtually all are dependent to some extent. Miller and coworkers

report that only 30 percent of those studied could care for themselves to a reasonable degree.[6]

6. For many, morale is low. Patients' feelings of hopelessness, lack of confidence, or fear of becoming more dependent may be exaggerated by the feeling that they have been rejected by their family or that the transfer from hospital to nursing home is "the end of the road." If physical dependence has come suddenly—as it does with the stroke patient—an acceptance of the limitations is hard to achieve, and negative or apathetic attitudes may develop. The problems the patient brings with him are intensified by the difficulties of adjustment to group living. It may be the patient's first experience in living away from his own home and family, in sharing a room or a closet, or in keeping his door open all of the time.

7. For most, rehabilitative measures can be expected to produce only modest increments to independent functioning.[7]

The Staff

The nursing home staff is largely short-trained, and their job commitment is often limited. The nursing home staff is part of the "case load" of the community health nurse more frequently than are the residents of the nursing home. It is to them that the nurse must direct her advice and teaching, and it is their efforts she is supplementing when direct patient care is provided by the community health agency.

The staff also represents a case load in the same way as does an industrial employee group: as a population, or a "patient," requiring care. Since many of the jobs are unskilled, the employee group will usually include workers recruited from the vulnerable low-income group. There will be working mothers and sick or pregnant workers who need educational or supportive nursing care. There may be special risks inherent in the work itself—such as exposure to infectious disease—that need attention.

In 1964 an estimated 299,900 persons were employed in nursing homes and related facilities, including geriatric hospitals; about 281,000 of these employees worked 15 or more hours a week.[8] The characteristics of this group were as follows:

1. Nonprofessional short-trained workers represented the vast majority of the nursing-home staff. In the survey, only 17,400 of the 281,000 full-time workers were registered nurses; 20,500 were licensed practical nurses. Nurse's aides, who represent the other employee group most directly concerned with patient care, numbered 120,000. Of the "other professional workers' employed, 20,700 of the 24,300 reported were administrators and, presumably, were only indirectly involved with patient care; the remaining 3600 represented such categories as physicians, dietitians, physical therapists, social workers, and speech therapists.

2. There appeared to be a high turnover rate among employees. Nearly 4 out of 10 employees had been in their current jobs for less than a year, and the median time on the present job was only 1.7 years. (It

should be noted, however, that this estimate did not take into account the time during which the home had been in operation.)

3. Few employees had any extensive training for their work. The study indicated that about 5 percent of the registered nurses and 6 percent of the licensed practical nurses had taken an accredited college or university sponsored course in nursing care of the aged; and about 5 percent of the registered nurses and 4 percent of the licensed practical nurses had taken such courses in mental or social problems of the aged or chronically ill.

Thus, the employee group may be described as largely short-trained workers who change jobs fairly frequently and who are for the most part without preparation, other than that received on the job, for the care they are providing.

The Visitors

The visiting population of the nursing home is a very real concern to the nursing-home administration and patient-care staff. It is important to the welfare of the patient that the physician who supervises the general medical care of patients be informed about the special needs of the home and about other community resources that might be used to extend the care the patient receives. It is important to patient morale not only that the family be concerned with his welfare, but also that they are skillful in showing this concern without upsetting the institution's plan for the patient's care; it is important that volunteers who contribute friendly services for the nursing home residents understand the rationale of care and also the need for community support in developing and controlling such care facilities. For the most part, the responsible nursing home administrator or the nurse who is directing and planning for patient care will provide such interpretation and, where necessary, training. In many cases, however, the community health nurse may be called upon to help when, for example, the physician responds to a patient's plea to be discharged to an incapable or resistive family or when some resources must be found to pay for the transportation of family members to the nursing home for visits with the patient. The community health nurse may also be able to suggest that nursing-home personnel engage more systematically in the education of the visiting group.

PROBLEMS OF THE NURSING HOME ENVIRONMENT

The nursing home represents a special population. It also represents a special environment with which this special population interacts and which influences in many ways the attitudes and the welfare of nursing-home residents. Even though the physical environment is of great importance to this accident-prone and infection-prone population, the psychosocial environment may have even greater impact. There is enormous variation in the environment of nursing homes, and each must be evaluated on its own merits.

The Institutional Physical Environment

Physical surroundings may be influenced by special patient needs or overexpansion. The particular needs of a nursing home population require adaptations in the physical environment that will reduce the environment's similarity to that of the patient's own home. The fact that many patients will be disoriented or confused means that the environment must provide for easy surveillance of patients, often at the expense of privacy. Limited mobility means that furniture must be designed with safety in mind, perhaps at the expense of a "homelike look." The severe economic strain imposed on most families by nursing-home care may mean that costs must be held to a minimum, and there will be an attendant sacrifice of space or privacy caused by a sharing of rooms or activity areas.

The escalating demand for nursing-home care has outstripped the available resources, and sometimes the community is faced with the decision of whether to maintain a nursing home that is frankly inadequate in its physical provisions or to have no facility at all. Outgrown hospitals, such as tuberculosis hospitals or obsolete general hospitals, may be converted into nursing homes. The facilities may be located at some distance from the main population center and may consequently be difficult for the family to visit. Often the remodeling that would be required to convert a facility into a nursing home is not done, and the result may be inaccessible activity areas or difficulty in maintaining adequate surveillance of patients. Marginal nursing home facilities are also frequent, especially in the proprietary home; an old residence may be converted to nursing home use, with makeshift arrangements and sometimes with minimal fire and accident protection. With such a rapidly expanding industry, there are apt to be fairly large numbers of relatively inexperienced administrators who may not be fully aware of the health and medical demands placed on the environment. Thus, attractively landscaped grounds may not be very useful to patients who spend most of their time in the much less attractive indoor environment.

The Unchallenging Psychosocial Environment

In discussing homes for the aged, Rosenblatt and Tavis use the term "total institution," which they define as a place in which individuals eat, sleep, play, and work in the same place under a single authority.[9] This description could certainly be applied to many nursing homes.

The psychosocial environment may therefore be monotonous and unchallenging and may impose severe limitations on the experience of the residents. Limitation of mobility for most means that their exposure is limited to the home itself and to the grounds. Visiting outside the institution is often not possible because of restrictions on the patient's mobility or because of sensory impairment or unavailability of family or volunteer personnel to provide for such experience. Personnel shortages are likely to preclude the use of staff for escort service.

In addition to the physical confinement that characterizes the world of the nursing-home patient, there is little excitement arising from changes in the group itself. For most, nursing home stay is measured in years instead of in days; and the same faces appear meal after meal, evening after evening. Furthermore, the homogeneity of the patient group with respect to age and disability permits even less variety in social association and may reinforce undesirable attitudes among the patient population.

The Highly Structured Operational Environment

The physical needs of nursing-home patients tend to be high, and the need to maintain supervision over activities is also great. As a result, in many instances a relatively rigid schedule and numerous regulations may be imposed in an effort to get the work done and to maintain some semblance of order. The reliance upon regulation and structure may be greater among nursing home administrators and staff who do not have any special preparation in the care of the aging patient or in situations where staff shortages make it difficult to meet the daily demands for care. There is no doubt that a highly structured environment makes life easier for the staff: if everyone must be in the dining room at 5 o'clock sharp, it is easier to serve the meals; and if bedtime is prescribed and early, demands on the staff are reduced. If the staff is not aware of the depersonalizing effects of regimentation and the contribution of depersonalization to ego diminishment and to unnecessary loss of function, they are obviously less likely to take the extra time and trouble to individualize care.

NURSING INTERVENTION AIMS AT CARE, COORDINATION, AND CONTROL

The community health nurse is concerned with three aspects of the nursing-home program: the improvement of the care afforded the patient, the optimum utilization of all available facilities for the benefit of the nursing home population, and the maintenance of required standards for the operation of nursing homes. These concerns are shared by many others: the nursing home staff, government organizations concerned with the licensure of and consultation to nursing homes, and the specialized staff in other health disciplines. The community health nurse's plan with respect to a particular nursing home is based not only upon an accurate assessment of the needs of the institution but also upon a firm understanding of the responsibilities and plans of others who are involved. The responsibility of the community health nurse may vary from providing very infrequent and incidental assistance in the care of patients to taking the major role in consultation and advisement of the nursing home staff. For example, there may be a nursing-home service team that includes professionals, such as a sanitarian, a physician, a nurse, and a dietitian, who visit nursing homes at regular intervals to assess the situation and to suggest improvements. This team may be in the agency in which the community health nurse works, or it may be in another agency, such as a department of welfare. It is important to know the purpose of such programs (whether they are related solely to licensure or primarily to consultation, for example) and the plans of these other workers in order to fit community health nursing in the nursing home into the total service pattern.

Improvement of Care

ASSESSMENT OF THE NURSING HOME SITUATION

As with care of a family or any other population group, a systematic assessment of the nursing home situation is an essential prelude to planning for nursing intervention. It is important to know the following:

1. The purpose of the nursing home: whether it is designed to provide skilled nursing care or essentially personal care with incidental nursing services or if it is designed to serve a special population group within the community.

2. The sponsorship and sources of support of the home: whether or not it is a government facility, a voluntary (nonprofit) venture, or a proprietary enterprise.

3. The characteristics of the patient population: age distribution, types of illness and degree of disability, cultural background, and closeness to or alienation from their families.

4. Provisions for medical supervision: whether there is a resident staff or an on call or part-time physician employed by the home; whether or not family physicians take major responsibility for medical supervision supplemented by some provision for emergency medical care and for medical advisement to those responsible for administration of the home.

5. The characteristics of the staff of the nursing home: numbers, preparation for their work, home and cultural background, stability of employment, and relationships among the various staff members. For the purposes of the community health nurse, volunteers participating in the care program are considered as staff.

6. The general pattern of administration of the home: whether or not there is a full-time professional administrator, a board of directors or advisory committee, or an organized administrative structure.

In some agencies there may be special record forms that are used in guiding and documenting services to nursing homes, and there may be a central filing facility where reports from various sources are combined so that there is the equivalent of a family record for each nursing home. In the absence of such aids to systematic assessment, the community health nurse will need to develop her own outline for collecting and analyzing data and her own scheme for securing information from others who are involved in advising the nursing home staff.

DEVELOPMENT OF SHARED GOALS

If the community health nurse is to be effective in improving the care of nursing home patients, there must be a sound foundation of goals that are shared by the nursing home staff, the patients and their families, and the community health personnel who provide services to the home. For the larger and more sophisticated nursing home, the establishment of nursing-care goals may be a familiar procedure, and the community health nurse can fit quickly into the process. For many homes, however, the staff will not be in the habit of thinking in these terms, or their concept of the scope of patient care may be exceedingly limited. In the latter case, more thought will need to be given to the process of interpreting the need for goals while avoiding methods of communication that make goal setting sound like an unrealistic or "academic" exercise.

The family and the patient must also participate in the development of goals for care and must understand and accept them. If the nursing home staff is trying to move the patient toward maximal self-help, whereas the family feels "everything possible should be done for the patient" and interprets the self-help regimen as patient neglect, the patient is apt to suffer.

Maximizing Functional Competence.   The goal of maximizing functional competence is central to the care of this age group. Many feel that the measure of an elderly person's health is the degree to which he is able to function in daily activities. There is a tendency on the part of those caring for aging people to overestimate the extent of disability.

Consequently, *an accurate assesment of the "can do" of the patient* is the first step toward this goal. The physician, physical therapist, nurse specialist, family, and community health nurse may all be involved in this estimation.

Once a realistic estimate is available, all of those in contact with the patient should *encourage the fullest possible use of the functional capacity* that the patient possesses. Sometimes habits of disuse are strong, and patient re-education is necessary to restore function. Obviously, overambitious plans for self-care or rehabilitation—measures that are beyond the capacity of the patient—will have a negative effect; but the likelihood of under-effort is usually much greater than is the likelihood of overeffort.

The proper use of functional aids helps to maximize function. The patient who is proficient in crutch walking or in negotiating a walker achieves a higher degree of mobility than would otherwise be possible. A properly functioning hearing aid and well-fitted glasses and dentures help the patient to do more for himself and make social contacts easier. It is important that sufficient time be taken to be sure that the patient understands how to use this equipment and to be sure that the equipment is in proper repair.

General health maintenance contributes to functional competence. Nutrition is an important aspect of health maintenance for the elderly. With increasing disability and limitation of activity, the amount of food needed may decline; however, the narrowing of life interests that takes place in the nursing home may lead to preoccupation with food, and mealtime may become the high point of the day. Food is important to the elderly patient, and eating activities are an important social event. One recurring problem is dentures. These should be checked to be sure they fit correctly and that dental restoration is adequate. The nutritionist may help deal with the problems of selection and preparation of foods that are acceptable to and suitable for older persons. Finding variety and allowing maximum choice in foods may encourage better eating habits.

Intellectual stimulation and orienting activities may help combat mental deterioration. The decline in mental ability is felt by many to be as much the effect of previous intellectual habits and of disuse as it is of physiologic change. Busse has pointed out that highly intelligent persons with good educational background show considerably less decline in mental ability than do those from low-income groups or those who have low academic achievement.[10] Opportunities for reading, for readers or records for the blind, for discussion groups, for participation in management of the nursing home, or for volunteer activities may help to keep patients alert and interested. Visits from younger people are sometimes effective in stimulating elderly patients and offer a valuable experience in voluntaryism for the young citizen.

For confused or disoriented patients, orientation can be promoted by providing clocks, newspapers, or calendars to help people to "place" themselves. Listening to a radio or watching television, especially news broadcasts, may also help.

Minimizing the Effects of Illness and Injury.   The goal of minimizing the effects of illness and injury takes an important place in the care of the nursing home population. In a recent study of over 600 nursing home patients in Massachusetts, 47 percent were found to require skilled nursing care.[11] When one considers the many additional patients whose needs are for personal care rather than for skilled nursing and the importance of such personal care in preventing decubiti or impairment of functional capacity, it becomes apparent that nursing care in the traditional sense is a very important component of the nursing-home program. The care required may be continuing or intermittent care for chronic illness or intermittent care for acute illnesses.

In the nursing home, as in the family home, much of the care required will be provided by nonprofessional personnel. The community health nurse may be requested to provide care in special instances, but for the most part her task will be to interpret and to teach to others the essentials of the care of the sick and elderly patient. The importance of such nursing measures as positioning, maintaining the electrolyte balance, and conscientious adherence to medication and exercise regimens may need to be interpreted to the staff. Even more important, perhaps, is the need for personalization and T.L.C. What Barbara Huber calls the "crime of immobilization" must be a constant concern.[12] Handling problems of incontinence are one example of an activity in which physical and social care assume equal importance.

The community health nurse may also be called upon to assist in the nursing diagnosis of a particular patient, to help decide what level of nursing care is required, and whether the staff of the home are indeed able to provide the care that is needed. In some instances, she may also suggest or arrange for other sources of nursing or related health care, such as the nurse specialist, nutritionist, or social worker, to supplement that which the nursing home can provide. In this setting it is particularly important to ascertain the source and adequacy of the medical supervision provided.

Controlling Infection and Accidental Injury. The goal of controlling infection and accidental injury involves both environment control and procedural surveillance. The physical environment should be safe for the elderly patient. Lighting should be adequate, stair railings present and sturdy, and equipment in good repair. A systematic check for accident hazards might be useful when there is no provision for regular inspection of the premises by an environmentalist.

Equally important are the care patterns and habits of residents and personnel. Handwashing facilities that are close to activity as well as to sleeping areas, habits of covering coughs and sneezes, the handling of dressings, and supervision of crutch walking are only a few examples of the many directions that must be taken in controlling accident and infections. There should be a specific plan for handling emergencies.

Screening programs may be afforded to nursing home residents. These programs will help identify possible sources of infection and also identify those at special risk because of sensory impairment or mental confusion. General health maintenance measures are also useful in reducing these special risks, in particular, unnecessary stress.

Improving Patient Motivation. The goal of improving patient motivation will contribute to all other aspects of patient care. The strength of the patient's will to achieve maximum function will depend upon his feeling that it is worthwhile to maintain function and that it is possible for him to do so.

The "want to" aspect of motivation grows out of attitudes, self-concept, social orientation, and the viability of support mechanisms. Attitudes may be brought to the nursing home by the patient, or they may grow as a result of group care. The patient who feels hopeless, discouraged and tired of trying so hard for small results, and desolate at the loss of a spouse will not be likely to progress unless these attitudes can be reversed. The patient who feels that he is "a worthless old man" for whom others can have but scant respect or that he is a nuisance to everybody is not likely to approach self-help activities with enthusiasm or confidence. The patient who feels alienated from those about him may be immobilized by this lack of social orientation. The patient who feels deserted by his family, ignored by his friends, and uncared for by the staff of the home is equally handicapped in taking positive steps on his own behalf.

Recognizing that for some, the very fact of admission to a nursing home represents a validation of these negative feelings, the community health nurse must join all others concerned with patient care in modifying these factors. The family may turn over the care of the patient to the institution too completely and fail to provide the letters, the visits, and the holiday remembrances that are such an important part of the patient's life. Visits that are frequent at first may tend to taper off. The community health nurse can do much to promote frequent contact between patient and family, pointing out to the family that the patient may be aware of the visit even though he may appear not to notice the visitor and that their support is an important ingredient in patient care.

If there is no family or if it is impossible for the family to fulfill its social obligation to the nursing-home resident, the community health nurse may help the staff of the home to locate family substitutes in the form of community volunteers who are willing to undertake such friendly services.

Sometimes symbolic activities help to reverse negative attitudes and feelings: the insistence that patients get up and dress when they are able to do so rather than go about in night clothes like invalids; participating in work activities as well as in recreational activities; or holding to a modicum of social graces at mealtimes are examples.

In other instances, an intensive, planned program for the remotivation of a particular patient may be indicated; all of those involved in care must attempt to bridge the gap between the patient and the world about him.

A "can't do" attitude on the part of the patient may arise from a previous unhappy, unsuccessful experience or from a lack of self-confidence. The patient who at one time tried to walk, fell, and was forced to wait some time for another person to help him get up may be forgiven if he is slow to try again. The patient who has had relatively inexpert care at home may have been persuaded by zealous relatives that he is incapable of doing anything for himself. The patient who is characteristically fearful and anxious will take longer to gain the confidence to try when he feels success is not certain. For many, the process of building self-confidence is a long one of slow progress that is punctuated by regression.

Staff attitudes or policies may affect patient motivation directly or indirectly. A nursing-home staff that has a cheerful, optimistic, and helping attitude; that makes clear that they believe patients are people worthy of dignity and respect and not merely childlike creatures; that can accept the inevitability of death and the right to a dignified exit from this world, and that takes the time to communicate with a patient whose speech is impaired inspires patients to do more for themselves. The staff that is willing to take the time for simple measures, such as a glass of warm milk or a backrub, to relieve discomfort and sleeplessness rather than to immediately offer a sleeping pill, tends to encourage more persistent patient effort.

Excessively rigid policies governing visiting, too great an emphasis upon an orderly appearance in the institution, or patterns of care that interfere with the development of close patient–care giver relationships (as, for example, when many individuals give fragments of care to the same individual in the course of a day) can also create conditions that may rob the patient of confidence in his capabilities.

Coordinated Use of Available Facilities

The coordination of care requires productive interagency and interpersonal relationships. As has been mentioned previously, the nursing home is only one link in the chain of services for the elderly incapacitated population. The community health nurse, because of her experience in working with a wide variety of community agencies, can be particularly helpful to the nursing-home administrator or staff in developing links between the nursing home and other sources of care. She may serve as an informal liaison agent, introducing or interpreting the home personnel to personnel in the community agency. The community health nurse may also assist the nursing home in locating and using informal community resources. She may, for example, suggest that the students in the "learn and earn" high school program or those in special classes might be suitable for certain nursing home jobs. She might suggest sources for volunteers to supplement the work of the paid staff of the home.

The community health nurse can also do much to strengthen the relationship between the family and the nursing home. She may encourage the family to accept the need for nursing care when it is indicated, explaining the effect of delay on the patient's ability to benefit from the nursing-home care and the importance of balancing the needs of the patient and those of the family. The danger of building up feelings of alienation and resentment by prolonged or inexpert home care and the negative effect of these feelings on the patient may also need to be emphasized. Specific anticipatory guidance with respect to handling their own feelings of inadequacy and guilt or the patient's overt or subtle recriminations also helps to support the care the nursing home gives.

At the same time, the nurse may interpret to the family that the nursing home is an adjunct to, not a substitute for, the supportive care that only the family can provide. The decision to seek nursing-home care does not free the family from the opportunity and the obligation to participate in the overall care of the incapacitated member.

The community health nurse, in collaboration with the physician, may help the family to select a nursing home, referring them to available resources for a preliminary visit and suggesting a list of observations they might make.[13] She can alert the family to look at the atmosphere, as well as at the tidiness of the home; at the activities provided for patients, as well as at the furniture and decor; at the availability of a telephone (hopefully with amplification for the hard of hearing) and rehabilitation equipment, as well as at a beautifully landscaped yard. She can alert them to the meaning of a full, as compared to a provisional, license and to the sources of information about community reimbursement for care. She can point out that impulsive placement in a home above the family's economic capability may be a real disservice to the patient who may later have to face transfer to another institution.

Maintenance of Standards

Control programs involve licensure, certification, and surveillance. Nursing homes are regulated by state provision for licensure or certification that are based on legislative requirements or on regulations deriving from legislation. The state agency responsible for implementing this legislative requirement is most often a department of health, but it may be another state unit such as a department of welfare or a special licensing branch. In addition, the federal government has set conditions for the participation of nursing homes in federally funded programs of Medicare.

Requirements for licensure and the provisions for checking and enforcing compliance with prescribed regulations differ greatly from state to state, and local communities may have regulations that amplify the state provisions.

The legislation that governs the operation of nursing homes usually includes a definition of a nursing home, the conditions for licensure, the penalties for noncompliance, and, often, criteria for approval of a nursing home.

It is important for the community health nurse serving nursing homes to familiarize herself with the specific provisions in her own state and locality and to clarify with her agency the role she is expected to fill in this service area. She will want to distinguish between licensure, which is a legal requirement for operating a nursing home, and accreditation, which is a voluntary activity. The major accrediting body for nursing homes is the Joint Commission on Accreditation of Hospitals, sponsored by the American College of Physicians, the American College of Surgeons, and the American Hospital Association. Accreditation is based on surveys made by experts in the field.

The nurse should familiarize herself with the conditions, criteria, or guides that exist. One example of such requirements is the statement developed by the Social Security Administration of the Department of Health, Education and Welfare regarding extended care facilities certified for reimbursement under the provisions of Medicare. An extended care facility, as defined in the basic legislation, is:

> An institution (or a distinct part of an institution) which has in effect a transfer arrangement ... with one or more hospitals. It is primarily engaged in providing to inpatients (a) skilled nursing and related care for patients who require medical or nursing care or (b) rehabilitation services for the rehabilitation of injured, disabled, or sick persons. (Public Law 87-89.)

About half of the skilled nursing homes in the country were participating in the Medicare program by June 1967 (one year after the program was launched), and by that time over 200,000 patients had been cared for in these institutions under Medicare provisions.[14] The conditions of participation that guide the states required to certify nursing homes as eligible for such participation specify that there be:
1. Written policies, developed by a group of professional personnel, governing the care provided.
2. A physician, registered professional nurse, or medical staff for carrying out these policies.
3. Round-the-clock nursing service with at least one full-time registered or licensed practical nurse.
4. Adequate records.
5. Adequate control of drugs.
6. Specified physical facilities in the plant.
7. A periodic "utilization review" to assure that patients are in the appropriate type of care facility.[15]

When nursing observations are to be used in determining eligibility for licensure or certification, it is important that they be supported by explicit documentation. For example, if the nurse feels nursing care is unsafe, the report should include an accurate and detailed account of precisely what was observed: the way the dressings were handled or the methods by which medications were dispensed, for example. Sometimes the agency provides forms for such notations.

When the nurse is not responsible for licensure or certification activities, she may still be called upon to provide some backstopping services. She may be asked, for example, to follow-up a survey team visit to see whether or not the nursing home operator understood and was able to comply with the recommendations made, or she may help the nursing-home staff to get ready for a survey visit and to understand the nature and intent of the licensure or certification process.

When or not she is engaged in any formal way with the licensure or certification, the community health nurse may visit the nursing homes in her community on a regular basis, maintaining some general surveillance over the adequacy of the nursing care provided and providing consultation as needed. Thus, much can be done to control the quality of care through persuasion and example rather than by the force of law.

These efforts of the community health nurse, being a blend of inspection and consultation, require very careful management of nurse-agency relationships. Such an interchange can be fruitful only when there is trust and confidence on both sides and when the nurse can appreciate and understand the problems of the nursing home staff while recognizing her obligation to protect the patient.

CAREFUL PLANNING IS ESSENTIAL

The nursing home offers an almost unlimited opportunity for the community health nurse. However, there are limits to the amount of help an institution can absorb at a given point in time, and there are also limits in the amount of community nursing time that can be allocated to this function. The frequently extensive help provided from other sources must be taken into account in planning what should be done by the community health nurse. For these reasons, planning for the nursing home aspects of the nursing program assumes considerable importance.

Explicit Goals

Goals for community nursing service should be clear. The community health nurse cannot expect to change the world of the nursing home in a few short visits, but she may hope to improve the personal care skills of nurse's aides or to increase the proportion of time spent by nursing home staff on rehabilitative or psychosocial problems as compared to physical care problems. Goals that are explicit, feasible, and acceptable to the nursing home establishment are guides, as well as goals, for action.

Selection of Approaches

Selecting among alternative approaches and methods will affect the time required for service and may affect the outcome of service. Among the many possible action alternatives are:

1. Providing direct care to selected nursing home patients or to their families.
2. Teaching, demonstrating, or participating in the supervision of the nursing home staff.
3. Consulting with nursing home personnel on nursing-care problems or arranging for consultative help.
4. Participating in inspection or licensure surveys.
5. Visiting the family of an institutionalized patient in order to provide support.
6. Arranging for or conducting group sessions with nursing home patients.
7. Assisting the nursing home supervisor or administrator with the development of record systems.
8. Conducting record surveys or special studies to determine the special needs of the nursing-home populations.
9. Arranging for multi-agency case conferences when indicated.
10. Visiting the home on a regular basis to check on problems and assist when necessary.
11. Interpreting health licensure regulations to the nursing-home staff and interpreting nursing-home problems to the health or licensing agency staff.
12. Arranging for, or participating in, screening programs for patients and employees.
13. Arranging for, and participating in, the implementation of immunization services (influenza vaccination, for example) or other preventive services.
14. Interpreting the needs of nursing homes and of nursing home patients to the public.
15. Locating special resources and, when necessary, serving as a liaison for such resources. Examples of special resources are physical therapist or occupational therapist services; special consultation in geriatric, psychiatric, or tuberculosis nursing; friendly visitor services; casework or welfare services; hospital personnel familiar with reactions of drugs that have been prescribed for nursing-home patients.
16. Keeping the nursing home staff informed of short courses or other educational opportunities.
17. Explaining special diets to the nursing home cook.

Here, as in any nursing venture, the objective is to pick the content and the approach that are most acceptable to the recipient of the service, that are the least time-consuming for the results likely to be obtained, and that are best suited to the particular problem.

Accurate and Complete Recording Keeps the Plan on Course

The nursing home, like the family, is a unit of service. As such, it is important that there be a precise statement of the condition of the "patient," the reaction to this condition, the nursing problems engendered by the situation, the reaction of the recipient to the care provided, and the observed outcomes of care.

The record of the nursing home focuses on the nursing home as an operating entity—as a population group functioning in a special environment. It is distinct from the records of individual patients who constitute the nursing home group or for whom the community health nurse has some special responsibility. The record might include:

1. An account of the characteristics of the nursing home patient population, their illnesses and impairments, their patterns of interaction with each other and with the staff, and their response to the environment of the nursing home.
2. A description of the nursing home staff, including characteristics and patterns of interaction.
3. An analytical statement of the problems in the nursing home environment that suggest a need for nursing intervention; this statement should include the staff's, as well as the nurse's, estimation of the problem.
4. A statement of goals for a specified period of time.
5. A statement of the nursing action taken and the results of such action.
6. An estimate of the effectiveness of the service provided; specific outcomes should be quoted wherever possible.

THE ULTIMATE CRITERION OF SUCCESS IS THE CARE AND SAFETY OF THE PATIENT

There will be many measures of success in the nursing home service program. Some indirect measures of success include an increased interest in learning about nursing care of the aged on the part of the nursing home staff; more frequent reference to psychosocial, as compared to physical, problems of patients in records and in case conferences; more effective nursing-care procedures; and more inclusive patient-care records. However, the ultimate criterion must be the care of the patient in the comprehensive sense. Careful collection of baseline data on patient and staff behavior will provide the basis for notation of change. The proportion of patients that is up and dressed during the day, the proportion engaged in some form of recreational or work therapy, and the proportion that is able to maintain a close relationship with their families may constitute helpful measures of success. Evidence of good physical maintenance of patients—provision for support of limbs, frequency of changing the patient's position in bed, presence or absence of decubiti—are further indices of the quality of care provided.

The community health nurse may also want to look for evidences of her own acceptability to the nursing home staff. The degree to which discussions of problems are initiated by the staff, the kinds of questions that are asked, the persistence shown in questions, and the following of suggestions designed to increase compliance to standards or to improve their own performance are examples of such indices.

Working with nursing homes does not require any esoteric information or unusual abilities on the part of the community health nurse. Much of the help provided the nursing home staff parallels that offered in the family situation. Yet, working with nursing homes does offer a special satisfaction, since the quality of nursing provided to residents of these institutions is such a potent contribution to patient welfare.

There have been many horror stories about the inadequacies and the "inhumanity" of nursing homes, and there has perhaps been too little mention of the great strides being made in turning nursing homes into places where the elderly and the incapacitated can find a safe haven and the challenge and the support to live life fully and in dignity. In this renaissance of concern for those whose need is great but whose potential for improvement or for increased productivity is small, the community health nurse can play a responsible and challenging role.

REFERENCES

1. Employees in Nursing and Personal Care Homes. U.S. Department of Health, Education and Welfare, Social Security Administration, U.S. Government Printing Office, Washington, D.C., 1967, p. 3.
2. Public health nursing services in nursing homes. Nurs. Outlook, 10:687, October, 1962.
3. Miller, M. B., et al.: Nursing in a skilled nursing home. Amer. J. Nurs., 66:321, February, 1966.
4. Ibid.
5. Solon, J., et. al.: Nursing Homes: Their Patients and Their Care. U.S. Government Printing Office, Washington, D.C., 1957.
6. Miller, et al.: loc. cit.
7. Kolman, H. H.: An experiment in rehabilitation of nursing home patients. Public Health Rep., 77:366, April, 1962.
8. Employees in Nursing and Personal Care Homes. May-June 1964. U.S. Department of Health, Education and Welfare, Center for Health Statistics, U.S. Government Printing Office, Washington, D.C., 1967.
9. Rosenblatt, D., and Tavis, I.: The home for the aged: theory and practice. Gerontologist, 6:165, September, 1966.
10. Busse, E. W. M.: The early detection of aging. Bull. N. Y. Acad. Med., 41:1090, 1966.
11. Kelliher, Rita P., and Shaughnessy, Mary E.: Fact Finding Survey of Massachusetts Nursing Homes. Boston College School of Nursing, Boston, 1963, p. 279.
12. Huber, Barbara: I chose to serve in a nursing home. Ohio's Health, 17:10, October, 1965.
13. Larson, L. G.: How to select a nursing home. Amer. J. Nurs., 69:34, May, 1969.
14. Medicare Newsletter. Social Security Administration, Washington, D.C., June 16, 1967, p. 3.
15. Conditions of Participation for Extended Care Facilities. U.S. Department of Health, Education and Welfare, Social Security Administration, U.S. Government Printing Office, Washington, D.C., 1966.

SUGGESTED READINGS

Amburghy, P. T.: Environmental aids for the aged patient. Amer. J. Nurs., 66:2017, September, 1966.

Anderson, W. F.: Practical Management of the Elderly. F. A. Davis Co., Philadelphia, 1967.

Baltz, F., and Reardon, R. A.: Medicare and nursing homes. Nurs. Outlook, 14:55, June, 1966.

Characteristics of Nursing Homes and Related Facilities. U.S. Department of Health, Education and Welfare, PHS Publication No. 930, U.S. Government Printing Office, Washington, D.C., 1963.

Cowdry, E. V.: The Care of the Geriatric Patient. 3rd ed., The C. V. Mosby Co., St. Louis, 1968.

Cumming, Elaine, and Henry, W. E.: Growing Old: The Process of Disengagement. Basic Books, Inc., Publishers, New York, 1961.

Federal Aid for Nursing Homes. U.S. Department of Health, Education and Welfare, U.S. Government Printing Office, Washington, D.C., 1963.

Framm, Erick: Psychological problems of aging. Journal of Social Rehabilitation, 32:10, September-October, 1966.

Kelman, Howard R.: An experiment in the rehabilitation of nursing home patients. Public Health Rep., 77:356, April, 1962.

Kemp, R.: Diagnosis of old age. Lancet, 2:515, September, 1962.

Larson, Laura G.: How to select a nursing home. Amer. J. Nurs., 69:1034, May, 1969.

Levy, S.: Planning for nursing homes. Nurs. Outlook, 15:46, November, 1967.

Linn, M. W.: Who goes to nursing homes? J. Amer. Geriat. Soc., 14:647, June, 1966.

Miller, Michael B., Keler, D., Liebel, Edward, and Meirowitz, I.: Nursing in a skilled nursing home. Amer. J. Nurs., 66:321, February, 1966.

Mitchell, D. L., and Goldfarb, A.: Psychological needs of aged patients at home. Amer. J. Public Health, 56:1716, October, 1966.

Moody, Mary L.: Another "family" for the public health nurse. Nurs. Outlook, 13:46, January, 1965.

Moss, Bertram, and Kent, Fraser: Caring for the Aged. Doubleday and Company, Inc., New York, 1966.

The Nation and Its Older People. Report of the World Health Conference on Aging. U.S. Department of Health, Education and Welfare, U.S. Government Printing Office, Washington, D.C., 1961.

Newton, Kathleen, and Anderson, Helen: Geriatric Nursing. 4th ed., The C. V. Mosby Co., St. Louis, 1966.

Nursing Care of the Aged: An Annotated Bibliography for Nurses. U.S. Department of Health, Education and Welfare, PHS Publication No. 1603, U.S. Government Printing Office, Washington, D.C., 1967.

Nursing Home Standards Guide. U.S. Department of Health, Education and Welfare, PHS Publication No. 827, U.S. Government Printing Office, Washington, D.C., 1963.

Nursing Home Fact Book. American Nursing Home Association. Washington, D.C., 1969.

Portraits in Community Health, Aging Center in Sinai Hospital. U.S. Division of Chronic Diseases, PHS Publication, 1965, p. 1344-2.

Positive Health of Older People. National Health Council, New York, 1960.

Preston, Florence: Improving county home care in Wisconsin. Amer. J. Nurs., 65:85, September, 1965.

Psychiatry and the Aged: An Introductory Approach. Group for the Advancement of Psychiatry, New York, 1965.

Public health nursing services in nursing homes. Nurs. Outlook, 10:687, October, 1962.

Rostow, Irving: Social Integration of the Aged. The Free Press, New York, 1967.

Shaughnessy, Mary E.: Nursing in nursing homes. Whose responsibility? Nurs. Clin. N. Amer., 1:399, September, 1966.

Shock, Nathan: Public health and the aging population. Public Health Rep., 76:1023, November, 1961.

Smith, Emily: Services for the aged in housing projects and day centers. Amer. J. Nurs., 65:72, December, 1965.

The Social Components of Care. American Association of Homes for the Aging, New York, 1966.

Solon, Jerry, Roberts, Dean, Krueger, Dean, and Baney, Anna: Nursing Homes: Their Patients and Their Care. Public Health Monograph No. 46, U.S. Government Printing Office, Washington, D.C., 1957.

Taylor, Josephine, and Gaitz, Charles: Obstacles encountered in the rehabilitation of geriatric patients. Nurs. Forum, 8:64, 1961.

Tibbitts, Clark: A Handbook of Social Gerontology. University of Chicago Press, Chicago, 1960.

Whitehouse, F. A.: Stroke: some psycho-social problems it causes. Amer. J. Nurs., 63:81, October, 1963.

The Community Health Nurse in the Early Discovery of Disease and Abnormality

The community health nurse's traditional responsibility for "case finding" has assumed a new look with the dramatic extension of, and the methodological advances in, screening and survey methods for early detection of disease. Increasing concern not only with disease entities but also with health conditions or behavior that are considered likely to result in disease or lowered vitality, has broadened the scope of services to the presumably well population. The standardization or automation of many diagnostic or screening measures has produced a vastly more sophisticated approach to early identification of disease or proneness to disease.

EARLY DETECTION OF DISEASE

The early detection of disease has assumed increasing importance both in private medical practice and in community health programs; it has, in fact, become a basic health service. This undoubtedly reflects the more hopeful and aggressive approach to preventing or moderating the effects of illness, especially longterm illness.

Major Approaches to Detection

SCREENING

Screening was defined by the Commission on Chronic Illness in 1951 as "the presumptive identification of unrecognized disease or defect by the application of tests, examinations or other procedures which can be applied rapidly. Screening sorts out apparently well persons who probably do have disease from those who probably do not."[1] It should be noted that screening does not include diagnosis; rather, screening identifies those who need more definitive study.

Screening is a valuable measure in that it can reach large numbers of people at a low cost and, for the most part, does not demand the services of the already scarce physician. In some cases, as with the irrigation smear for detection of cancer of the cervix, the patient takes the responsibility for securing the specimen and for submitting it for analysis.

Screening measures may be directed toward a single disease or health condition, such as tuberculosis or food intake; or it may be *multi-phasic* — that is, directed toward several diseases or health conditions. The American Public Health Association has endorsed the use of multiphasic screening as part of community health programs and has emphasized its particular value in the detection of chronic illness and its usefulness as a practical supplement to the more complete periodic medical examination, which, at present, reaches only a small proportion of the population.[2]

Screening measures may be directed toward the population as a whole (mass screening), or they may be aimed at selected groups within the population. Tuberculosis screening, for example, may be primarily directed toward low-income groups or other groups at special risk; screening for cervical cancer is directed toward women in the age group 25 years and over; and vision and auditory screening may be directed at preschool and school-age children.

MEDICAL EXAMINATION

The medical examination (checkup) is usually accompanied by laboratory or other technical diagnostic procedures and, increasingly, is given along with health counseling by the physician, nurse, or other designated associate, such as a social worker or nutritionist. This procedure offers a more comprehensive health assessment than does screening. The examination may be undertaken by the family physician, by an organized clinic group or research team, or by a physician in a particular setting (*e.g.,* the industrial or school physician). In 1947, the American Medical Association established standards for the physicians' examination and suggested a schedule for such examinations throughout life:[3]

Prenatal	Monthly to biweekly examinations
First 6 months	biweekly examinations
Second 6 months	monthly examinations
1 to 2 years	quarterly examinations
2 to 5 years	semiannual examinations
5 to 15 years	examination every 2 to 3 years
15 to 35 years	examination every 2 years
35 to 60 years	annual examinations
60+ years	semiannual examinations

It is obvious that many in the population will probably not fulfill this schedule.

Since 1947, a great variety of schedules have been proposed for school-age children, for industrial populations, and for the general public. For the most part, subsequent recommendations proposed wider spacing of examinations. However, the change appears to have been based upon feasibility rather than on need factors. As Breslow says, "However desirable as an ideal, health examinations represent only a partial solution to the problem of early detection of disease."[4] He cites limitations in the number of physicians available and the high costs of the examination as reasons for this point of view.

Regular medical examinations may be provided on a "selected population" basis for those in hazardous jobs in industry, for vulnerable families, for low-income populations, or for others at special risk. In the detection of handicapping conditions in children, a "risk register" or a "special service register" may be used. Under this system, those factors associated with high risk are identified; and for each family, designated health workers record the presence or absence of these risk factors. Those exposed to risk factors are entered on the special register and are seen more frequently than are the others in that age group. A WHO working party estimated that about 20 percent of the children born might be expected to fall into this special risk group and that about 80 percent of the children with disabilities would be found within this 20 percent.[5] The trend is definitely toward a broad-spectrum health examination with high reliance on laboratory tests and on the observations of the physician and of other professional personnel. Wright, in discussing the executive health examination, points out the need for assessing what he calls the "personality–environment" equation in order to understand why the patient is sick as well as to determine from what disease or disability he is suffering.[6] Experiments with family clinics suggest that family interaction at the time of health examination may also offer significant clues to health.

INTERVIEW OR QUESTIONNAIRE SURVEY

Individual or household interviews or questionnaires may also be used as a measure of securing data on the probable presence of illness, presymptomatic disorders, or prejudicial health conditions or behavior (such as smoking). These interviews are, for the most part, "structured"—that is, designed to cover specific content in a uniform way, although Wright describes the benefits of a "free ranging" interview as part of history-taking.[7]

Self-administered health questionnaires are sometimes used either as a self-screening device or as an adjunct to medical examination. Follow-up counseling is provided to those whose questionnaire returns indicate problems; referral to medical care is made when indicated.

In addition to the use of this approach as a measure for individual health assessment, such interviews may be administered to a probability-sample in the population at large or to special groups, such as a school population, in order to establish the prevalence of specified conditions.

CONTINUING SURVEILLANCE

Continuing observation by physician, teacher, nurse or other professional worker, or by others sensitized to make pertinent observations is
also an effective disease detection measure. For example, observation of
the young child, undertaken by the parent and monitored by the nurse,
may reveal symptoms of impaired hearing: difficulty in waking the child
without shaking him, a lack of response to speech, or ignoring a ringing
telephone. The teacher's observation of a child who appears to block out
the outside world and to retreat to nonresponsive indifference may lead
to early recognition of psychiatric disorder.

EARLY DETECTION OF ABNORMALITY

Discovery of unrecognized disease is a focal concern of early detection measures, but it is not the only purpose served. The uncovering of
developmental irregularities, predisease conditions, or poor health practices may be less dramatic but sometimes equally important findings. In
particular, many health workers feel that the discovery of a slight eleva-
tion of blood pressure, a heightened cholesterol level, or obesity may
indicate a higher than normal risk of specific disease and that these signs
suggest treatment that may lessen the risk. Overcompetitive work habits
or a beginning dependence on alcohol may be as important to executive

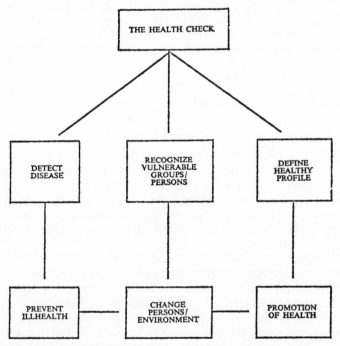

FIGURE 15.   The many uses of the health check. (Courtesy of Hart, John D.: The health
check and the general practitioner. Royal Soc. Health J., 88:259, September-October,
1968.)

health as is diabetes; the overanxious parent may be as much a danger to her child as is the mother who has tuberculosis.

Early detection measures may also yield important data regarding prevalence and incidence of specific health conditions. Perhaps the most notable development of such data is the continuing household interview and health examination program of the National Health Survey. Through the use of representative sampling units of the population, the survey provides data that make possible an estimation of characteristic health patterns and trends for the population of the country as a whole.

Since early detection measures start with presumably well populations, they contribute to the accumulation of data that are necessary to more clearly define what is "health" and what is "normal." At present there are large areas of borderline illness: conditions that do not warrant a diagnosis of disease but that are of sufficient impact to reduce one's effectiveness in meeting family or work responsibilities or to suggest a threat of illness.

Lastly, early detection measures may serve an important health education or health promotion end. Inquiry about smoking or inadequate sleep may lead to changed behavior; inquiries and tests for specific diseases may lead to a greater awareness of the symptoms of these diseases, more prompt self-reporting should these symptoms occur, or the institution of regular self-inspection, such as regular self-examination of the breast. Figure 15 shows the many uses of the health check.

THE OUTCOMES OF DETECTION PROGRAMS VARY

The outcome of a specific program will vary with the program's purpose and the population served. "Executive screening"—the examination of presumably well men, usually in the 40 to 65 age bracket and in salaried positions in industry—is expected to produce a relatively high yield of previously unknown disease and of predisease conditions, especially if laboratory support is liberally provided.[8] Glaucoma screening for those over 35 years of age is also likely to yield a high number of new cases, since the incidence of glaucoma is great (about 2 percent in the over-35 age group) and the onset of chronic glaucoma (which constitutes about 85 percent of the total cases) is insidious and not easily recognized.[9]

If persistently undertaken, screening for cervical cancer gives promise of discovering the disease at the preinvasive, and hence more treatable, period. Even when the number of new cases uncovered is small, as in PKU testing of infants, if the possibility of treatment is bright, the savings to the individual and to the community may be great.

However, screening measures are not always indicated. For example, nutritional surveys might be expected to be quite effective in identifying previously unknown nutritional deficit in low-income communities; but this detection measure is too expensive for the high-income community where a smaller yield is likely.

Yankauer and associates have shown that school health examinations uncover few cases of previously unrecognized disease. He points out, however, that other purposes of the examination, such as education in and motivation toward the use of preventive health care, may make the procedure worth-while.[10]

It is important for the nurse, as a participant in or supporter of early disease detection programs, to know what outcomes the sponsors of the program expect.

THE ROLE OF THE COMMUNITY NURSE IN DETECTION PROGRAMS

The community health nurse has an important role; she directly or indirectly does much to support and implement programs for early detection of disease.

Motivation of Participants

The community health nurse motivates families and groups to use available resources. A persistent and troublesome problem in using early detection methods as a measure of health improvement is assuring that those who should receive the benefits of screening or other measures actually do receive them. In settings such as school and industry, utilization of preventive care facilities is encouraged by the organization's sponsorship and by the pressures to conform to the behavior of the majority. In some instances these procedures may be required as a condition of admission to school or the retainment on a job. Community sponsored programs, on the other hand, tend to be unevenly utilized. Fink and others, for example, found that participation in a breast cancer screening program was related to demographic characteristics of the population and also to individual perceptual and motivational differences. Those with higher educational achievement, those younger in age, those of Jewish faith, and those with habits of high utilization of other health services were most likely to take advantage of the opportunities for preventive care.[11]

Borsky and Sagen, however, found that cooperation was more likely from low-income groups and nonwhites in health examinations for survey purposes. The attitudes affecting participation were belief in the potential benefits, the importance of furthering medical research, and the reasonableness of the arrangements.[12]

The differences between the results of these two studies may reflect the nature of the invitation to participate in the screening program and also the difference in the nature of the examination offered. In the case of screening for cancer, it is likely that fear of discovering the disease may have been more operative. Studies such as these suggest that motivation may be a very individual thing and that the community health nurse's role may be to help the susceptible group to recognize and deal with the barriers to seeking such care. Steps that appear useful are:

1. Use all channels to inform families, groups, sources of referral (doctors, schools), and the community as a whole of the opportunity provided and of the advantages of participation.

2. Make special efforts to reach the most vulnerable groups with the message; inform and enlist local leaders, and "reach out" to families most in need through special home visiting and group discussions in the school or the community.

3. Try to anticipate and deal with hang-ups, such as fears of finding out about disease or a dislike of using public health care facilities.

4. Make participation easy or, at least, possible by making provisions for such needs as child care or transportation.

5. Offer help to private physicians in the required, more definitive follow-up care for his patients.

6. Identify those who do *not* participate and try to uncover the reasons for their nonparticipation. This information will be most helpful in the preparation of future programs.

The Nurse May Be the Screener

Nurses are expanding their role in patient care with startling speed, and in many instances this role expansion involves taking on certain screening responsibilities. Nurses in schools and in industry have traditionally provided considerable screening service, aided by teachers and other health personnel. For many years, nurses in rural or inaccessible areas have served as screening agents. In some localities, nursing clinics to which patients come for a variety of tests — as well as for nurse counseling — have functioned for several years. In the past these responsibilities were undertaken usually because there was no other professional worker available. At present, however, there is considerable pressure for nurses in urban areas to take on expanded screening functions. Even though physicians are available, there is a feeling that the community health nurse is by training and temperament well adapted to the provision of such screening and that it may be easier for the family to deal with the nurse, especially if the nurse-family relationship has been a close one. The problem of follow-up care is simplified when the nurse, backed by laboratory services, takes a central role in the actual screening.

In most instances when the nurse's role in screening is to be enlarged, the agency will make the decision as to which procedures can be safely delegated, and it will arrange for such additional training as the nurse may need to absorb this new responsibility. If the nurse is working in a setting where such administrative support is not available (for example, if she is the only nurse in an independent project setting), she must take the responsibility that any professional worker would take in the control of his own practice. She must be sure that she is not assuming responsibilities that either contravene medical or nursing practice acts or that require a level of skill or judgment for which her professional training has not prepared her. If she is unsure of herself or does not know sources for special training, the nurse may want to seek the help of the city or state nursing consultant, the local nurses' association, or the nurse administrator in a larger agency in the community.

Recruitment and Training of Screeners

Screening may be done by the nurse herself or by paid or volunteer workers who are trained for this function. Whether screening is on a continuing basis (as with self-examination of the breast or with teacher observations of school children) or on a periodic basis (as with school or industrial health examinations), the community health nurse may be expected to recruit some or all of the members of the screening team — or in the case of individual self-screening, enlist the individual in this effort — and to provide for any needed training.

Recruitment of screening agents must be based on getting those who have sufficient commitment to follow through with the task once it is undertaken and to appreciate the necessity for accuracy and consistency in following the recommended procedures. It is well to recruit a few stand-by helpers to fill in if someone else must be absent. Consideration should also be given to enlisting the help of the consumer group as a measure of increasing interest and commitment to the project. Sometimes ready-made groups may be used, such as members of the parent-teacher association or graduates of a Red Cross home nursing class.

Timing of the screening service and of the training sessions should be consistent with the other demands made upon the screening team. If, for example, teachers are to help with screening procedures, the times should be worked out with the responsible administrator in order to interfere as little as possible with regular teaching duties. If parents are the screeners, a time of day that will not conflict with home responsibilities may be a primary consideration in arranging schedules.

A review of content and procedure may be necessary. The nurse should allow herself enough time to be sure her own content is up-to-date and accurate. If necessary, the content and procedures of the program may be checked with a nurse consultant or with material in the library. When the screening involves the use of equipment, manufacturers may be able to provide assistance.

A training program, with a mini curriculum, will have to be developed. This program should allow for:

1. The definition and interpretation of the purpose of the screening effort.
2. The presentation and discussion of the basic principles or concepts involved.
3. The explanation of the procedures involved.
4. The demonstration and practice of the procedures.

A plan for supervision of trainees must also be developed. This may involve observation of the screeners at work and review conferences with individuals or groups. In most instances, questionable or negative findings are checked by another screener with more experience.

The plan for recording, reporting, and follow-up care should be built into the training program.

Sometimes the community health nurse is responsible only for arranging for the use of screening personnel that have already been fully trained either by a voluntary association, such as the Society for the Prevention of Blindness, or by the agency. If this is the case, the nurse's responsibility for teaching and supervision will be limited.

The Nurse May Be the Interviewer

When interview data are the basis of a survey or study, the community health nurse may be the interviewer. In this case, the primary purpose is not to secure change but rather to secure information.

Sometimes the interview is focused on a single individual who can provide information about his own symptoms, experience, plans, or feelings. He may be the "index case"—that is, the person first reported for care—he may be someone closely associated with the patient (a contact) who may also have the disease, or he may be a parent. Sometimes the focus of the fact finding is the household, and data are secured regarding all members residing in the household.

In this responsibility, as in the whole fabric of nursing practice in any setting, the general skills of interviewing are exceedingly important. Emphasis will be placed here on those aspects, or characteristics, of interviewing that are of particular importance for this type of interview.

The purpose of the fact finding interview may be to describe events, behavior, values, perceptions, or feelings. There are three types of fact finding interviews with which the community health nurse may be involved:

1. The epidemiologic investigation, in which the purpose is to assemble relevant information about the onset and course of the disease, the possible sources of the disease, others who might be affected, and the presence or absence of factors that may be associated with the occurrence of disease.

2. The individual or household survey interview, which is designed to secure data on the incidence and prevalence of health or health-related conditions or behavior and demographic or personal data that may be related to the occurrence of these conditions.

3. The in depth interview, which is designed to describe an occurrence or a situation in detail and from several viewpoints.

The purposes of the interview will determine the type of interview and the methods that are used.

The fact finding interview may be integral to nursing care or separate from it. In some cases, the fact finding interview is undertaken in the course of providing care to the family and may be used not only as a means of securing information but also as a vehicle for explanation or teaching. This is often the case in the care of communicable disease.

In other instances, the fact finding interview may be purposely divorced from care. This is important when the interview is part of a study, and it is essential that the responses be obtained under uniform conditions. The interjection of service, advice, or comment may in itself influence the nature of the responses. To provide even incidental assistance might make the findings unreliable.

THE INTERVIEW MAY BE STRUCTURED OR UNSTRUCTURED

The Structured, Standardized Interview. The structured, standardized interview aims to collect data under uniform circumstances in order to minimize differences in response that might be caused by the bias or the manner of the interviewer or the way in which the question was asked. Thus the structured interview attempts to subject each respondent to precisely the same stimulus. An interview schedule is developed and tested; each question is spelled out in detail, even the introduction of the interviewer is prescribed. It is extremely important that the interviewer ask the questions exactly as they are written and in exactly the order in which they appear in the schedule, since the timing of "sensitive" or of "recall" questions may affect the answer. If the question is not answered, the interviewer should not explain or probe for an answer unless the directions specifically permit this; and the interviewer should respect any limitations that might be set with respect to "probe" questions. Care must be taken not to suggest a "correct" answer by tone of voice or by expression.

Questions unrelated to the interview should not be answered until after the interview has been completed. If advice or services are requested, the request should be noted and another time should be set for such care, since the interposition of service may affect the answers supplied.

The Unstructured, Unstandardized Interview. The unstructured, unstandardized interview is generally used when the effort is not to compare responses but to use the responses as a means of understanding or explaining a situation. This type of interview is more exploratory and depends on the skill of the nurse in asking questions that encourage adequate response and in recognizing verbal and nonverbal clues that suggest that a different line of questioning might produce useful information. The content of the questions, the method of the questioning, and the timing and arrangement of various facets of the inquiry are matters left to the interviewer. This kind of interview allows for great flexibility in adapting to differences among individuals.

Many fact finding interviews fall between these two extremes. Richardson and coworkers, for example, describe a "non schedule standardized interview" in which the interviewer is provided with a list of the information to be obtained. The interview itself may take many different forms, since the interviewer uses his own judgment in formulating the questions in order to make them understandable and acceptable to the respondent.[13]

The nurse's general interviewing skill will come into play in the unstructured, unstandardized interview. The intuitive responses to observations of subtle changes in the appearance or manner of the interviewee—the delayed response, the "closed down" expression, or the flicker of interest and response that signals an interpersonal breakthrough—are important elements in fact gathering. The skill of the nurse in the timing and wording of sensitive questions—the matter of fact tone of voice or the prior sanction of a negative response by such remarks as "Do you find it hard to remember to take all of yours pills?"—will influence the quality of response.

THE EPIDEMIOLOGIC INTERVIEW

The epidemiologic interview usually combines both structured and unstructured approaches. Usually there is a form that indicates just what information the epidemiologist will need in his assessment of the situation. However, these forms may be rather general, in which case the nurse may want to supplement them by reminders to get information related to the particular disease being investigated. In any event, she should refresh her memory of the nature of the disease and its transmission before proceeding to the interview. There is more freedom in the way the questions are asked than there is in the structured interview, and probing is not only permissible but highly desirable when information is not forthcoming.

For example, if the patient suffering from salmonella infection can't recall eating anything other than what was eaten by other and unaffected members of her family, questions might be raised about visiting with the neighbors, an unremembered between-meal snack, or "just a taste" of something. If the unanswered or incompletely answered question is a sensitive one, as when the inquiry concerns sexual contact, the nurse may go to other questions for a while and rephrase the delicate question later in the interview when a greater degree of trust has been developed. When the reply involves recall of something that happened some time ago, there may be need for a "check" question; for example, if the mother reports the onset of disease in a child as occurring on Tuesday, the nurse might check by asking later, "Did Johnnie go to school on Monday?"

Subjective observations or comments may be a helpful supplement to the interview data, if this practice is consistent with the study design. For example, even in the structured interview, the nurse interviewer might express some doubt about the validity or completeness of responses by a recorded comment such as "the respondent appeared over-anxious to give the right answers and reiterated several times that she was doing exactly what the clinic told her to do," or "the respondent appeared reluctant to answer the question, although she did not refuse to do so," or "the respondent was preoccupied and anxious about a son who has just been hospitalized following an automobile accident."

THE SURVEY

A survey is as good as its sample. Most interview surveys are based on securing information from a sample that is representative of the whole population. The selection of those to be interviewed is carefully made to assure this representativeness. However, if a substantial number of the sample group is not located or refuses to participate or provides only partial or obviously unreliable answers, the findings will be much less useful. The nurse interviewer can make a valuable contribution to the study by using her ingenuity to find all of those in the sample group and to encourage those in the sample to participate in the study.

The Nurse May Be the Organizer

Sometimes the community health nurse is the one responsible for arranging for the screening or examination activity. She may, for example, plan for the medical examination of school children or of employees. When this is the case, it is likely that there will be available for her guidance a manual or a set of directions that indicate the necessary steps and governing regulations. In general, it is important to:

1. Notify the eligible population (or, in the case of minors, their parents).
2. Interpret the purpose and limitations of the procedure to the eligible population and, when indicated, to other community sources of care such as family physicians.
3. Secure the necessary authorization. This includes getting parental permission for the examination or procedure and clearing the general plan and schedule with appropriate authorities (*e.g.*, school personnel or the medical director of health).
4. Recruit and train volunteer assistants.
5. Schedule the activities and post and announce the schedule well in advance of the date.
6. Arrange for anticipated follow-up activities.

Follow-Up Care

The community health nurse is inevitably involved in follow-up activities. Follow-up activities of the nurse will include:

1. The provision of health counseling.
2. Referral to sources of further study or care.
3. The interpretation to the public of the meaning of the screening or the examination.
4. Reporting on follow-up outcomes and other data useful in evaluation of the screening activity.

POST-SURVEY HEALTH COUNSELING

Provision for post-survey health counseling requires that the nurse be thoroughly acquainted with the survey or screening procedure that has been used and with the meaning of the findings. In particular, the nurse should be able to answer the following questions:

1. How *sensitive* and how *specific* were the tests used? In other words what is the likelihood that those *with* the disease or abnormal condition would be identified by the test used? If, for example, there are a large number of false negative results, it is important that the family not be overconfident of wellness and that they continue to be alert to any symptoms that might appear. If the tests are likely to yield a large number of false positive results, the family should know of this likelihood and not worry unduly. Above all, the community health nurse should emphasize that no screening system is foolproof and that continuous observation for, and reporting of, any unusual development is necessary.

2. What are the criteria for referral for care? In screening or survey procedures there are usually a significant number of instances in which there is no disease but in which there are predisposing conditions, such as obesity, high cholesterol level, marginal hearing, or vision disabilities. The responsible screening or survey team will decide the level at which

referral will be made and to what extent those with predisease conditions will be encouraged to seek further diagnostic work-up or anticipatory care.

3. What can be done to deal with the disease or predisease condition discovered? There will be some instances in which nurse counseling may be indicated—for instance, mild obesity or poor habits of daily hygiene. There may be community resources available for anticipatory or definitive care. Unfortunately there will be some conditions in which little can be done to improve the situation or for which community resources have not been developed. In these instances, general supportive measures may be all that can be given.

REFERRAL

In making referrals to other sources of care, the community health nurse may need to locate new resources or to strengthen ties with sources of help not frequently used. Local chapters of voluntary health agencies, such as the American Heart Association or the National Tuberculosis and Respiratory Disease Association, may be helpful in locating resources for care. When referral is to the family physician, the community health nurse may need to acquaint him with the survey or screening procedure that was used, and she also may need to offer her own help in follow-up care either by working directly with his patients and their families or, when there is a nurse in his office, by providing her with information and materials.

Evaluation of the Detection Effort

The community health nurse's accurate and prompt reporting of the action taken by those referred for further study is important to assure adequate care for each participant; it is also a means of evaluating the screening effort. In the long run, it is the number of persons who receive care, not the number of persons discovered to have disease or abnormality, that tests the usefulness of the screening measure.

Response to the screening program and the degree of effort required to implement the recommendations for postscreening care are useful in evaluating the methodology used. The nurse's observations or judgments concerning the reasons families had for using or for not using the screening opportunity can be a valuable contribution to the evaluation of the acceptability of the methods used and to the improvement of planning for future programs.

It is obvious that follow-up activities for screening programs will require a substantial amount of nursing time. This time requirement must be taken into account when planning the screening program.

There seems to be every indication that organized early-disease-detection methods will continue to expand and that methodologies will be further refined. The community health nurse will inevitably be involved with these activities; through her involvement, she can increase her ability to contribute to preventive health care.

REFERENCES

1. Chronic Illness in the United States, vol. 1: Prevention of Chronic Illness. Commission on Chronic Illness, Harvard University Press, Cambridge, Mass., 1957, p. 45.
2. Policy Statement on Multiphasic Screening. American Public Health Association, Amer. J. Public Health, *59:*174, January, 1969.
3. Periodic Health Examination: A Manual for Physicians. American Medical Association, Chicago, 1947.
4. Breslow, Lester: Chronic disease and disability in adults. *In* Rosenau, Milton J.: Preventive Medicine and Public Health. 9th ed. (Kenneth F. Maxcy and Philip Sartwell, eds.), Appleton-Century-Crofts, New York, 1965, p. 534.
5. Early detection of handicaps in children. WHO Chron., *22:*16, January, 1968.
6. Wright, H. B.: The executive health examination. Roy. Soc. Health J., *88:*251, September-October, 1968.
7. *Ibid.,* p. 254.
8. Sharpe, J. C., and Marxer, W. L.: Physical examination of well persons. Calif. Med., *96:*32, January, 1962.
9. New York State Department of Public Health Weekly Bulletin. *31:*133, August, 1968.
10. Yankauer, A., Frantz, R., Drislane, A., and Katz, S.: A study of case finding methods in elementary school: methodology and initial results. Amer. J. Public Health, *52:*656, April, 1962.
11. Fink, Raymond, Shapiro, Sam, and Levinson, John: The reluctant participant in a breast cancer screening program. Public Health Rep., *83:*479, June, 1968.
12. Borsky, P. N., and Sagen, O. N.: Motivation toward health examination. Amer. J. Public Health, *49:*514, April, 1959.
13. Richardson, Stephen A., Doherwend, Barbara S., and Klein, David: Interviewing: Its Forms and Functions. Basic Books, Inc., Publishers, New York, 1965, p. 45.

SUGGESTED READINGS

Collen, M. F.: Value of the multiphasic health checkup. New Eng. J. Med., *280:*1072, May, 1969.
Guthrie, R., and Susi, A.: A simple phenylalanine method for detecting phenylketonuria in large populations of newborn infants. Pediatrics, *32:*338, September, 1963.
Hays, Una: A Developmental Approach to Case Finding with Special Reference to Cerebral Palsy, Mental Retardation and Related Disorders. Childrens Bureau Publication No. 449, U.S. Government Printing Office, Washington, D.C., 1967.
Health Care of the Preschool Child. Currents in Public Health, Ross Laboratories, Columbus, Ohio, vol. 5, April, 1965.
Hoenig, Leah: A hearing program for school children. Amer. J. Nurs., *63:*85, May, 1963.
Horn, Daniel: Current smoking among teen agers. Public Health Rep., *83:*458, June, 1968.
Kegeles, S. S., Kirscht, J. P., Haefner, D. P., and Rosenstock, I. M.: Survey of beliefs about cancer detection and taking Papanicolaou tests. Public Health Rep., *80:*815, September, 1965.
Kurlander, Arnold B., and Carroll, Benjamin: Case finding through multiple screening. *In* Lilienfeld, Abraham, and Gifford, Alice (eds.): Chronic Diseases and Public Health. The Johns Hopkins Press, Baltimore, Maryland, 1966, p. 163.
Martin, Marguerite M.: Diabetes mellitus: current concepts. Amer. J. Nurs., *66:*510, March, 1966.
McDonald, Glen W., Fisher, Gail F., and Pentz, Phillip C.: Diabetic screening activities July 1958 to June 1963. Public Health Rep., *80:*163, February, 1965.
Moore, Mary Virginia: Diagnosis: deafness. Amer. J. Nurs., *69:*297, February, 1969.
Multiphasic screening (policy statement). American Public Health Association. Amer. J. Public Health, *59:*174, January, 1969.
Naguib, Samir M., Geiser, Patricia B., and Comstock, George W.: Response to a program of screening for cervical cancer. Public Health Rep., *83:*990, December, 1968.
The nurse and the multiphasic exam. Nurs. Outlook, *16:*40, September, 1968.
O'Sullivan, John B., Wilkerson, Hugh L. C., and Krall, Leo P.: The prevalence of diabetes

mellitus in Oxford and related epidemiologic problems. Amer. J. Public Health, 56:742, May, 1966.
Preschool Vision Screening. Currents in Public Health, Ross Laboratories, Columbus, Ohio, vol. 3, November-December, 1963.
South, Jean: Tuberculosis Handbook for Public Health Nurses. National Tuberculosis Association (Now, the National Tuberculosis and Respiratory Disease Association), New York, 1965, pp. 1-7.
Tabenhaus, Leon, and Jackson, Anne A.: Vision Screening in Preschool Children. 2nd ed., Charles C Thomas, Springfield, Illinois, 1969.
Thorner, R. M.: Whither multiphasic screening? New Eng. J. Med., 280:1037, May, 1969.
V.D. — Today's VD Control Program: A Joint Statement Sponsored by the American Public Health Association, The American Social Hygiene Association, and The American Venereal Disease Association. The American Social Hygiene Association, New York, 1969, pp. 51-54.
Savitz, Roberta, Reed, Robert, and Valadean, Isobel: Vision Screening of the Preschool Child. U.S. Department of Health, Education and Welfare, Children's Bureau Publication No. 414, U.S. Government Printing Office, Washington, D.C., 1964.
Wallace, Helen: Health Services for Mothers and Children. W. B. Saunders Company, Philadelphia, 1962, p. 200.

The Community
Health Nurse in
Disease Control

The control of disease is a central concern of community health agencies. Originally centered primarily on the control of communicable diseases, public health agencies have broadened their concerns to include the control of many other diseases and, in particular, the control of chronic illness.

The incidence of acute communicable diseases has been dramatically reduced as sanitary measures and new immunizing agents have become available. Smallpox, diphtheria, and poliomyelitis, for example, have been brought to very low levels in developed countries; and there is every indication that measles and rubella will soon be equally rare. However, occasional outbreaks do occur, and vigilance is still necessary until these diseases are completely eradicated. Venereal disease and tuberculosis continue to present problems.

The control of noncommunicable disease is a much more complex problem than the control of communicable disease. For many diseases, knowledge about causation is scanty, and the role of the multiple contributing factors is not clear. Furthermore, much of the required care is provided by family physicians, and their aid must be enlisted if control is to be achieved.

METHODS OF DISEASE CONTROL

The control of disease is a dynamic process; it is a problem in which the pieces of the puzzle are being constantly rearranged. The distribution of disease may change as social and economic conditions change.

New methods of prevention and cure continue to be discovered at a rapid pace, and incidence rates may fall precipitously over a very short period (as was true after the introduction of penicillin). Acceptance of the concept of multiple causation of disease opens an almost inexhaustible range of intriguing lines of inquiry in which it sometimes appears that nonmedical forces outweigh the medical forces as a factor in change. Thus the problem of disease control in populations must be a constant process of study, action, and restudy. Control programs enhance efforts to define the nature and distribution of disease in the population, to institute the preventive measures that are available, and to secure prompt and adequate curative and rehabilitative care.

Define the Nature, Extent, and Distribution of Disease

Obviously, it is vital to know the incidence and the prevalence of specific disease entities in the population in order to judge the size of the problem with which the health system must deal. A knowledge of trends in incidence and prevalence is essential as a basis for planning programs for the future.

Knowledge of the distribution of the disease among various segments of the population is essential in developing more precise measures for control and for gaining increased insight into the nature of the disease itself. Knowledge of the age, socioeconomic, or occupational groups that are particularly affected provides valuable clues to causative or influencing factors in the disease; these data also provide a basis for case selection and for program direction.

Define the Determinants and Consequences of Disease

A knowledge of the determinants and the consequences of disease is essential to the control of disease. The search for the determinants of disease has moved from a narrow focus on the specific causative organisms or on the event without which the disease or condition *cannot* occur, to a wide-angle look at the multiple factors that determine whether or not the disease actually *will* occur. For example, infection with tubercle bacillus is *necessary* for tuberculosis to develop in an individual, but it may not be *sufficient* to cause the disease. Stress, poor nutrition, crowding, or poor health practices or facilities for health care may be equally important in explaining why, with the same degree of exposure to the causative organism, some people respond by contracting the disease and others do not.

Thus it may be important to know not only the disease state of the population but also the pattern of predisease states or of disease-associated conditions. For example, it may be useful to estimate the nutritional levels, immunization status, birth weights, or smoking habits of the population; these indices help to elucidate the nature of the disease experience and to suggest the relative vulnerability of specified populations.

Knowledge of the health or social consequences of disease is also an essential for control of disease, since it provides an index of the urgency for the control measures and a means of determining the value of the program to the community.

Primary and Secondary Preventive Measures

Preventive measures may be primary or secondary and have varying levels of specificity. Some measures, such as measles immunization or abstinence from smoking, are expected to prevent the occurrence of the disease. Other measures, such as early detection of disease or programs of rehabilitation that maximize functioning of the disabled, are expected to minimize the effects of the disease once it occurs.

Preventive measures in common use vary widely in the degree to which their utility has been validated. For example, smoking is almost certainly implicated in the development of certain respiratory diseases, and "tender loving care" by parent or parent surrogate is quite clearly associated with the infant's ability to thrive. Other preventive measures—such as health education measures as a means of reducing the incidence of venereal disease or counseling services as a measure for reducing emotional stress among college students—are more speculative.

When the means of prevention are not known, reliance must be placed on secondary preventive measures and the alleviation of the effects of the disease. When the causes of disease are multiple, as is the case with tuberculosis, and when there is a lack of precise information about the reinforcing effect of contributing conditions that exist concurrently, prevention may involve many components; the value of a specific component cannot be singled out from the value of any of the others, and consequently, effort is directed toward doing all of the things that might help.

In some instances, then, "instituting preventive measures" may indeed represent a clear-cut, obvious program; the current efforts to immunize children against rubella in order to protect their mothers from infection that may endanger future offspring is one example. In other instances "instituting preventive measures" may imply a concerted attack, including such things as efforts to reduce the stress factors in the physical or social environment, to provide nutritional guidance to increase the hemoglobin level, to institute welfare services to support a more adequate level of living, and to refer to a marriage counselor to reduce stress arising from domestic difficulties.

Prompt and Adequate Care

Prompt and adequate care means more than the provision of care facilities. Prompt and adequate care requires that the condition be put under care as soon as the need arises and that the care encompass secondary prevention and rehabilitation, as well as curative, content. It implies that the recipients are willing to accept the care provided and that the professionals providing the care are adequate in number and competency. It also implies that the facilities are both adequate to permit the professionals to work efficiently and accessible and acceptable to the users. Thus "prompt and adequate care" is as much a responsibility and a function of the individual who is ill as it is of the community that is obligated to see that the necessary care is available. It is as much a function of the consumer — be he patient or taxpayer — as it is of the health professional.

The provision of direct therapeutic intervention must be combined with measures designed to produce an informed and highly motivated population, an adequate supply of professional personnel of appropriate levels of preparation, and an action program that develops the facilities and the procedures necessary to reach those who require care.

Prompt and adequate care in the present-day context must also encompass provisions for social and environmental, as well as medical, action.

NURSING IS A UBIQUITOUS FORCE IN DISEASE CONTROL

Control Through Ongoing Activity

The community health nurse has many opportunities for disease control action in the course of her daily work. The alert community health nurse discovers many disease problems other than those conditions for which service was initiated. The visit to a preschool child may uncover an older member of the family with fatigue, cough, and listlessness that suggest possible disease. The routine visit to the school may turn up information about an increase in the number of sore throat or gastrointestinal upsets among the pupils and teachers and suggest the need for an epidemiologic investigation. For patients who have a longterm illness and who are cared for at home, the community health nurse may be a major observer of changes that suggest intervention to prevent secondary complications.

The ongoing educational activities of the nurse also do much to further the disease control program. These may extend from general public education designed to alert the public or a large segment of the population to a particular problem to the intensive family teaching that occurs in the home care of the stroke patient. Education may be directed toward others in the professional community (such as nurses working in physician's offices or in industry) in order to increase their contribution to disease control efforts. It may be directed to those who have, or are at special risk of having, a specific disease, such as inactive tuberculosis patients or families in which diabetes has appeared. Education may be directed toward the "deciders" in a particular community, such as elected officials, labor leaders, or clergymen. These leaders may sanction or encourage a particular course of action and thus build community commitment to the program.

The ongoing health promotional activities of the nurse contribute to the improvement of the general condition of the population and to increasing their resistance to disease or to improving their capacity to cope with disease, physically and emotionally, when it occurs. For example, the child who has learned the value of handwashing in school may be less likely to pick up infections transmitted from hand to mouth;

the well-nourished expectant mother may be at less risk during pregnancy; the person who has learned to deal realistically with life problems
and who has established an "emotional reserve" may be better equipped
to handle catastrophic illness should it occur. Although not all "good"
health behavior can be shown to have a direct influence on disease
occurrence or severity, the assumption of a relationship is usually made
as a working hypothesis, as a basis for planning control programs. Much
further research is needed to document or disprove these hypotheses.

A major contribution of the community health nurse, then, is to nurse
the families and groups to which she is assigned, armed with the
knowledge of existing disease and other diseases that might be expected
to occur in particular situations. She should cultivate a high degree of
alertness to anything that is unexpected.

Anticipatory Guidance

A second large contribution that is made in the course of the nurse's
daily work is the anticipatory guidance that is provided when the risk is
known to be high. This might be called the "special alert" aspect of
nursing. Thus, when a family is known to have a member suffering from
diabetes or tuberculosis, a special anticipatory guidance effort will alert
the family to early symptoms of trouble and to the value of periodic
screening for the disease. The high-strung mother may be armed with
specific knowledge about symptoms of illness in order to reduce her
undue stress from imagined ills in the child and also to reduce the
consequent stress build-up in the family as a whole. In areas where
teenage pregnancies are high, the school nurse would herself be particularly alert to symptoms of pregnancy among the group she serves; she
might also encourage referral by others in teaching and counseling positions and arrange with teachers to include in the general health instruction program a strong component on the recognition of pregnancy, the
dangers of nonmedical or illegal abortion, and sources of help for expectant mothers. When it is consistent with school and community policy,
the availability of contraceptive advice and the conditions under which
this advice can be obtained may also be included. All of these measures
have the potential for securing early and adequate care of disease. They
are not special activities of nursing; rather, they are just the application
of good nursing practice.

Reinforcement of Nursing Knowledge Is Imperative

The disease conditions with which the community health nurse deals
will cover a very wide range of diagnoses. Many of the conditions are
not commonly encountered in the hospital because of their minor nature.
Other conditions with which the community health nurse deals will be at
various points in the progress of the disease and will take quite different
forms of nursing intervention than those needed during the more acute
phases when the patient is in the hospital. For example, the nursing

problems of patient and family at the time of an acute cardiac episode are quite different from the nursing problems encountered in the maintenance phase of care.

The hospital-based nurse is able to keep pace with rapid changes in therapy much more easily than can the community nurse. The hospital-based nurse tends to have a smaller range of diseases with which she must deal, and she also has more avilable sources of advice and reference. If the community health nurse is to participate effectively in the detection and control of disease, she may need to develop regular channels of information or quick sources of reference. These supports may be in the form of agency manuals, up-to-date reference materials, or periodic publications pertinent to her work. The sources of reference may also be people such as the agency personnel, physicians, social workers, or others working in community services. Such reinforcement of nursing knowledge should be considered to have a legitimate and imperative claim on the community health nurse's time.

The Community Nurse Is a Member of the Epidemiologic Team

The concept of epidemiology has broadened considerably in recent years. Originally conceived rather narrowly as concerned with the natural history and cause of disease in populations, epidemiology is now regarded as the study of the distribution and dynamics not only of disease but of health states and conditions as well.[1] As a result of this change of focus, traditional epidemiologic methodology has expanded to encompass methodologies from many fields, in particular from the social and behavioral sciences. The distinctive characteristic of epidemiology is the focus on health in *populations* as distinct from the health of *individuals*.

Epidemiologic investigations may be *descriptive* — that is, they may center on describing the occurrence and distribution of disease or health states among different segments of the population, in different communities or settings, or in trends over time; or they may describe observable phenomena such as the clustering of cases or the patterns of epidemics. They may be *analytic,* seeking out statistical associations that help to explain the occurrence and pattern of disease. They may be *experimental,* designed to test an hypothesis and using rigorous research techniques. Thus, epidemiologic investigation takes many forms, may involve many methodologies, and may engage many different types of practitioners.

The community health nurse working with the epidemiologist and the biostatistician may participate in epidemiologic investigation through the following activities:

1. Serving as an advance intelligence officer regarding conditions that merit epidemiologic study. The community health nurse may notice that within a low-income area, one certain neighborhood or cultural cluster tends to seek care and to adhere to recommended medical procedures, whereas other groups, subject to the same economic pressures, fail to do

so. A study of the characteristics of this phenomenon may lead to a better understanding of the factors associated with compliance and may cause the modification of care practices.

2. Collecting data essential to epidemiologic analysis. This may be done as part of an organized study in which an epidemiologist or research officer has designed a study or developed formal interview schedules or report forms for securing and transmitting required data. The fact finding interview described in the preceding chapter is a major tool in this effort. On other occasions the community health nurse may be on her own, collecting data to be submitted to the epidemiologist as a basis for his decision on the best way to evaluate the situation. Here, the nurse's knowledge of disease and disease processes is vitally important, since the need is not for information *per se* but for information relevant to the particular disease or situation.

3. Participating in the design of epidemiologic investigation by identifying relevant areas of information not already included or possible nonmedical factors that might be significant in the analysis of data. For example, the nurse might point out that absence patterns in industry appear to be related not only to the worker's characteristics but also to the supervisory style of the worker's immediate superiors.

4. Motivating and assisting subjects of epidemiologic investigations to cooperate in disease investigation and control. The person with tuberculosis may find it difficult (or sometimes, of course, impossible) to identify the probable source of his infection or to admit that he did not take the prescribed medications. The willingness of each patient to try to provide required information and to "level" with the study personnel will influence the amount of knowledge that can be accumulated about the disease and its treatment. The busy mother of a small infant may find it difficult to find time to talk with a household interviewer about her childbearing experience and her feelings about the professional care she received unless she can see the ultimate benefits of the study. The nurse's own conviction of the importance of learning more about disease and disease-related conditions and her understanding of the importance to the study of the cooperation of those being studied will undoubtedly influence the quality of data secured. There is an increasing use of longterm projective studies of factors associated with disease or health behavior, often involving the use of study cohorts that are followed over many years. In this case, maintaining the integrity of the study group is extremely important. Keeping families "in the study"—having them return for periodic tests or interviews, report frequently, or maintain specified dietary records or practices—may be of major concern to the investigator. This may become a nursing assignment in itself, with the nurse assigned wholly to the project to maintain contact with the family and to encourage and assist them in their part of the study. In some instances, investigators have offered comprehensive nursing care as a bonus for participation. Thus a community health nurse assigned to a longterm follow-up project for brain damaged children might provide general nursing support to the family. Establishing such a service-oriented and close relationship may lead to the family's identification with the purposes of the project and increase their willingness to participate fully over an extended period of time.

5. Using the results of epidemiologic investigation as a springboard for the improvement of community health nursing practice. The findings of epidemiologic studies may help to pinpoint the nursing needs of population groups, to identify the crucial components of the care required, or to suggest areas of investigation in nursing practice.

The Nurse May Implement Regulations for Control

The community health nurse may be involved in the implementation of regulations for the control of disease. The nurse may support the efforts of the disease control program to secure adequate reporting of disease. She may facilitate reporting by private physicians or others required to report. She may be called upon to report breaches in the observation of required practices of individuals who are afflicted with a communicable disease or to explain and interpret the nature of the constraints imposed upon the patient by the regulations that do exist. Thus the school health nurse must be prepared to interpret and support regulations regarding exclusion from school for medical reasons and the requirement for hospitalization for the tuberculosis patient who has persistent positive sputum and who lives where there are small children.

The nurse will want to have readily available the regulations regarding the reporting of disease and the public safety practices required of the family and of others associated with the patient. The community agency usually provides the nurse with such guides; if it does not, she may need to secure the information from the local or state health department.

CONTROL OF COMMUNICABLE DISEASE POSES SPECIAL PROBLEMS

As has already been said, the impact of communicable disease on the health of the public has been sharply reduced. However, the problem of communicable disease control still persists, although to a lesser degree than formerly. The problem may be the more harassing to the community health professional because it is so often preventable.

Goals Change with Changing Technology and Resources

Payne states that the goal of communicable disease control is "to reduce the incidence of the disease to a tolerable level as quickly as possible within the resources available."[2] The "tolerable level" depends on the degree to which the disease can be prevented or ameliorated and on the community's ability to take the required action. In some diseases — tuberculosis, malaria, and syphilis, for example — it is felt by many that the complete eradication of the disease is a feasible goal. In other instances, where the determinants are complex and the treatment less well defined, the goal of eradication may be unrealistic. In the case of gonorrhea, for instance, the nature of the determinants and the limitations of present diagnostic methods is such that control is difficult and eradication probably not possible, even though treatment methods are well advanced. Furthermore, diseases wax and wane in occurrence and in virulence. As some diseases are brought under control, others, such as hepatitis and influenza, continue to baffle; and newly emerging viral diseases challenge the health professional. Gregg expresses the problems in these terms: "Infectious disease is the final expression of interaction between a progressively changing and aging host population, an endlessly adaptable parasite, and a constant pressure from a man made environment".[3]

THE ROLE OF THE COMMUNITY HEALTH NURSE

The community health nurse has a dual role of care and control. The nursing care of a patient with communicable disease is no less important than it is for any type of illness. The emphasis here will be upon the control measures, but this should in no way be considered as minimizing the focal role of personal care.

Disease control measures have special emphasis when the disease is communicable. The general methods of disease control are, of course, pertinent to infectious, as well as to noninfectious, diseases. However, certain aspects of the control procedure may be emphasized.

Reporting Disease

In establishing the prevalence and incidence of disease, reporting is of prime importance. All states and most local communities have regulations requiring the reporting of communicable diseases not only by the physician who is responsible for the diagnosis but, in many instances, also by householders or others having knowledge of, or reason to suspect, the existence of a communicable disease. Reporting is carried out at all levels of government in order to maintain an epidemiologic intelligence system that facilitates control. Local intelligence is relayed to states; states give the information to the appropriate national agency; and the national agency informs the World Health Organization. The specific diseases to be reported are established by each government unit, but all listings include the diseases designated by the World Health Organization as those reportable internationally.

The community health nurse may be involved in several ways in insuring adequate reporting. First, she may educate the public concerning the importance of securing care for what may be a communicable disease. If parents feel a disease is a natural occurrence in childhood and fail to seek medical assistance, the disease is not diagnosed and is not reported. The nurse may assist the family physician in reporting by seeing that he has the necessary regulations and forms and by reminding him of the need to report. She may report any suspicious symptoms she herself observes, such as an increased number of reported gastrointestinal upsets; and she may request a visit by the epidemiologist if her observations suggest that further disease investigation is required.

Maintaining a Safe Level of Immunization

The community health nurse contributes to the achievement of a safe level of immunization in the population. The need to intensify the immunization effort has been recognized nationally, and impetus for the extension and improvement of immunization for preschool children was provided by the passage of the Vaccination Assistance Act of 1962 and the 1965 amendments to this act (Public Law 89-109). Essentially, this legislation provides assistance in planning for and organizing immunization programs, for the purchase of immunization materials, and for the development of studies to determine needs. Immunization needs are not limited to children. Protection against such diseases as influenza, tetanus, or cholera may be recommended under certain circumstances for adults: for travelers, employees with high exposure to disease, elderly people, pregnant women, or those living in groups (such as nursing home residents). Booster shots are currently recommended on a regular basis for smallpox at five to ten year periods or, when traveling abroad, at three year intervals.

The nurse should familiarize herself with the immunization measures that are available in her locality, for whom they are recommended, at what ages or intervals, and under what conditions and at what cost they can be secured. Textbook information in this area must be supplemented by more current sources because of the rapid development of new immunizing agents and methods.

The nurse may be called upon to give immunizations, to interpret the need for them to potential users, and to inform others who may influence potential users. She may be called upon to organize special immunization clinics or special programs for immunizing special groups.

The community health nurse should get whatever information is available on the immunization level of her community and determine how close this level comes to the "epidemic safe" 85 percent level for the more important diseases. This information may be available from the local health department, or it may be estimated on the basis of records of children entering school, of industrial populations, or of clinic groups.

The sharp decline in diseases for which specific immunizing agents are available may lead to overcomplacency about the immunization status of the population. Surveys all too often indicate that the level of immunization among some segments of the population is far below a satisfactory level. In one state-wide survey in a state with well-established and effective health programs, it was found that 22 percent of the children under five years had had no "baby shots," which should have been started at two or three months and that whereas 97 percent of the children in school were vaccinated against smallpox, only 54 percent had been vaccinated before the age of five; 30 percent of the population were not adequately protected against poliomyelitis, and only 12 percent of the population of all age groups had had a smallpox vaccination within the past four years.[4] Other surveys have shown similarly disturbing results.

Failure to receive such protective care varies greatly with socioeconomic status, even when immunization is available without charge. In one recent study, the presence of measles in the community was considered a phenomenon of low-income groups.[5] The community health nurse can do much to even out these differences.

Controlling the Spread of Infection

The community health nurse contributes to the control of the spread of infection by the following three measures:

1. Monitoring the care provided for those who suffer from an infectious disease and who are being cared for in a nonhospital setting.
2. Securing compliance with regulations affecting those with communicable disease or those who have been exposed to communicable disease. Regulations may include exclusion from school or from specified occupations and the observance of reasonable precautions in protecting others from infection.
3. Inculcating personal health behavior that prevents the spread of communicable disease.

Home care of communicable disease is for the most part limited to minor communicable diseases or to longterm illnesses that are considered under reasonable control. The major effort, of course, is to assure the safety and the comfort of the patient. Whether the nurse is providing a major part of the care or whether the family is providing care under the general direction of the nurse, provision should be made for adequate daily care, for the maintenance of nutrition, and for the relief of the patient's boredom and stress. In particular, efforts should be made to have the patient continue to feel a part of the family despite his isolation and the avoidance of close contact.

Isolation measures become much less restrictive as more is known about the spread of infection and as treatment becomes more effective in controlling infectivity. For example, the effectiveness of chemotherapy in producing a negative sputum and the knowledge of the great importance of the airborne droplets in the transmission of infection has made it possible to dispense with much of the strict isolation, with the boiling of dishes, and with the burning of materials handled by the patient in favor of simple separation of the patient from the stream of family traffic and from very close contact with others, of soap and water cleaning, and of covering the mouth when sneezing or coughing.

It is the nurse's responsibility to know the methods by which the disease is spread and the measures that must be taken to prevent the transmission of the disease. She must be satisfied that the person who gives care in her absence thoroughly understands the principles on which these measures are based. The procedures should be as simple as possible, since the home situation is much different from that in the hospital. The nurse's skill in estimating the family's capability with respect to care is an important element in determining the way in which this information will be transmitted.

The nurse should also be aware of groups that might be particularly susceptible to infection and that consequently require special protection, such as the very young child or the elderly person.

In most instances the agency will provide a quick reference guide to communicable diseases that indicates the symptoms, incubation period, method of transmission of the disease, and principal control measures. If a guide of this type is not available, the nurse should be sure to secure a source for such information that can be kept for ready reference.

Exclusion from certain types of occupation or from school may be necessary to protect other vulnerable groups. The nurse can do much to encourage patients not only to follow the required exclusion regulations but also to act in advance of the need. For instance, mothers may be encouraged to keep small children home from school when they have symptoms of an upper respiratory infection. The nurse should be familiar with the regulations and should be prepared to explain the reason for their existence.

The inculcation of health habits that prevent transmission of disease play an important part in disease control. The school nurse, the visiting nurse, and the nurse in the clinic setting can incorporate such teaching into their ongoing services to patients in many ways.

In the whole area of disease control, as in all other areas of the health program, the nurse has an important function. Perhaps her most important contribution is the provision of "just good nursing" to those she serves.

SYPHILIS AND GONORRHEA ARE PERSISTENT PROBLEMS

It is believed that syphilis can be eradicated. Yet in 1968 in the United States, 20,182 cases of primary or secondary syphilis were reported, and the findings of a national survey sponsored by the American Social Health Association, the American Public Health Association, and the American Venereal Disease Association indicate that the true incidence was probably about 75,000 cases.[6] Although the reported rate has declined somewhat since 1962, when the rate was 11 cases per 100,000 of the population, and since 1968, when the rate was 10.3, there is still concern because of the large number of unreported cases and also because of the possible longterm costly effects of the disease.

There were 431,380 cases of gonorrhea reported in 1968; and on the basis of the survey referred to above, it was estimated that this incidence represented almost 1.5 million cases. The reported incidence represents a dramatic increase between 1962, when the rate was 142.8 per 100,000, and 1968, when the rate was 219.2.[7]

The reasons given for this increase are many; among them are the ease of cure, the greater sexual freedom, and a more widespread knowledge of contraception. Incidence varies greatly from locality to locality and by age group; teenagers and young adults comprise the majority of those affected.

In 1967, for instance, the overall reported rate for gonorrhea was 206.9 cases per 100,000 of the population. The rate for those in the age group 15 to 19 was 531.0, and the rate for those 20 to 24 years of age was 1088.9.[8] Between 1966 and 1967 the incidence of gonorrhea increased in the overall population by 15.1 percent, whereas among teenagers the rate increased 20.2 percent during the same period.[9]

Although very different in manifestation and in occurrence, these two diseases have certain characteristics in common that influence the kind of action that is required for their control:

1. Both diseases are endemic in the population; small outbreaks that affect ten or more people occur frequently.
2. The roots of the problem are social-behavioral rather than biologic, and they are difficult to control. Furthermore this behavior is not likely to be helped by repressive legislation. Prostitution still plays a part in the occurrence of venereal disease, but this source of infection probably accounts for only a small proportion of the infections.[10]
3. Reported incidence does not tell the whole story. Many cases are cared for by private physicians, and a large number go unreported.
4. Venereal disease, especially gonorrhea, is a disease of youth. In 1967, 1 in 200 teenagers had reported gonorrhea, and if the same proportion not reported but actually infected and receiving treatment pertains as in the 1966 survey, the ratio would be 1 in 50.
5. The private physician is the major provider of care. It is estimated that about 75 percent of the venereal disease care is provided by private physicians.

The Role of the Nurse

The community health nurse contributes to the venereal disease control program through case finding, through case management, through assisting others in the control team, and through education.

CASE FINDING

The nurse contributes to case finding in three ways:
1. By contact tracing and cluster identification.
2. By direct or delegated general case finding measures in vulnerable populations.
3. By participating in mass or crash programs or screening measures.

Contact Tracing.   The highest new-case yield comes from the investigation of those who have been exposed to the infection by a known case, and the backbone of the case finding program must be contact tracing. The success of such a venture must in the long run rest with the index case's willingness to divulge the names of those who might be contacts. Experienced investigators indicate that patients rarely provide a complete list of contacts during the first interview and that in most instances follow-up re-interviewing is essential if the list is to be complete. Contact interviewing must be of a high quality in order to motivate the individual not only to get treatment himself but to get others under care as well. Sensitivity and timing are of the utmost importance in achieving this end.

Cluster Identification.   Recently, emphasis has been placed on cluster approaches—that is, bringing in for interview and diagnosis those people with whom the patient is closely associated but who are not necessarily named as contacts. If the patient is fully convinced of the need for his own care, he may be persuaded of the importance of naming those among his acquaintance that might have been exposed and enable them to secure prompt treatment. In some instances prophylactic treatment may be prescribed for contacts who do not show clinical or serologic symptoms in order to abort the disease if it is incubating.

General Case Finding.   General case finding measures include incorporation of venereal disease content into all services provided to groups that are particularly vulnerable and maintaining a high alert to the possibility of venereal infection. It must be remembered that venereal disease is no respecter of social class; outbreaks have occurred frequently in "good" schools and in "highly respectable" families. However, the incidence does tend to be greater among mobile groups in the population, such as agricultural migrant workers, among those with inadequate family life or other problems of social adjustment, and among those living in areas with poor homes and few recreational facilities.

CASE MANAGEMENT

The nurse contributes to venereal disease case management in several ways. She may, of course, provide therapeutic care in treatment centers. She may use therapeutic and counseling interviews with patients and their contacts to increase their understanding of the disease and its treatment and to promote their active participation in their own care and in safeguarding others. The person who has a venereal disease is in many instances upset about it: he may feel embarrassed or stigmatized or that he has been wronged by the source of his infection. His feelings of self-respect and personal worth may be damaged, and an already poor self-image may be even more depressed. Properly used, this experience may be constructive and may build, rather than diminish, responsibility and self-respect.

In the case of minors, it is possible in some states to treat the child without parental consent or knowledge. It may be possible for the professional worker to notify the contact of the possible infection without involving or naming the patient who identified the contact. This may be the easy way to accomplish the job; it is not easy for a teenager to face his family with the fact of his infection or for a young person to tell on another. However, when it is possible for the patient himself to explain his plight or to bring in a friend for treatment, he is being given an opportunity for responsible behavior that may accomplish much more than case finding *per se.*

In her contacts with patients, it is especially important that the nurse come to terms with her own feelings about venereal disease and sexual behavior and realize how her own feelings may influence her ability to help. Sometimes it is not possible for a particular nurse to get through to a particular patient. When this is the case, the nurse may want to seek help from a more experienced interviewer; and if she still finds difficulty, she may suggest that someone else try.

In all work with venereal disease, it is, of course, especially important not to violate a confidence. All information should be kept in locked files, and all personnel working with this patient group should be fully briefed on the confidentiality of all record or interview content.

Interviewing has been used intensively and extensively with the patient who has syphilis. It has been much less frequently used for those with gonorrhea. This is partly because of the overwhelming number of cases and the shortage of interviewers and partly because the extremely brief period of treatment does not lend itself to a counseling approach. The question could be raised as to whether or not the failure to use this powerful tool is hampering the control effort.

ASSISTING OTHERS IN THE CONTROL TEAM

The community health nurse may support others in their care of patients with venereal disease. She may work with a venereal disease investigator, a disease control officer, or a nonmedical epidemiologist, all of whom may also function in this program. These workers may have backgrounds that vary from on-the-job training to master's degrees in public health. All will have had some training in interviewing and in epidemiologic investigation. They may participate in field investigations, in contact tracing, and in other case finding measures and may carry treatment responsibilities. When there is such a member on the service group, it is obvious that there will be much sharing of responsibility between him and the nurse. Each can do much to support the other's activities; however, frequent conference and exchange of information is vital to effective activity.

The community health nurse can be of particular help to the family physician or specialist providing care for venereal disease. In most instances he will be dealing with a relatively small number of cases of this type and will welcome the assistance of the nurse. The community health nurse might provide him or his office nurse or receptionist with materials or information, or she might work directly with his patients and their contacts. The health department will usually provide for epidemiologic follow-up for all reported cases, but the nurse can offer more patient-focused care in addition to this. The nurse may also reassure the physician, as well as the patient, that the patient's right to privacy will be respected.

EDUCATION

Far too little attention has been paid to the ability of teenagers or others to deal themselves with the problems of venereal disease. The use of peer group motivation toward responsible behavior may be a powerful influence, and group work an effective method.

School counselors or administrators may also need help with problems of venereal disease or venereal disease education. Many schools do provide instruction in venereal disease in the curriculum of the junior or senior high school, but this practice is by no means universal. The nurse may be instrumental in convincing education authorities and, more importantly, parents of the need of young people to know the facts so that they can secure care promptly.

Finally, the nurse may support parents and communities as they try to establish a climate in which children can grow and develop the ability to establish values that have meaning for them. Parents must be encouraged to help their children develop a normal and responsible sexuality; to find ways, if not to bridge it, at least to attain a reasonable coexistence with the generation gap; and to find opportunities for freedom with responsibility in the context of family life. Communities may be encouraged to find useful ways in which young people can find expression for their need to help. This may seem to be a far cry from the control of syphilis and gonorrhea until one reads Deschin's study of urban teenagers with venereal disease. She reported that there appeared to be no particular factors related to socioeconomic condition, to education, or to broken (as differentiated from intact) homes that were characteristic of these children. What she did find was that the group was characterized by a sense of drifting, a lack of purpose, and a lack of knowledge of sex in more than the physical sense. Of the 600 youths interviewed, when asked what they did in their spare time, 509 replied, "Nothing."[11]

TUBERCULOSIS IS STILL A THREAT

Tuberculosis is also a disease that many consider possible to eradicate. It is a disease that is far less likely to appear in industrialized countries than in developing countries. Yet in this affluent country in 1966, there were 47,767 new active cases of tuberculosis reported; this is only slightly less than the 49,016 cases reported in 1965.[12] The rate was higher for males than females and higher for nonwhites than for whites, as has been true for several years. In 1966, the rate for nonwhite males was 3.5 times that of white males, and the rate for nonwhite females was 5 times that of white females.

Special Characteristics of Tuberculosis

The community health nurse's approach to the care of tuberculosis is governed by the nature of the disease and its distribution in the population. The following points are pertinent to the care of tuberculosis:

1. There is at present no generally applicable means for the prevention of tuberculosis.
2. Although tuberculosis cannot occur without infection by the tuberculosis bacillus, there is great variation in resistance to the disease. Malnutrition, poor personal and environmental hygiene, occupational exposures of various types, and emotional conflict and stress are all implicated in the development of the disease. Poverty greatly increases the risk of a primary infection becoming a demonstrable disease.
3. Specific treatment is available, but it requires prolonged and largely patient-controlled adherence to a prescribed drug regimen.
4. Long and sometimes lifelong surveillance is required for those who have inactive disease and for some especially vulnerable contacts.
5. Tuberculosis may appear anywhere and in any age group, but it is essentially a disease of adults, and it is concentrated in metropoli-

tan areas. About half of the cases are in 77 large metropolitan areas.[13]

6. Tuberculosis is essentially an airborne disease; the infective agent is transmitted by means of droplets.

7. Tuberculosis is usually accompanied by considerable stress for both patient and family and, in many instances, requires substantial reorganization of individual and family life.

The Care of Tuberculosis Is a Family Affair

By far the greatest part of care for the patient with tuberculosis is provided at home. The hospital, once the major treatment center, is now usually only used for those phases of care that require the facilities of the hospital or for those persons who do not have a home to which they may go. Thus the motivation and education of the family, as well as of the patient, become crucial in securing the long and regular care that is required. It is important that the patient and family understand the elements of care.

The family should understand *the primacy of the drug* in the curative regimen. Several recent studies indicate that many patients and their families still believe such general measures as rest, fresh air, and food as most important in care and consider the drug as having secondary importance.[14] It is important that they know the need for sustained and regular drug taking—that it is not possible to skip several doses and then to make up for it by taking an extra amount. They must know that the efficacy of the drug may be impaired by intermittent use. They should be familiar with any side effects that may occur and how and when to report them.

The family needs to understand *the method by which the organism is transmitted* and the ways in which they may protect themselves from droplet infection. The importance of ventilation and of covering coughs and sneezes cannot be overemphasized.

The family needs to understand *the level of isolation* that is required at given points and that the minimal procedures that are proposed are indeed safe. The family can alienate the patient by too great an emphasis on isolation.

The family should understand *the increased susceptibility* of young children, of those who have inactive disease, and of those who are undernourished, overfatigued, or under stress.

If *prophylactic treatment* is ordered, the family should understand the rationale for such care and be reassured of the safety of the treatment even though the disease is not present.

They should understand *the importance of a thorough evaluation of all family members or friends* who have been close associates of the patient. They need also to understand why surveillance may need to go on for a considerable time after the disease has become inactive.

Families may serve a very useful community function if they understand the part they can play in "licking TB" by encouraging others to report symptoms promptly.

The Role of the Community Health Nurse

DIRECT CARE

The community health nurse may be involved in active care of tuberculosis patients and their families in clinics or in the home. Since, for the most part, patients will be ambulatory, the primary service is surveillance and education. Since reliance must be placed on the patient for taking the prescribed drugs, instruction must be painstaking and thorough. The nurse may also want to find ways of judging whether or not the drugs are in fact taken. This may be done by estimating the number of pills delivered to the patient and asking that the bottle with the remaining pills be returned when a new supply is needed. In this way it is possible to estimate how many pills have been used (assuming, of course, that they have not just been thrown out!). Urine tests may also be used to determine whether or not the drug has been taken. Simply asking the patient, using good interviewing techniques that make him feel free to give a negative answer, may also provide a measure of drug taking.

Prophylactic treatment may be ordered in specific cases.[15] The exact schedule recommended will vary from community to community, and the nurse should be fully informed in order to interpret the procedure correctly.

The nurse may also participate in vaccination programs, although vaccination is used only infrequently in this country. However, when exposure is massive and unavoidable and medical supervision is not readily available, vaccination may be used. One major disadvantage of vaccination is that it sensitizes the individual to tuberculin and consequently makes it impossible to use the tuberculin test as an indication of infection; when the incidence of positive reaction to tuberculin tests is low, this may be a real disadvantage. In the United States as a whole it is estimated that only about 3 percent of the population up to age 25 are positive reactors, compared to about 75 percent of those 65 or older.[16]

PLANNING FOR HOSPITAL CARE

When hospital care is indicated, the community health nurse can do much to help the family with the necessary adjustments. Both patient and family need to understand the place of the hospital experience in the total care plan and the special opportunity the hospital provides for determining the patient's response to the drugs prescribed and for him to learn about his disease and its care.

The family should understand the importance of protecting the patient from problems that might arise as a consequence of his absence from home. They may need to be helped to use community resources or other family members for advice and support. They may need help with economic aid or with child care.

At the point of discharge from the hospital, the community health nurse may again support the family as they readjust to having the patient back home. There may be a public health nurse or liaison nurse in the hospital to help with this planning. Sometimes the community health nurse will have to take the initiative and with the hospital, the family physician, and the family for a smooth transfer from hospital to home care. Even though the nurse may have provided intensive care prior to hospitalization, it is still likely that some reinforcement may be needed at this point.

TUBERCULIN TESTING PROGRAMS

The community health nurse may participate in tuberculin testing programs. The nurse may give tuberculin tests as a regular part of her work in schools or clinics, or she may give such tests when special programs are set up for this specific purpose. Ordinarily the nurse will administer and read the tests, reporting those whose reaction is great enough to suggest the need for further study and those that convert from negative to positive status. The tests most often used in screening are the Tine or Heaf tests, both of which are frequently administered by nurses.[17] When nurses are assigned this responsibility, the agency provides for the necessary training in the procedures. A joint committee of the American Academy of Pediatrics and the American College of Surgeons recently recommended that all children have a tuberculin test at 6 to 12 months, before vaccination for measles and chickenpox.[18]

CONTINUING SURVEILLANCE OF HIGH-RISK GROUPS

Certain groups of patients or tuberculin reactors require intensive and longterm follow-up. Inactive patients have been found to be at great risk of re-infection.[19] For this reason, follow-up care is usually recommended for at least five years, and some urge lifelong follow-up.[20] Positive reactors to the tuberculin test, particularly young children, are usually also followed over a long period of time; again there are some who propose lifelong surveillance. Such longterm supervision may serve not only as a disease control measure but also as an opportunity for sustained family health education.

PLANNING FOR CARE IS IMPORTANT

Even though the number of tuberculosis patients in the case load of any one nurse is likely to be small, these patients have a genuine claim on nursing time because of the possibilities for prevention and amelioration. Attention in case finding might well be concentrated in groups where the incidence is likely to be high: low-income neighborhoods, migrant labor groups, places where homeless men congregate, or those in occupations that increase the risk of tuberculosis.

Individual case planning also becomes important. The periodic, multidiscipline case review is particularly useful for those under care for long periods of time. In addition, careful planning by the nurse and the family she visits is important, since the visits may be spaced at wide intervals and the problem of maintaining a good working relationship may be difficult.

Whether in the field of cancer, of influenza, of tuberculosis, or of venereal infection, the disease control program represents an engrossing area of the nurse's work. It is a phase of the work that requires the full use of every facet of nursing practice, where the results are likely to be commensurate with the energy expended and where the satisfactions are deep.

REFERENCES

1. See, for instance, Morris, N. N.: The Uses of Epidemiology. The Williams and Wilkins Co., Baltimore, 1964, p. 52.; Mustard, S., and Stebbins, E. L. (eds.): Introduction to Public Health. 4th ed., The Macmillan Company, New York, 1968, p. 107. Rosenau, Milton J.: Preventive Medicine and Public Health. 9th ed. (Kenneth F. Maxcy and Philip Sartwell, eds.). Appleton-Century-Crofts, New York, 1965, p. 1.
2. Payne, A. M. M.: Approaches to communicable disease control. WHO Chron., 22:3, January, 1968.
3. Gregg, Michael R.: Communicable disease trends in the United States. Amer. J. Nurs., 68:88, January, 1968.
4. Janney, John H., Robbitt, Wayne R., Jr., and Murphy, Shelley: Maryland's immunization project. Maryland's Health, 39:4, July-September, 1967.
5. Dandoy, Suzanne: Measles, epidemiology and vaccine use in Los Angeles County, 1933 and 1966. Public Health Rep., 82:659, August, 1967.
6. Today's VD Control Program, A Joint Statement of the American Public Health Association, The American Social Health Association, and the American Venereal Disease Association. The American Social Health Association, New York, 1969, p. 953.
7. Ibid.
8. Ibid., p. 48.
9. Ibid., p. 25.
10. Ibid., p. 15.
11. Deschin, C.: Venereal disease and the adolescent personality. Amer. J. Nurs., 63:58, November, 1963.
12. Reported Tuberculosis Data, 1966. U.S. Department of Health, Education and Welfare, PHS Publication No. 638, pp. 1, 5.
13. Annual Report, 1968. National Tuberculosis and Respiratory Disease Association, New York, 1968, p. 3.
14. See, for instance, A Survey of Tuberculosis Patients in the South Bronx. New York, The Community Service Society, New York, 1966; or Kuemmerer, J.: Adherence to a Prescribed Oral Medical Regime for Tuberculosis. Doctoral thesis, School of Hygiene and Public Health, Johns Hopkins University, 1968.
15. Blomquist, Edward T.: Program aimed at eradication of tuberculosis. Public Health Rep., 78:897, October, 1963.
16. Tuberculosis in the Early Sixties. U.S. Department of Health, Education and Welfare, Public Health Service, U.S. Government Printing Office, Washington, D.C., 1963, p. 16.
17. South, Jean: Tuberculosis Handbook for Public Health Nurses. 4th ed., National Tuberculosis Association (Now The National Tuberculosis and Respiratory Disease Associaton), New York, 1965, p. 47.
18. Planning Eradication of Tuberculosis. Currents in Public Health, Ross Laboratories, Columbus, Ohio, 7:2, June, 1967.
19. Comstock, George W.: Untreated inactive pulmonary tuberculosis: risk of reactivation. Public Health Rep., 77:461, June, 1962.
20. Perkins, James E.: Tuberculosis—a special health problem. In Porterfield, John D. (ed.): Community Health. Basic Books, Inc., Publishers, New York, p. 40.

SUGGESTED READINGS

Blomquist, Edward T.: Program aimed at eradication of tuberculosis. Public Health Rep., 78:897, October, 1965.
Calafiore, Dorothy C.: Eradication of measles in the United States. Amer. J. Nurs., 67: 1871, September, 1967.
Comstock, George W.: Untreated inactive tuberculosis: risk of reactivation. Public Health Rep., 77:461, June, 1962.
Control of Communicable Diseases in Man. 11th ed., American Public Health Association, New York, 1969.

Curry, F. J.: A new approach for improving attendance at tuberculosis clinics. Amer. J. Public Health, *58:*877, May, 1968.

Dandoy, Suzanne: Measles epidemiology and vaccine use in Los Angeles County. Public Health Rep., *82:*659, August, 1967.

Deschin, Celia J.: VD and the adolescent personality. Amer. J. Nurs., *63:*58, November, 1963.

Douglas, Gordon W.: Rubella in pregnancy. Amer. J. Nurs., *66:*2664, December, 1966.

Gray, Robert M., Kesler, Joseph P., and Moody, Philip M.: The effects of social class and friends' expectations on oral polio vaccination participation. Amer. J. Public Health, *56:*2028, December, 1966.

Gregg, Michael R.: Communicable disease trends in the United States. Amer. J. Nurs., *68:*88, January, 1968.

Hall, Madelyn: Immunization practices in large health agencies. Nurs. Outlook. *13:*42, September, 1965.

Kogan, B. A., *et al.:* Mass measles immunization in Los Angeles County. Amer. J. Public Health, *58:*1883, October, 1968.

Kriegman, Saul: Rubella: new light on an old disease. Amer. J. Nurs., *65:*126, October, 1965.

Lester, Mary R.: Every nurse an epidemiologist. Amer. J. Nurs., *57:*1434, November, 1957.

Morris, J. N.: The Uses of Epidemiology. 2nd ed., The Williams and Wilkins Co., Baltimore, 1964.

Moulding, Thomas: New responsibilities for health departments and public health nurses in tuberculosis—keeping the out patient on therapy. Amer. J. Public Health, *56:*416, March, 1966.

Moulding, Thomas: Realized and unrealized benefits of chemotherapy for tuberculosis. Public Health Rep., *82:*753, September, 1967.

Payne, A. M. M.: Approaches to communicable disease control. WHO Chron., *22:*3, January, 1968.

Perkins, James E.: Tuberculosis—a special health problem. *In* Porterfield, John D. (ed.): Community Health Services, Basic Books, Inc., Publishers, New York, 1966, Chapter 4.

Raska, Karl: National and international surveillance of communicable diseases, WHO Chron., *20:*315, September, 1966.

Richie, Jeanne: The tuberculosis patient who refuses care. *In* Stewart, D. M., and Vincent, P. A. (eds): Public Health Nursing. William C. Brown Company, Publishers, Dubuque, Iowa, 1968, Chapter 37.

Riley, Richard: Air borne infections. Amer. J. Nurs., *60:*1240, September, 1960.

South, Jean: Public health nursing services in the tuberculosis control program. Nurs. Outlook, *15:*46, January, 1967.

South, Jean: Tuberculosis Handbook for Public Health Nurses. 4th ed., New York, National Tuberculosis and Respiratory Disease Association, New York, 1965.

Swayne, James B., and Tepper, Leo: Tuberculosis contact follow up in the Los Angeles Health Department. Amer. J. Public Health, *54:*1270, August, 1964.

Terris, Milton: The scope and methods of epidemiology. Amer. J. Public Health, *52:*1371, September, 1962.

Today's VD Program: A Joint Statement of the American Public Health Association, the American Social Health Association, and the American Venereal Disease Association. American Social Health Association, New York, 1969.

CHAPTER
25

Excellence – The
Sine Qua Non

For the nurse who is a true professional, the urge to excellence is compelling, unremitting, and lifelong. For society, excellence in its helping professions is a necessary protection against the misuse of a powerful social force. For the recipient of community nursing service, excellence in the nurse is that intangible something that makes the nurse "special" and the service "great."

Excellence in community health nursing is not an "extra," nor is it a matter of choice. It is becoming more and more clear that without excellence in practice, the process of helping can degrade the human spirit even while catering to the physical needs of patients; care may stifle independence and sap vigor through the very act of loving, but unknowing, ministration.

Community health nursing touches the lives of people over long periods of time. This sustained relationship, coupled with the human values attached to nursing skills, means that the social impact of nursing is great. For this reason, the search for excellence must be seen as a mandate rather than an opportunity.

CRITERIA CALL THE TUNE

The "think slim" concept in dieting calls for a focus on the desired effect – a mental image of the "you" that will emerge. The "think slim" outline of professional development is the set of criteria that distinguish excellent from mediocre community health nursing practice. The "think slim" body is the configuration of personal values and style through which the criteria are met.

The Criterion of Relevance

If one were forced to choose a single criterion for excellence, it is likely that the criterion of relevance would serve. Relevance implies a goodness of fit between worker and work that should maximize both efficiency and effectiveness. In community health nursing practice, the concept of relevance might be discussed in the contexts of relevance to purpose, relevance to people, and relevance to program.

RELEVANCE TO PURPOSE

Relevance to purpose requires congruence between both the services provided and the method by which these services are provided and the purposes of nursing, the purposes of the health movement, and the purposes of the specific action unit in which the nurse is functioning.

Thus, if the purpose of nursing is to help families cope with their problems, practice must give evidence of extending family capability through teaching and guidance and of sharp identification of and dealing with the real problems of real people.

If the purpose of the health system is to provide care for the whole community, the nurse's program must be developed within this same context of concern. Nursing service that provides exquisite care to a small segment of the population but no service at all to the rest of the population is not relevant in terms of the health system's purpose; less exquisite, but better distributed, care may be closer to the ideal of excellence.

If the purpose of a particular agency is to reach out aggressively to unserved groups, a traditional service not particularly geared to the needs of the low-income group would fail to meet the criterion of relevance, whereas unconventional activities that may not even appear to fall within the realm of nursing may be very relevant indeed.

RELEVANCE TO PEOPLE

Relevance to people implies congruence between nursing action and the needs, the expectations, and the desires of the people served. A concept of needs that is directed toward disease-related care or to standard preventive procedures is unlikely to meet this measure of relevance unless it also allows for meeting the basic human needs of security or recognition or achievement.

Relevance to people must also take account of the degree to which nursing is supporting and meeting the needs of other workers in the health effort. For example, a community health nurse might use a home health aide in such a way as to provide for the continuing growth in responsibility and competence in the aide, or the nurse may manage to have the aide provide excellent care to patients while stifling any moves of the aide toward taking initiative or experimenting with new ways. The failure to support coworkers may also detract from the value of the nursing effort.

Another facet of "people relevant" practice is congruence with the ways in which people are accustomed to act. Nursing referral patterns that do not take account of the local dependence upon the aid of the family physician or of interagency communication by memo in a highly informal interagency setting are examples of irrelevant nursing behavior.

RELEVANCE TO PROGRAM

Program relevance has to do with the degree to which nursing is integrated with other ongoing health and welfare programs. For example, one nurse might hear that a new community mental health center is developing and respond by immediately seeking a conference to know how to modify nursing to support this new venture; another—and less relevant—nursing action would be to just do nothing until asked.

The Criterion of Maximum Actualization

Excellence in community health nursing is characterized not only by relevance but also by a high level of actualization—that is, by the achievement of the greatest possible effect for the amount of nursing time and competence expended.

One great enemy of productivity is nonservice time: time spent in travel, in visits made to families that are not at home, and in routine preparations or reports not directly involved with service itself. Case and service reports or telephone or mail contacts with physicians are essential to the service provided; and even though all possible economies should be effected in completing these activities, the time so spent should not be called nonservice time. Time spent in the routine checking of supplies or in visits made simply to secure information may be considered nonservice time. Such nonservice time should be constantly analyzed to see if it can be reduced—if telephoning in advance might reduce not-at-home calls or if the use of aides might release nursing time spent in accounting for the laundry in the clinic.

Actualization is greater if the services provided are of sufficiently high *impact* to produce the changes or the action that is desired. A large number of very brief parent contacts may do little to influence the parents' concept of good child rearing practices. whereas a much smaller number of well planned and leisurely conferences might be very effective in exploring and changing ideas; a visit made to a discharged psychiatric patient who has been home from the hospital for six months will almost certainly have little impact, but a nursing visit may have been welcomed and highly effective if made shortly after his discharge from the hospital. Timing, method, and content all affect the degree of impact.

Maximum actualization is also related to the wise *choice among alternative courses of action.* Unfortunately, far too much nursing care is provided in a follow-the-book manner—visits are made at specified times to families in which tuberculosis is present; group work is provided for expectant mothers or parents but not to other groups with similar problems; nursing contacts are equated with home visits, so that telephone contacts are not counted as service accomplishments but as "office time." The result may be that nursing service is organized with too little attention paid to possible alternatives. Thus, selection among alternative courses of action must include discovering new alternatives as well as the selection among those already in use.

Maximum actualization supposes that nursing time is not used to do those things that can be done as well or better by some other available or potentially available resource. Much has already been said about the unused potential of those served by community health agencies: the capacity of individuals and groups to make health decisions, to plan action for health care, to seek out and refer those needing community health services, and to teach and support one another. There is no doubt that nursing effort could be much more effective if these resources were fully used.

Volunteer or paid nurse assistants may also represent an underused resource; this kind of help is presently limited to jobs far below the level of decision and independent action of which these workers are capable. For example, the volunteer or clinic aide may be useful in planning and evaluating the program, as well as in handling routine tasks; moreover such participation may enhance the nurse's efforts in this area.

In the foregoing italicized sentence it is important to note the phrase "available or potentially available resource." Even though the school teacher may be able to do many things ordinarily undertaken by the community health nurse, the teacher may in fact not be an "available" resource for weighing and measuring children (unless such activity has been incorporated as a teaching measure) because of the demands of her work. The mental health clinic might be more able to help parents deal with a rebellious, handicapped adolescent than is the community health nurse; but if the clinic has a waiting time of several months, the nurse might feel that this clinic is not in fact an "available" resource.

The Criterion of Growth

Excellence is characterized by a continuing increment in the skills of professional practice and in the scope of professional influence. Such growth is as important to the seasoned nurse as it is to the novice.

Growth in professional skills may be indicated by an increase in technical and professional knowledge and process and also by the development of specific personal skills that are basic to professional practice. Thus the nurse in community health may need to improve her knowledge of modern care of the cancer patient or of the legal implications of emergency care in industry, or she may need to develop her ability to work with people of a cultural background that is different from her own.

The "growing nurse" is constantly increasing the impact of her interchange with recipients of nursing service, constantly broadening the range and the complexity of the decisions she is making, and constantly experiencing an increment in the degree to which she assumes a leadership stance.

The Criterion of Creativity

Of all traits considered desirable in today's world, the capacity for creativity or innovation is perhaps most valued. Creativity isn't something that exists apart from the "nitty gritty" of the daily work. It is only as one has wrestled with these daily problems and worked with the facilities and people available that the problems that need resolution can be identified; and it is with these real problems that an innovative and creative approach is demanded. The nurse who never toys with a way-out idea or who never takes time to speculate on what would happen if the system could be changed is unlikely to go far in original thinking and action. On the other hand, innovative thinking must also be geared to the "can do" answer; there must be at least some chance that the idea is feasible. The habit of challenging the establishment appears to be common among young (and some that are not so young) people today, and this is a valuable habit for one who wants to live creatively; but the true test of creativity is to use the same degree of energy and persistence in seeking new answers to right what is wrong.

The Achievement of Excellence Takes Time and Planning

The achievement of excellence within the nursing service as a whole is a primary concern of the supervisory and the consultant staff. In the long run, however, it is the nurse herself who must set both the goals for her own development and the course of action for meeting these goals.

Goals Give Direction

If excellence is to be achieved, it is important to know just what kind of change is desired. This will be related to one's career goals and life commitments. For some nurses, work will be an interlude between school and marriage; for others, it will be an absorbing career; and for many nursing will fall somewhere between these two points. For some the quiet victory of doing a good job in a small sphere and at the direct service level—to do tangible good—is the exciting challenge. For others, the challenge lies in exerting a different kind of influence—to develop something new, to lead others to greater achievement, or to influence public policy or social action on a broad front. Goals will be different, and the courses of action to achieve excellence will be different; but in every case the contribution of excellent nursing has the potential for bettering the situation in which nurses work.

As with service goals, goals for self-improvement will come in systems. There will be long-range goals to fit one's self for leadership or to continue to deepen the quality of practice in a direct care situation. Within these long-range goals there will be other goals, such as to improve one's capacity to deal with groups, to strengthen one's content knowledge in tuberculosis or in psychiatric nursing, to gain greater assurance in working with members of other disciplines, or to start some small field studies that are both compatible with full-time employment and sound in concept and technique.

Assessment Shapes the Plan

It is important to know by what route these goals for self-improvement are likely to be realized and by what means achievement can be

measured. An accurate reading of the present status is a necessary basis
for estimating the needs for change and for measuring progress. Part of
this evaluation of needs and progress may come from the supervisor's
periodic evaluation of performance. Most of the evaluation, however,
must come from an honest and thoughtful comparison of present performance with one's own concept of ideal professional behavior.

Improvement must rest on a clear understanding of the barriers to
progress, whether the barriers be a lack of knowledge, a lack of personal
or interpersonal skills, or administrative restrictions that interfere with
change. Often nurses feel that their jobs do not allow sufficient freedom
to try out new ideas. This may be true in some instances. However, this
perception may be an excuse rather than an actual reason for a lack of
action; it is sometimes surprising how far a regulation can stretch if one
just asks! For example, one nurse who wanted to try evening visits to
families was told that regulations did not allow for overtime and that the
agency could not take responsibility for workers being out during the
evening. When it was explained that the nurse wanted an opportunity to
talk to the fathers of the household, it was found that visits on Saturdays
would accomplish this purpose and be quite compatible with the regulations.

The study of one's performance should not stop with estimating how
well things are working under the present system for providing care; it
should also include speculation as to whether or not a result would have
been better if the problem had been approached differently. For example, the nurse who is achieving good response from expectant
mothers in a one-to-one relationship of a home visit might ask if perhaps
results would be even greater if a group approach were used.

Helping Resources

Nursing has a great advantage over many professions in that the uses
of supervision have been developed over a long period of time; as a
result, there is almost always available some more experienced person to
whom the worker may turn for help in evaluating performance or improving practice. In addition to the designated supervisor, there are
many other resources that can be tapped for the diagnosis or improvement of community health nursing practice. The nursing supervisor will
be the key adviser in the improvement program.

Neophyte community health nurses sometimes have difficulty ad-
justing to supervisory assistance available in the community setting.
Nurses who come directly to community health nursing from basic
educational programs must adapt from the role of student to the new
role of worker. During the student's basic training, the attention of
clinical instructors and other supervisory personnel was focused on the
student's learning. The responsibility for facing the limitations, the frustrations, the inevitable compromises that must be made in the real life
situation are all too often not a part of the student's experience. The new
staff member may, for example, fail to understand why services are not
provided freely to alcoholic patients; the concept of balancing their
needs against the needs of the rest of the population and the small

likelihood that nursing will make much difference in this situation are new to her. She is apt to hold on to the idea of one-by-one treatment and feel that any patient must receive care.

The problem of establishing communication may be a difficult one, since each generation of professionals seems to develop its own patois; moreover, the supervisor may have come from quite a different type of basic education than that of the staff nurse. Sometimes the supervisor is under such pressure that she is not as receptive to new ideas as she might be if the situation were a bit more relaxed, and the new nurse may feel rebuffed when she comes up with a world-shattering idea and finds no audience waiting breathless to hear it. Sometimes the supervisor is indeed unaware or is rigidly set in patterns that have congealed years ago and that are not very well adapted to the present situation.

The nurse who truly wants to increase her competence must learn to work within the supervisory style of the supervisor she has and not expect a supervisor to be a clinical instructor. The supervisor hopefully will try to understand and to use the fresh ideas that the younger members of the staff can bring to this situation.

Consultants come in many styles, and the supervisor will help the nurse to locate and use the ones that are most useful for her particular situation. Such consultation may come from the agency itself, from the state or federal health agency, or from other agencies in the community. Thus, the consultant in a tuberculosis case might come from the state department of health: the nurse in the cardiac service in the local teaching hospital might serve as a consultant in cardiac care at home; or the community organizer in the local Office of Economic Opportunity may advise in the use of indigenous aides.

Representatives of other disciplines in the agency (or in another health agency in the community) may also provide useful consultation assistance. The sanitarian may have excellent ideas about school safety, or the director of geriatric services may advise on matters relating to nursing home supervision.

The community health nurse should apprise herself of the ways in which consultation is secured in the agency in which she works. In some instances all arrangements for consultation go through the nurse supervisor; in other situations the nurse supervisor provides general direction, but each nurse is free to get help without immediate supervisory clearance; in still other instances, the nurse may be pretty much on her own in finding and using consultant help.

EXCELLENCE IS A WAY OF LIFE

Many suggestions can be made about ways in which the quality of professional performance can be brought to the excellence level, but the achievement of excellence really requires the adoption of a consistent and persistent way of life that is based on analysis, challenge, and innovation.

The habit of analyzing failures alone, with others who are more experienced, or with those that can give an objective "outside" viewpoint is perhaps the most valuable habit of all. It is failure analyses that make possible the identification of factors that require different approaches, personal skills that need strengthening, and the things that appeared *not* to influence the outcome. For example, in caring for a coronary patient at home, the family may appear unwilling or unable to change the family life style to the degree necessary to support the patient. Without careful analysis, the nurse may try to meet the situation by providing more of the same—more intensive instruction, more home visits, more exhortation. Analysis will help determine that information is entirely adequate and that the family is fully aware of the nurse's availability and willingness to provide support; the difficulty instead lies in the efforts of the family to deal with a demanding adolescent: in order to keep her at home, they have been, in effect, setting up a noisy junior canteen in the home.

Cultivating habits that lead to exposure to new ideas is also an important way to move toward excellence. The habit of professional reading, of attending professional meetings, and of sitting in on meetings of other groups provides stimulation for new ideas and new approaches.

The habit of making experience work for development is also valuable. For some people, working for five years is the same as repeating one year of experience five times. For others, it is a continuing opportunity for growth. To achieve excellence in practice is a professional obligation, and the quest for excellence can be an exciting and rewarding personal adventure.

Index